The Tools of Neuroscience Experiment

This volume establishes the conceptual foundation for sustained investigation into tool development in neuroscience. Neuroscience relies on diverse and sophisticated experimental tools, and its ultimate explanatory target—*our* brains and hence the organ driving *our* behaviors—catapults the investigation of these research tools into a philosophical spotlight.

The chapters in this volume integrate the currently scattered work on tool development in neuroscience into the broader philosophy of science community. They also present an accessible compendium for neuroscientists interested in the broader theoretical dimensions of their experimental practices. The chapters are divided into five thematic sections. Section 1 discusses the development of revolutionary research tools across neuroscience's history and argues to various conclusions concerning the relationship between new research tools and theory progress in neuroscience. Section 2 shows how a focus on research tools and their development in neuroscience transforms some traditional epistemological issues and questions about knowledge production in philosophy of science. Section 3 speaks to the most general questions about the way we characterize the nature of the portion of the world that this science addresses. Section 4 discusses hybrid research tools that integrate laboratory and computational methods in exciting new ways. Finally, Section 5 extends research on tool development to the related science of genetics.

The Tools of Neuroscience Experiment will be of interest to philosophers and philosophically minded scientists working at the intersection of philosophy and neuroscience.

John Bickle is Professor of Philosophy and Shackouls Honors College Faculty at Mississippi State University and Affiliated Faculty in the Department of Neurobiology and Anatomical Sciences at the University of Mississippi Medical Center. He is author of four academic books and editor of *The Oxford Handbook of Philosophy and Neuroscience* (2009).

Carl F. Craver is a Professor in the Philosophy Department and the Philosophy-Neuroscience-Psychology Program at Washington University in St. Louis. He specializes in the Philosophy of Science and has continuing research activity in the neuropsychology of memory. He is the author of *Explaining the Brain: Mechanisms and the Mosaic Unity of Neuroscience* and (with Lindley Darden) *In Search of Mechanisms: Discoveries across the Life Sciences.*

Ann-Sophie Barwich is Assistant Professor at Indiana University Bloomington (Department of History and Philosophy of Science and Medicine; Cognitive Science). She specializes in olfaction as a model for theories of mind and brain. Barwich is the author of *Smellosophy: What the Nose Tells the Mind* (2020).

Routledge Studies in the Philosophy of Science

For more information about this series, please visit: https://www.routledge.com/Routledge-Studies-in-the-Philosophy-of-Science/book-series/POS

The Tools of Neuroscience Experiment

Philosophical and Scientific Perspectives

Edited by
John Bickle, Carl F. Craver,
and Ann-Sophie Barwich

Routledge
Taylor & Francis Group

NEW YORK AND LONDON

First published 2022
by Routledge
605 Third Avenue, New York, NY 10158

and by Routledge
2 Park Square, Milton Park, Abingdon, Oxon, OX14 4RN

Routledge is an imprint of the Taylor & Francis Group, an informa business

Library of Congress Cataloging-in-Publication Data
A catalog record for this title has been requested

ISBN: 978-1-032-12799-6 (hbk)
ISBN: 978-1-032-17011-4 (pbk)
ISBN: 978-1-003-25139-2 (ebk)

DOI: 10.4324/9781003251392

Typeset in Sabon
by codeMantra

Contents

Foreword

Stuart Firestein

The comic Emo Phillips has a very wry comment about the brain. He muses that he always thought his brain was the most wonderful organ in his body. Until one day he asked himself, "Wait a minute, who's telling me that?" Who indeed. This quip points out the hopelessness of understanding the brain by introspection. Indeed, having a brain may be the biggest obstacle to understanding it. Not that the organ is not smart enough to understand how it works, but that the first-person experience of having a brain, what it feels like it's doing, is rarely a very good indication of what is actually happening up there. In fact, it is usually dead wrong.

Thus, there is the need for instruments to visualize the structures of the brain, to measure the activity of the brain and to probe its working at every level from single molecules to the whole buzzing, whirring 3.5 pounds of electrified pate. These instruments allow us to have a kind of third-person disinterested view of the brain that is not as likely to be swayed by its pernicious self-promoting propaganda. Or such would be the ideal.

Of course, there always lurks the danger that the choice of measuring device will reflect the answer we expect to get. As the geneticists warn, you always get what you screen for. As neuroscientists, if we use electrodes and amplifiers we will see the brain as a fundamentally electric organ and believe we can understand it by recording voltages and ion currents. The chemists and pharmacologists on the other hand will be measuring neurotransmitters and binding kinetics revealing a picture of a massive chemical factory. Then the anatomists with their golden rule – function follows structure – will convince you that it's all in the connections and the vast parts list. And so it goes.

A hopeful solution to this is to take a pluralistic approach – not wholistic – but pluralistic. Recognizing that the brain is a subject (or is it an object?) that can be examined at many different levels and from many different perspectives. It is important to recognize that these multiple perspectives are not likely to add up to a complete picture. Indeed, they are more likely to maintain a very fragmented view of the brain. I for one believe this is the correct view of the brain. It will not be summed up in a neat formula or model. Its very interest lies in its multiplicity.

When I first began in Neuroscience there were no departments of neuroscience at any major university. There were loose confederations of faculty whose research was focused on the brain, but they all had their primary appointments in various departments – anatomy, molecular biology, physiology, evolution, psychology, computer science, electrical engineering – all over the campus. Not to strike a nostalgic note here, but there was something particularly correct about having brain research distributed in that way. I'm still a bit uneasy about the proliferation of institutes dedicated to BRAIN RESEARCH, as if that was some monolithic endeavor like building pyramids or cathedrals. It does seem like something a brain would be very pleased about – and that may not be good.

An alternative and more positive view of this concentration of brain scientists into single departments or institutes is that neuroscience may now find outreach to other fields even more beneficial. And those other fields could even be outside the traditional scientific silos. They might include philosophy, literature, law, the arts, economics, sociology – indeed many of these sorts of overtures are already in existence. Writers or artists in residence at Neuroscience institutes have become more common; books on music and the brain have proliferated; there are conferences on ethics and law in the light of neuroscience findings. Perhaps counterintuitively neuroscience has become more pluralistic by becoming more monolithic. After all, what we do with this brain is just as important to understand as to how the parts fit together. The importance of instruments and technology in driving the evolution of neuroscience both as science and cultural phenomenon is the main subject of this collection, so I will not go any further with this argument and allow the authors herein to make it more thoroughly.

The pleasure of this volume is the inclusion of so many and varied ideas about the brain, not only from practicing neuroscientists but also philosophers and historians of neuroscience, all grounded in a wealth, an abundant wealth, of technical, intellectual and instrumental approaches that provide a wonderfully complicated view of this miraculous organ. But who's telling you that?

Editors' Introduction

*John Bickle, Carl Craver and
Ann-Sophie Barwich*

The brain is science's most photogenic organ. Glossy covers of modern science journals routinely feature mesmerizing fluorescent neurons and intricately woven cell structures with multicolored connections. And increasingly, these figures are matched by the ability to intervene into brain systems with drugs, electrical currents, magnetic fields and light, to change them and bring them into line with our projected ideals. The brain's visual appeal mirrors the substantial insight that research on the brain has advanced throughout the last century and beyond, as well as our hopes and dreams for a future in which this central organ of control is itself responsive to direct human commands.

The research tools of contemporary neuroscience have provided vectors of access to brain structure and function that would have flabbergasted the pioneers of the field just 70 years ago. Tools are the most conspicuous feature of neuroscience research, visible the moment you walk into the lab: the scanner, the stereotactic surgery rig, the microscope, the laser pointed at fixed tissue, the magnetic coils positioned over localized regions of the brain, are themselves objects of our wonder and vehicles of our imagination. These technologies drive progress in neuroscience by opening new avenues by which we can "peer into" and act upon brain systems. Through these technologies, we image active brain areas, listen in on neurons talking to each other, and make mice stop or go, feed or go wild, all with the flip of a switch.

Some have criticized neuroscience for its overreliance on technology and fancy gadgets at the expense of theory, that neuroscience is "data rich but theory poor." Is neuroscience overwhelmed by the data generated by its research tools? And does this fixation on technology and the data-collection it inspires explain why neuroscientists still lack a general theory of how the brain makes the mind? This is a genuine concern. Contrasted with physics, chemistry and evolutionary biology, neuroscience does not yet offer a global theory of brain function. And a fascination with tools can, in fact, become a distraction from the hard work of experimental design and theory building. Indeed, in his classic *Advice for a Young Investigator*, first published in 1897,[1] Santiago Ramón

DOI: 10.4324/9781003251392-1

y Cajal described "instrument addiction" as one ever-present form of malaise threatening to derail the career of the young investigator.

Yet, even if we acknowledge Ramón y Cajal's concern, there can be no scientific theory of the brain or mind without the existence of instruments that hone and refine our ability to intervene in and measure brains and behavior. Good theory requires good data, and good data requires instruments that work. Ramón y Cajal, himself a pioneer and devotee of his own instruments (in his case, stains and light microscopes), would surely acknowledge that nobody can understand contemporary neuroscience or its history without attending to the arsenal of tools neuroscientists use to probe nature — to, in words often attributed to Francis Bacon, "twist the lion's tail."

Specific research tools inform each of neuroscience's many "levels" of investigation, from the designer pharmacology used to study molecular activities in intra- and inter-neuron signaling to the electrophysiology rigs used to probe individual neuronal activities, to the functional imaging modalities used to study neural systems, to the tasks and protocols used to study behaving organisms and their cognitive processes. Indeed, the often ambiguous notion of "levels" in neuroscience is closely tied to the observational affordances of experimental tools and their heuristics. Sometimes the localization of a particular event or item to a given level is merely shorthand for describing the research tools and techniques employed to study it.

Some contend that every landmark discovery of contemporary neuroscience can be tied directly to the development and ingenious use of one or more research tools (see Bickle this volume). Perhaps this claim is exaggerated, but if so, only slightly. This centrality of research tools in current neuroscience practice even motivates one of today's most well-funded and influential government-private enterprise partnerships, the BRAIN Initiative. Its name is the acronym for Brain Research through Advancing Innovative Neurotechnologies®, and it aims explicitly at "revolutionizing our understanding of the human brain… [b]y accelerating the development and application of innovative technologies," (https://braininitiative.nih.gov). The aim is to revolutionize neuroscience by funding research into the development of new research tools and instruments. The sheer dollar amounts associated with this initiative speak volumes about neuroscientists' recognition of the importance of new research tools in their professional activities. Through 2019, BRAIN Initiative research awards already exceeded 1.3 billion US dollars (https://braininitiative.nih.gov/about/overview).

Neuroscience is not unique in its reliance on experimental tools. Many landmark discoveries in other sciences can likewise be tied directly to their innovations and developments. Telescopes guided Galileo's heliocentrism, the microscope was crucial to the development of the germ theory of disease, and Rosalind Franklin's X-ray crystallography led directly to the double helix model of DNA, to name just a few of the most obvious examples. However, there is one crucial difference between neuroscience and other tool-reliant sciences: the target of inquiry. Neuroscience's ultimate explanatory target is *our* brains, the organ driving *our* behaviors. This target catapults the investigation of research tools in neuroscience into a brighter philosophical spotlight.

Philosophers are well suited to join neuroscientists in reflecting on the development and use of research tools. Increasingly, young philosophers are acquiring backgrounds in neuroscience as part of their undergraduate, graduate, and postgraduate training. Acquiring this background often involves using the tools involved in neuroscience research. Still, sustained philosophical attention to the development and uses of experiment tools in neuroscience remains rare. When new functional neuroimaging technologies such as positron emission tomography (PET) and functional magnetic resonance imaging (fMRI) developed toward the end of the twentieth century, there was a flurry of philosophical interest in how these techniques worked and were being used in experiments in the then-new cognitive neurosciences (e.g., Bogen, Roskies, cited in these chapters). Unfortunately, those earlier discussions remained relatively self-contained, as philosophers often linked their analysis of these new techniques primarily to orthodox philosophical questions about the nature of mind. Around that same time, the science-in-practice movement across all of philosophy of science was successfully directing more philosophical attention to aspects of day-to-day scientific activities and away from philosophy of science's traditional focus on the justification of scientific theories and the relationship between theory and world. Many philosophers of neuroscience came to count their research as part of the broader science-in-practice movement, or the "practice turn." Philosophers of neuroscience have also been at the forefront of recent broader interest in the philosophy of experiment. Nevertheless, the published literature from this important refocusing on practices and experimentation still has one glaring lacuna. It has not yet addressed systematically how the tools of scientific experiment come to be, how they are justified, adopted, and proliferated, and finally how our theories change through the uses of these tools, leading to cycles of change in the ability to intervene into and detect brain function. In addition to epistemic and pragmatic considerations about their application, another emerging question concerns the explicitly cognitive role of tools in this context. Just *how* do tools facilitate new thinking in scientific practice?

This gap in the philosophical literature presents philosophers with a rare opportunity: to contribute fresh and novel ideas by reflecting on how these research tools provide access to the brain and nervous system. Furthermore, such philosophical contribution can play a notably *active* role in the ongoing neuroscientific debate, given the dynamic nature of the field and the relative recency with which many experimental tools have entered the brain sciences. (After all, fMRI is a child of the 1990s.) Making such an active contribution will require detailed knowledge of tool use in neuroscience practice. The project calls for *collaborations* between philosophers and neuroscientists. Moreover, the work of the handful of philosophers who have wandered onto this topic must eventually be combined into a coherent research program. This is what we are trying to facilitate with this volume. As reflected in the chapters of this volume, the work of a cadre of philosophers and philosophically interested neuroscientists has begun to coalesce. We showcase their work here in an effort to spawn more effective collaboration, to encourage more consolidation into a recognized research area, and to instigate discussions and arguments that, we believe, will contribute meaningfully and uniquely to our understanding of science as practiced.

The idea for this volume developed over the past half-decade. When a handful of us first noticed our shared interest in a new tool in 21st-century neurobiology, two of the editors of this volume (Bickle and Craver) joined up with two other philosophers of neuroscience (Sarah Robins and Jacquiline Sullivan) to organize a submitted session on "optogenetics" at the 2016 Philosophy of Science Association meeting. Coincidentally, neuroscientist Stuart Firestein, who wrote the Foreward to this volume, and the third editor, Barwich, were in the sessions' audience. Attention to those discussions on the nature of new technologies in the brain sciences seemed to persist, so Bickle and Craver co-organized two recent professional workshops on tool development in neuroscience; Barwich presented her research at both. The first was held in Pensacola Beach, Florida, in September 2019. We expected 10–12 submissions to our Call for Abstracts; by the submission deadline, we had received 25. We held two ten-hour days of presentations and discussions. The second conference was an Early Career Workshop on Neurotechnology, hosted by the Center for Philosophy of Science and the Center for the Neural Basis of Cognition at the University of Pittsburgh in January 2020 (fortunately, just before the Covid-19 pandemic shut down in-person conferences). Bickle and Craver co-organized this second workshop with Colin Allen and two History and Philosophy of Science Ph.D. candidates at the time, Mahi Hardalupas and Morgan Thompson. Although the general topic of this second workshop was broader than just research tool development, that theme was prominent in our call for submissions. In the end, we accepted eight submitted abstracts for presentation, each was assigned a senior commentator; we invited four keynote speakers and held a poster session. This workshop likewise comprised two full days of presentations and discussions. And here our focus explicitly was to promote work by junior investigators, the philosophers and scientists who will be working on these topics for the next three to four decades. These workshops, just like this volume, reflect the youth and diversity of the philosophers and scientists who've taken interest in this topic. The philosophy of neuroscience is fortunate to have attracted not only highly talented scholars but an impressively diverse group as well.

Those events led to this volume. Our fundamental goal is to promote sustained investigations into tool development in neuroscience by philosophers *and* neuroscientists. We hope this volume encourages more researchers to reflect and perhaps extend this discussion to other sciences. In these essays, broad epistemic considerations juxtapose seamlessly with practical concerns. New insights emerge about the special place of research tools in science, the norms of experimental practices, and the strategies experimentalists use for teasing out nature's secrets about that wonderfully complex organ of thought, affect, and consciousness, the human brain.

We've divided the 15 chapters in this volume into five sections. The first section, *Research Tools in Relation to Theory*, has chapters organized around several case studies of tool development, some historical, some recent. Each chapter discusses the development of revolutionary (or potentially revolutionary) research tools across neuroscience and supports different conclusions concerning the relationship between new research tools and theory progress. *Bickle* describes the late-1950s development of the metal microelectrode for single-cell neurophysiology and the late-1970s development of the patch-clamp. He argues that the historical details of these cases show that theory in neurobiology is doubly dependent, not only on new research tools but also on atheoretical "laboratory tinkering" through which these tools developed. *Johnson* looks at examples of tools Bickle has stressed previously, especially gene targeting and optogenetics. He finds a much less tidy picture than Bickle's "tools-first" account proposes, and one that reflects an important ambiguity in the claim that "theories depend on tools." He argues that sometimes theories and tools work in tandem, while in other cases, tools are "first" and theory has little or no role in the investigation. *Atanasova, Williams, and Vorhees* recount the process of the designing and continuous refinement of the Cincinnati water maze, a tool utilized in the study of rat egocentric learning and memory. This case study exemplifies the interplay between toolmaking, experiment, and theory where tool availability often determines the kinds of experiments performed in a certain laboratory. The authors introduce the notion of theories as interpretative devices to capture cases in the practice of neuroscience in which multiple experiments precede, rather than succeed, the theory for which they provide empirical support. *Barwich and Xu* present a first-hand account of Xu's recent application of a new tool, SCAPE microscopy, which uncovered a new mechanism of mixture coding at the olfactory periphery. SCAPE (Swept, Confocally-Aligned Planar Excitation) microscopy allows for fast three-dimensional, high-resolution imaging of entire small organisms (e.g., larvae) or large intact tissue sections (e.g., in mice). Barwich and Xu illustrate how technologies facilitate a broader and different theoretical perspective by being an integral part of the thinking process itself and by co-creating mental structures. *Hardcastle and Stewart* show how "tinkering" with 19th-century manual "handheld" autopsy techniques led to discoveries about otherwise puzzling "brain fog" reported in some advanced cases of COVID-19 infection. This revamped technology enabled researchers to get around CDC (and common sense) restrictions on using aerosol sprays in brain autopsies of COVID patients and to find in infected brains a class of large platelet-producing cells normally found in the bone marrow. In this case, the "tinkering" with tools has led to new implications about the blood-brain barrier, viral activity and the relationships between nervous and other bodily tissues.

We title the second section *Research Tools and Epistemology.* It includes chapters that show how a focus on neuroscience's research tools and their development transforms some traditional, much-discussed epistemological issues in the philosophy of science, including the dissemination of knowledge, the integration of knowledge across fields of neuroscience, and the relationship between explanation and prediction. *Silva* argues that the power of a new research tool to capture scientists' interests depends not only on its ability to reveal new and transformative phenomena, but also on its ease of use and transferability across labs. He illustrates these dual(ing) concerns by discussing recent developments of "miniscopes," miniaturized head-mounted fluorescent microscopes capable of recording from hundreds of cells for days or weeks in freely-moving, behaving animals. Besides their potential impact on science, miniscopes are also inexpensive, require no previous experience with *in vivo* recordings, and can even be manufactured in the lab at very low costs. How exactly do these epistemic and practical concerns interact in daily laboratory science? *Craver* uses the early history of optogenetics technologies to study the norms governing the evaluation of new interventionist technologies. Craver integrates this discussion with James Woodward's much-discussed manipulationist view of causal relevance and lays out some foundational assumptions for an epistemology of intervention. Craver calls attention to crucial normative distinctions between those (the modelers) who use new tools for the purposes of exploring the brain and those (the makers) who use those tools to engineer brain systems for our own ends, arguing for some significant epistemic differences between these two groups of scientists. *Tramacere* analyzes various cases of triangulation, where multiple tools have provided both discordance and concordance of evidence. She argues that the use of two or more measurement techniques (such as electroencephalography (EEG), magnetic resonance imaging (MRI), and functional MRI (fMRI)), has proven useful to minimize the limitations of each tool and to refine experimental hypotheses about the role of the brain in cognition. Finally, she argues that triangulation, especially *within the same experimental setting*, is helpful with the integration of data and findings, contributing to the understanding of how the mind works. *Nathan* examines neuroimaging techniques in cognitive neuroscience and their use in "reverse inferencing" psychological states from locations or patterns of brain activity. Using these strategies the measured neural states predict psychological features, but provide no causal-mechanistic explanations of the psychological processes. This aspect of contemporary cognitive neuroscience investigations, which Nathan also finds in other human brain-mapping endeavors, does not sit easily with traditional philosophy of science's related treatments of explanation and prediction. He suggests a "black-box" solution, according to which prediction and explanation are grounded in the same underlying causal network, but require different degrees of mechanistic detail.

Section 3 concerns *Research Tools, Integration, Circuits and Ontology*. New research tools in neuroscience speak to the most general of philosophical questions about how we characterize the nature of the portion of the world that neuroscience addresses. The chapters in this section cover three such questions: do research tools help or hinder attempts to integrate the many fields and "levels" of neuroscientific investigation (or both)? The great increase in the contents of neuroscience's "toolkit" over the recent decades seems not yet to have yielded comparatively great explanatory increases in uncovering the mechanisms of behavior in even our simpler animal models. Is this because new tools need the coincidental development of new neuroscientific concepts? How do our research tools help us characterize the correct set of basic categories, the "ontology," of the brain and its activities? *Colaço* discusses CLARITY, a tissue clarifying tool that extends the scale at which optical microscopy can be used and so has successfully contributed what he calls "local" integrations. However, his analysis of CLARITY also addresses why the constraints and productivity of a research tool can contribute to the difficulty, acknowledged by philosophers and neuroscientists alike, of "systematic integration" of methods, data and explanatory schema across neuroscience's numerous fields. *Parker* considers the use of experimental tools to understand neural circuits. In the last 25 years, the range of tools available for these analyses has increased markedly, but he argues that neural circuit understanding has not increased significantly despite techniques that allow us to examine more components with greater precision and in more detail than before. He considers whether we will have to develop tools that will allow us to address aspects of neurobiology that have not been considered in traditional circuit approaches. *Burnston* investigates recent novel data-analysis tools that some have proposed to offer illuminating explanations of how mental functions are realized in the brain. He rejects this conclusion and instead insists that results with these new tools recommend switching to a "task-based cognitive ontology" of neuroscience's basic explanatory target.

Section 4, *Tools and Integrative Pluralism* explores how new computing technologies have combined with more standard neuroscientific wet-lab and behavioral laboratory tools and protocols to yield powerful new approaches that integrated laboratory and computational methods in exciting new ways. We organize these two chapters historically. *Favela* presents Hodgkin and Huxley's Nobel Prize-winning work as an instance of research constrained by both technological limitations and mathematical assumptions. He then argues how the discovery of scale-invariant neuronal dynamics required both technological and mathematical advances, and points out how these cases conflict with the priority on technological dependence that some philosophers of neuroscience have urged. *Prinz* describes the dynamic clamp technique, which interfaces living neurons and circuits with computational models in real-time and at multiple levels, ranging from models of cellular components and synapses to models of individual neurons to entire circuits. This technique creates hybrid *in vivo-in silico* systems where living brains and computer models directly "talk to each other," to take advantage of combining experimental investigation of living neural systems with the precise, theoretically-guided control over neural, synaptic, and circuit parameters that computational models provide.

We end the volume with a section on *Tool Use and Development Beyond Neuroscience*. Neuroscience is hardly the only scientific endeavor driven by its research tools. And yet none of the philosophies of specific sciences has emphasized explicitly the place of tools in that science's activities or the implications tool use and development hold for philosophical reflection on its practices and products. Our hope is that this volume spurs philosophical interest in research tools across all of science. To illustrate that potential, in our final chapter *Baxter* investigates biologists conducting loss of function experiments, where they often single out the genes they manipulate to explain the observable differences these manipulations produce. She notices that the logical structure of the resulting explanations vary in a regular fashion and argues that the types of experimental tools that biologists use to intervene on genes account for this variety.

Our broader goal of introducing a new concern into the philosophy of neuroscience predates our specific interests in neuroscience's research tools. In mid-February 2008, two of us (Bickle and Craver) were invited speakers at a one-day "Symposium on Neurophilosophy" hosted by the then-new Ludwig-Maximilians-Universität Munich Center for Neuroscience. Rather than immediately fly back to the States, we spent the weekend at the Tegelberg in southern Bavaria. On the train back to Munich late Sunday evening, before a long day of air travel back to the States the next day, we decided that the ruthless reductionism-mechanism disagreement we had both been so committed to fighting for nearly a decade was growing stale. (That was just as the issue of mechanisms was becoming the clearly dominant view in the philosophy of neuroscience.) We wanted to find a new topic, perhaps even one on which we could agree. It took us a while to find tool development; it was another seven years after that first discussion until the idea for the optogenetics symposium at PSA 2016 took shape. But it was fun to see a new topic attract the attention of two longtime philosophical antagonists (and personal friends), especially one that also captured the attention of Barwich and this outstanding collection of contributors from philosophy and neuroscience.

By integrating these pluralistic approaches and interdisciplinary works on tool use and development in neuroscience, we hope with this volume to give this emerging research further momentum and to facilitate growing interest in this area.

We thank Andrew Weckenmann, editor of the Routledge Studies in Philosophy of Science series, for his interest in pursuing a volume of essays that seeks to introduce a new topic for further investigation, and for the speed with which he and Routledge got our project into press. We also are thankful for the helpful and positive comments of two anonymous reviewers on the book's proposal.

Note

1 And recently made available in paperback by MIT Press (Cambridge: MIT Press/Bradford Book, 2004).

Research Tools in Relation to Theories

1 Tinkering in the Lab

John Bickle

1 Putting Theory in Its Place

Progress in neuroscience is driven by its research tools. Nervous systems are complicated and delicate and don't readily reveal their machinations. Available research tools are and have always been our only means of revealing them. Philosophers have increasingly come to acknowledge this fact, starting with a spate of interest in the workings of whole-brain functional neuroimaging tools. More recently some have focused on research tools common in neurobiology labs, including optogenetics and DREADDs (Bickle 2016, 2018; Robins 2016, 2018; Sullivan 2018), gene targeting techniques (Bickle 2003, 2015, 2016, 2019, 2020; Sullivan 2009), and various behavioral paradigms for rodent models (Sullivan 2010; Atanasova 2015).

The general philosophical lesson I have stressed in my contributions to this growing literature is that in "wetlab" neurobiology, new tool development *drives everything else*. It is where progress in this science inevitably starts, and also where the bulk of attention in leading labs is focused. This lesson contrasts sharply with the theory-centrism that has characterized mainstream philosophy of science since its inception as a recognized field in the mid-20th century. While contemporary mainstream philosophy of science has certainly come to recognize the existence and importance of scientific practices other than theorizing—prediction, modes of observation, experimentation, to name a few—it still too often subjugates these extra-theoretical practices to the goal and service of theory progress and the confirmation of theory-world relations. Countering this mainstream theory-centrism was one explicit motive behind Ian Hacking's (1983) push for a "back-to-Bacon" movement. The still-advancing science-in-practice movement, which dedicates more attention to extra-theory aspects of science, has been a promising recent development. Still, a lot more needs to be done to square philosophy of science with science's actual day-to-day practices. More research on tool development and use in laboratory neurobiology is a useful next focus. A developer of one of laboratory neurobiology's most influential research tools, the high-impedance metal microelectrode (which you will

DOI: 10.4324/9781003251392-3

read about in the next section) once remarked that "our science seemed not to conform to the science that we are taught in high school, with its laws, hypotheses, experimental verification, generalizations, and so on" (Hubel 1996, 312). Okay! So what did their science "conform to"? Our philosophical view of what laboratory science is all about may hang in the balance of these investigations.

It is important to clarify a number of points at the outset. First, rejecting theory-centrism about science *is not* tantamount to claiming that theory *has no place* in wetlab sciences like neurobiology. Such a claim is not only preposterous but also conflicts with the simple observation that neuroscience's best-confirmed current theories are from wetlab neurobiology. The structure and function of ion channels and active transporters that underlie neural conductance of action potentials; the detailed molecular mechanisms of chemical neurotransmission in both pre- and post-synaptic neurons; the intra- and inter-neuronal signaling pathways leading to new gene expression, protein synthesis, and ultimately plasticity of structure and responses in individual synapses, neurons, circuits, and ultimately organism behavior; these are current neuroscience's experimentally best-confirmed theories. The rejection of mainstream philosophy of science's theory-centrism is instead an attempt *to put theory in its proper place*. Theory in wetlab neurobiology is dependent upon the development and ingenious use of new research tools. The genesis of every piece of theory just mentioned can be traced back directly to the development of some new research tools. Theoretical progress in this paradigmatic science of our times *is secondary to and dependent upon* new tool development, both temporally and epistemically. Not the other way around.

In this chapter, I will urge one more step away from theory-centrism through further reflection on research tool development in neurobiology. Theory progress therein is also dependent on what I will here call *atheoretical laboratory tinkering*. Theory progress in neurobiology is thus doubly dependent, and hence tertiary in both epistemic and temporal priority:

> atheoretical laboratory tinkering → new experiment tool development → theory progress.

My goal in this chapter is to argue for this additional step toward "putting theory in its place," in laboratory sciences like neurobiology.

Second important clarification: A common challenge to my attacks on theory-centrism has been: "Surely the development of these research tools presupposed theory! So how can theory be so dependent on them?" Of course, theory informed the work that produced these research tools. But as the detailed history of each tool shows, the theory progress that results didn't guide the tool's development. Here a distinction that emerged in the recent philosophical literature on "exploratory experimentation" is helpful. Franklin (2005) distinguishes experiments directed by both theoretical background and local theory about the specific objects being investigated from experiments directed only by the theoretical background. Burian (2007) distinguishes theory-*driven* experiments from theory-*informed* experiments depending upon whether or not the theory provides expectations about what experimenters will find. Like exploratory experiments, tool development experiments appear to be these latter types.[1]

A final clarification: Everyone concerned about the place of theory in science should embrace philosopher Wilfrid Sellars' quip, "the term 'theory' is one of those accordion words which, by their expansion and contraction, generate so much philosophical music" (1965, 172). I won't "provide an analysis" of "theory" here. Sellars' quip explains why any "analysis" will simply be an explication of one of any number of concepts that ambiguous word signifies. Instead, I'll pursue my usual metascientific approach (Bickle 2003; Silva et al. 2014) and present some little-discussed history of laboratory neurobiology, namely, the development of two of its most impactful research tools: the metal microelectrode for extended sessions of single-cell neurophysiology; and the patch clamp, the tool that opened the door to the molecular revolution that has guided mainstream neurobiology for the last four decades. The mainstream philosophical sense(s) of "theory" that I'm trying to "put in its (their) place" will hopefully become clearer in contrast with some historical details about the kinds of atheoretical solutions that developers of these laboratory research tools hit upon to get them to work.

2 Atheoretical Tinkering in David Hubel's Lab circa 1957

For a quarter century, from the late-1950s well into the 1980s, electrophysiology involving single-neuron recordings throughout the mammalian cortex was a mainstay of basic neuroscience research. Not just *in vitro*, in tissue slices, but *in vivo*, inside the brains of living animals. A then-new research tool, the high-impedance conducting metal microelectrode, made some of that research possible. Armed with this new tool, David Hubel and Torsten Wiesel (1962, 1965) found orientation-selective neurons and the hierarchy of simple and complex neurons in cat primary visual cortex. Each won a one-quarter share of the 1981 Nobel Prize for Physiology or Medicine for this work. A decade later Charles Gross and colleagues (Gross et al. 1972) and two decades later Robert Desimone and colleagues (Desimone et al. 1984) found face- and hand-selective neurons in the primate inferotemporal cortex. These neurons were real-world approximations of Jerry Lettvin's "grandmother" neuron, the fanciful neuron that fires a high rate of action potentials when and only when Granny is in its receptive field. Patricia Goldman-Rakic's group (Funahashi et al. 1993) found "working memory neurons" in the primate dorsolateral prefrontal cortex, whose activity coded for the spatial locations of stimuli that had been presented a few seconds earlier. And William Newsome's (Salzmann et al. 1992) and Ranulfo Romo's (Romo et al. 1998) labs transformed these recording metal microelectrodes into a microstimulation tool, using variants small enough to be inserted directly into cortical columns to activate tiny clusters of similarly-tuned cortical sensory neurons. These microstimulations altered monkeys' behavioral judgments about the character of the presented sensory stimuli. This shortlist of groundbreaking results just scratches the surface. (I'll have more examples of landmark results from metal microelectrodes later in this section.)

Less known is that David Hubel (1957) himself first perfected tungsten microelectrodes for cortical use, just a few years before he and Wiesel embarked on their Nobel Prize-winning research. As Hubel remarks in his Nobel acceptance speech, recording from single cells in the visual cortex was "potentially a gold mine" but "methods were needed that would permit the recording of single cells for many hours, and with eyes immobilized" (1981, 24). The standard glass micropipette electrodes of the mid-1950s, which Vernon Mountcastle and Stephen Kuffler had used to map the receptive fields of single neurons in primate primary sensory and motor cortices and retina, tended to break or bend at their tips during the much longer recording sessions required for exploring visual neurons' responses. Insulated metals were the obvious choice for developing durable electrodes, but tip dimensions necessary to resolve individual action potentials in single neurons ranged from 5 microns for extracellular recordings to 1 micron for intracellular recordings.[2] Achieving these tip dimensions in metal faced serious technological difficulties. As Hubel remarks in the *Science* publication introducing his technique, steel wire "becomes too fragile near the tip when thus sharpened, and also requires too thick a shaft" to resist breakage while being inserted through brain tissue (Hubel 1957, 549). Following a suggestion by physicist Leon Levin, Hubel chose tungsten as "by far the stiffest, easily available metal" (1957, 549). Notice the nature of these initial problems and solutions, as reflected in Hubel's word choices, "becomes too fragile," "requires too thick a shaft," "stiffest, easily available." He confronted *engineering* problems that required *practical* solutions.

Hubel's shift to tungsten only exacerbated his practical challenges. He quickly discovered that one of the then-standard techniques for steel electropolishing worked to generate tips of the required dimensions in tungsten wire.[3] Hubel consulted or appealed to no theory; he discovered this strictly by trial and error, working with then-standard electropolishing techniques. He also quickly discovered, by trial-and-error tinkering, that he could obtain almost any degree of taper in tungsten tips

by raising and lowering the wire during all but the final stages of electropolishing. However, insulating the tungsten microelectrodes proved
trickier. Hubel's autobiographical remembrances illuminate the kinds of
problems this posed and the solution he stumbled upon:

> I *tried every coating I could find* but nothing seemed *adherent
> enough or viscous enough.* Formvar did not adhere and in any case
> *was available only in tank-car amounts.* A solution of Lucite in
> chloroform *came close to working.* One day *while I was playing
> around with this* my neighbor in the next lab walked in *with a can
> of something called "Insulex" and said, "Why not try this?"* I soon
> found that when Insulex was thickened by evaporation *it became
> viscous enough to adhere to the wire,* and suddenly I had an elec-
> trode that was recording sensational single units.
>   (Hubel 1996, 303; my emphases)

The italics I've added emphasize the many practical considerations that
drove Hubel's discovery. These are the phrasings of a skilled tinker, not
a physical chemist.

Hubel's remembrances of inventing the hydraulic microelectrode ad-
vancer, required to drive the metal microelectrode to precise locations
in brain tissue *in vivo,* are equally revealing of the practical problems he
confronted and the tinkering solutions he found. "The problem was not
entirely simple ... a hydraulic system seemed to be the best bet, but one
had to make the piston-and cylinder compatible with a chamber closed to
the atmosphere" (1996, 304). A closed chamber was required to prevent
movements of the cortex caused by pulsations in an open environment,
which would alter the electrode penetration path. Hubel found himself
"having to continually mollify machinists" when he brought back their
"skillfully built ... latest model" and explained to them "why it couldn't
work" (1996, 304). His solution? "Finally I decided I must learn how
to operate a lathe, and went to night school in downtown Washington,
D.C.," (1996, 304). When all else fails, do it yourself (in Hubel's case,
on your own time and dime). Note that this attitude about tool development was from a future Nobel laureate.

Hubel's tinkering attitude likewise drove his (and Wiesel's) addition
to the histological "reconstruction technique" pioneered by Mountcastle for confirming the exact placement of the recording electrode where
single-neuron recordings were taken. "Our addition ... was the strategy of making multiple small (roughly 100 μm diameter) electrolytic
lesions along each track by passing small currents through the tungsten
electrodes" (1981, 37). Did "theory" inform Hubel's discovery of this
"addition"? Not hardly: "I worked out this method at Walter Reed by
watching the coagulation produced at the electrode tip on passing currents through egg white" (1981, 37). Tinkering redux.

And the rest really was history, in terms of progress in the neurobiology of vision. Hubel and Wiesel's work with Hubel's tinkering-generated metal microelectrode and hydraulic microdriver on single neuron responses in cat primary visual cortex (striatal, V1), then on into extrastriatal cortex (V2, V3), won them their shares of the 1981 Nobel Prize for Physiology or Medicine "for their discoveries concerning information processing in the visual cortex" (https://www.nobelprize.org/prizes/medicine/1981/summary/). The Press Release announcing the award ends by noting the principle of cortical organization based on individual neuron function that directed subsequent neuroscience research for the next quarter-century:

> By following the visual impulses along their path to the various cell layers of the optical cortex, Hubel and Wiesel have been able to demonstrate that the *message about the image falling on the retina undergoes a step-wise analysis in a system of nerve cells stored in columns. In this system each cell has its specific function and is responsible for a specific detail in the pattern of the retinal image.*
> (https://www.nobelprize.org/prizes/medicine/1981/press-release/;
> emphases in original)

The last sentence expresses the key theoretical concept of a sensory neuron's "receptive field," which soon found application in motor and even associational "cognitive" cortices. This experiment tool and approach not only informed neuroscientific research through the 1980s that I surveyed briefly at the beginning of this section, but its use also generated the "subway map" models of visual cortical processing, and the distinction between the "dorsal visual stream" through the posterior parietal cortex and the "ventral visual stream" through the inferior temporal cortex (a distinction first found in nonhuman primates using Hubel's metal microelectrodes). All of this has been textbook neuroscience for three decades. In his Nobel Award Ceremony Speech introducing Hubel and Wiesel, Karolinska Institutet physiologist David Ottoman compared the pair's "translation" of the "symbolic calligraphy of the brain cortex" to

> the deciphering of the hieroglyphic characters of the ancient Egyptians ... denoted as one of the greatest advances in the history of philology. By breaking the code of the enigmatic signals of the visual system you have made an achievement which for all time will stand out as one of the most important in the history of brain research.
> (https://www.nobelprize.org/prizes/medicine/1981/
> ceremony-speech/)

All of this ground-breaking and enduring theory ties directly to Hubel's catch-as-catch-can, make-it-work, trial-and-error-tinkering invention of a new experiment tool, and the new kinds of experiments it enabled.

3 More on the Theory and Its Influence Driven by Hubel's Metal Microelectrode

Hubel and Wiesel's shares of the 1981 Nobel Prize for Physiology or Medicine stem in large part from three joint publications (1959, 1962, 1965).[4] In these publications, the pair report their initial discoveries of the receptive field properties of single neurons in the cat visual cortex, both striate (Brodmann's area 17) and extra-striate (Brodmann's areas 18 and 19). They report their unexpected initial findings that bar stimuli at specific spatial locations and orientations, rather than the expected small circles drove activations in single neurons in area 17. This initial discovery itself was by accident, resulting from Hubel and Wiesel's attention as experienced bench scientists, not appliers of systematic theory. One of the only slides that initially evoked a consistently strong neuronal response in a single cortical visual neuron in a single cat happened to have a vertical crack near its bottom (see Hubel 1981, 27). Hubel and Wiesel noticed the anomaly in that slide and immediately tried presenting slides with bars oriented in various orientations instead of circles. Neurons across V1 suddenly began responding vigorously to these new stimuli.

Extended recordings from individual cortical neurons *in vivo* during the presentation of multiple stimuli, which Hubel's metal microelectrode permitted, led Hubel and Wiesel to their discovery that activity in these neurons takes a Gaussian shape. A given primary visual cortex neuron responds most actively (highest number of action potentials per time unit) to bar stimuli at one specific orientation, e.g., vertical; its response rate decreases systematically as bar orientations fall away from its most preferred orientation in either direction. The careful penetrations and follow-up histological techniques they refined and used with their new tool also demonstrated that area 17 visual neurons in a given cortical column shared receptive field properties (preferred spatial location and bar stimuli orientations), but that a neuron's exact rate of action potentials depended on its location in a specific cortical layer.

These three publications also introduced another of Hubel and Wiesel's contributions to subsequent neuroscience theory. They distinguished among "simple," "complex," and "hypercomplex" neurons, strictly on measured receptive field properties and anatomical locations. They speculated on circuitries obtaining between visual cortical neurons through which the measured receptive field properties might be generated. Their (1965) paper demonstrated the feasibility of using the metal microelectrode to explore receptive fields of individual neurons outside of the primary visual cortex, and as Hubel states in his Nobel Prize address, reported "the tendency toward increased complexity as one moves centrally along the visual path, and the possibility of accounting for a cell's behavior in terms of its inputs" (1981, 36). Single-cell work on the visual system also provided the experimental model for more detailed work on other sensory systems, motor systems, and various cognitive systems throughout the association cortex in all cortical lobes. The influence of those three Hubel and Wiesel publications has been enormous across all of the neurosciences; this influence is well reflected by these papers' citation numbers. Hubel and Wiesel (1965) has been cited 3,164 times; Hubel and Wiesel (1959) 5,447 times; and their most-cited joint publication, Hubel and Wiesel (1962) has 15,303 citations.[5] This number puts their (1962) among the most cited papers in the history of neuroscience.

4 Laboratory Tinkering by Erwin Neher and Bert Sakmann, circa 1974 ... to 1980!

In the opening paragraph of his Nobel Prize address from December 1991, German biophysicist Erwin Neher describes the state of the search for the mechanisms of neural conductance circa 1970. Alan Hodgkin and Alex Huxley had "provided the basis" of the neuron action potential nearly two decades before with their extensive experimental manipulations and quantitative modeling of the fast sodium ion (Na^+) influx, then the slower potassium ion (K^+) efflux across the axon membrane. But "the question of the molecular mechanisms underlying these signals was still open" (Neher 1991, 10). Hodgkin and Huxley (1952) speculated about a voltage-operated "gate" in their formal model, and by 1970 "the terms Na-channel and K-channel were used frequently ... although no direct evidence for the existence of channels was available from biological preparations" (Neher 1991, 10). Experiments throughout the 1960s using artificial "black-lipid" membranes as models for biological bimolecular lipid membranes had suggested that conductance changes were from "single pore-like structures," but in the biological membranes "similar measurements were not possible at that time" (1991, 10). Using then-current recording equipment, background noise levels greatly swamped currents of the sizes that were measurable in biological membranes by more than two orders of magnitude. However, "indirect evidence" suggested that channels with current conductances similar to those measurable in artificial membranes should be operative in both neurons and muscle cells. So:

> It was very tempting to think about *better methods* for recording currents from biological preparations. There was good reason to hope that *an improved technology* would reveal a whole 'microcosmos' of electrical signals in a multitude of electrically and chemically excitable cell types.
>
> (Neher 1991, 11; my emphases)

Neher's words and attitude should be very familiar by this point in this paper. A new experiment tool seemed the key next step to revealing the mechanisms. And solving a host of practical problems in building such a tool seemed to be the key first step: "an improved technology." Was this another job for laboratory tinkers?

The first task for resolving these tiny currents amidst extensive background noise was to isolate far smaller signal sources than that of the membrane itself: to isolate small "patches" of the cell membrane. Neher brought to this task his background in the spinning and use of glass suction micropipettes from his Ph.D. work in Munich. Bert Sakmann, fortuitously the scientist in the lab next door to Neher's at the Max-Planck Institut für Biophysikalische Chemie in Göttingen, had trained in Bernard Katz's lab and was experienced in treating cell surfaces enzymatically for precision current measurements. In the 1960s, working with modifications of the voltage clamp, Katz's lab had resolved macrocurrents from acetylcholine receptors from the end-plates of frog muscle cells, which form the muscle component at neuromuscular junctions (where motor neurons synapse onto muscle fibers). That work had provided the first direct experimental evidence of the "quantal" (step-wise) nature of chemical neurotransmission. With their scientific backgrounds Neher and Sakmann set to work to construct a "patch-clamp rig," a miniaturized variation of Kenneth Cole's quarter century-old voltage-clamp.

The basic idea of Neher and Sakmann's patch clamp is simple. A tiny hollow glass micropipette, filled with both electrolyte solution and a recording electrode connected to an amplifier, is attached to the isolated cell membrane being kept alive in a nutrient bath. "Tiny" is an understatement. The diameter of the pipette tip is in the single micron range (see footnote 1 above), with a smoothened rather than sharp tip surface. (At that time, sharp-tipped glass micropipette electrodes had been in use for nearly three decades, to puncture membranes for intracellular recordings.) A second electrode serves as a ground, completing a circuit. For such "cell-attached" recordings the electrolyte solution inside the pipette matches the composition of the nutrient bath solution. Often a standard voltage-clamp rig is attached to the cell or membrane, to maintain a fixed membrane potential or to change the membrane potential to precise values at specific times. Basic electrodynamics predicted that achieving seals between micropipette tip and membrane surface with resistances in the 10–100 gigaohms range should permit relatively noise-free recordings of currents across the membrane in the single picoampere range (1 ampere = 1,000,000,000,000 [1 trillion] picoamperes). The pipette-membrane attachment is viewed under a microscope. The entire rig is affixed to an anti-vibration table since the slightest vibration can weaken the pipette-to-membrane seal.

As is typical with many ideas that seem simple, actually building a functioning patch clamp rig was complicated. Neher and Sakmann had a prototype rig in operation by 1974. They used it first to measure currents from a variety of cell preparations that contained acetylcholine (Ach) receptors, as these were "probably the best-described channel in biological membranes" at that time due to Katz's ground-breaking work from the previous decade (Neher and Sakmann 1976, 800). However, as Neher later remarked, the pair "soon realized that it was not so easy to obtain a satisfactory 'seal'," and despite their complementary expertise and backgrounds on micropipette design and cell surface polishing, "our initial attempts failed" (1991, 13). Trial-and-error work on firepolishing micropipettes achieved the required smooth tips and reduced tip sizes to the 3- to 5-micron range. This continually decreased the size of the "patch" of the membrane the tool recorded from. Further refining various enzymatic treatments of membranes, especially to extra-synaptic portions of denervated hypersensitive frog muscle fibers known from pharmacological studies to be highly responsive to acetylcholine manipulations, eventually generated seals sufficient to block background noise and to measure square pulse waves of inward current of roughly 2–4 picoamperes from patches of tissue of roughly 10 square microns. A variety of properties of Ach receptors they observed in their measurements, predicted from Katz's and others' previous macroscopic recordings, led Neher and Sakmann to conclude "that the observed conductance changes are indeed recordings of single-channel currents" (1976, 801). Their first paper reporting the patch clamp method and these initial landmark but limited recordings was published in *Nature* in April 1976.

By the time their 1976 *Nature* publication appeared, Neher had spent parts of 1975 and 1976 in Charles Stevens' lab at Yale. He constructed a patch clamp rig there and noted, in the phrasings of a true experimentalist, that "the fact that similar records could be obtained both in our Göttingen laboratory and ... at Yale ... gave us confidence that they were not the result of some local demon, but rather signals of biological significance" (Neher 1991, 13). The square-wave nature of the measured currents was particularly important because it was "proof" of Katz's previous ground-breaking indirect macroscopic experimental evidence that channels in biological membranes "open and close stochastically in an all-or-none manner" (Neher 1991, 13; see also Neher and Sakmann 1976, 801 and Figure 3). The development of this new tool might have been laborious and piecemeal, but the excitement generated by its early results was palpable. "For the first time one could watch conformational changes of biological macromolecules *in situ* and in real time" (Neher 1991).

Despite their excitement, Neher and Sakmann knew their initial measurements were far from optimal. The big problem remained the excessive background noise, traceable to the weakness of the pipette tip-to-membrane seal relative to the tiny size of the currents. Too-weak seals also led to currents from channels located under the pipette tip to be recorded only partially. To strengthen the seal, preferably with internal resistance in the gigaohm range, the pair and their collaborators "made many *systematic* attempts to solve the seal problem" (Neher 1991, 15; my emphasis). These included what you would expect from scientists with Neher's and Sakmann's specific expertise and backgrounds: additional manipulation and cleaning of membrane surfaces, further miniaturizing of pipette tip sizes and formation of even more steeply tapered final tip lengths, coating pipette surfaces with different materials, reversing charges on glass surfaces, even developing a technique for mass-producing pipettes so that a new one could be used for each experiment, solving the problem of miniscule pieces of membrane left on the tips from previous experiments and weakening the seal (Neher et al. 1978; Neher 1991). In other words, the pair did everything that then-current theory suggested would strengthen the seal, yet all of this "with little success" (Neher 1991, 15). Despite this failure to achieve the desired seal, the new tool still proved useful for studying the properties of single channels, especially cholinergic channels in hypersensitive muscle tissue. But the patch clamp's promise still seemed so much greater, for resolving even smaller currents from other channels, if the gigaseal could somehow be reliably and sustainably achieved.

Yet seemingly that achievement was not to be. As Neher notes, "by about 1980 we had almost given up on our attempts to improve the seal" (Neher 1991, 15). Notice the date Neher mentions. That was after more than *four years* of working on the seal problem, virtually daily, since their first *Nature* publication appeared in April 1976. Then one day:

> we noticed by chance, that the seal suddenly increased by more than two orders of magnitude when slight suction was applied to the pipette. The resulting seal was in the gigaohm range, the so-called 'Gigaseal.' It turned out that a gigaseal could be obtained reproducibly when suction was combined with some simple measures to provide for clean surfaces, such as using a fresh pipette for each approach and using filtered solutions. The improved seal resulted in much improved background noise ...
>
> (Neher 1991, 15)

Later in 1980, the group published their initial recordings of Na^+ currents through the gigaseal-achieving patch clamp, through single acetylcholine receptors in rat muscle fibers (Sigworth and Neher 1980). By 1981 they published a full report of the improved new technique, including how to mass-produce patch micropipettes, procedures for reliably achieving gigaseals, recording circuits and designs for improving frequency responses, and improved procedures for preparing cell membranes and physically isolating patches (Hamill et al. 1981). That paper reported recordings using the improved technique from small-diameter cells, including Na^+ currents from single channels in bovine chromaffin cells. Resolving currents from these channels had been impossible due to too-weak seals, because of the currents' tiny size and short duration. The trial-and-error atheoretical tinkering attitude I am stressing is apparent in Neher's remarks quoted above ("by chance," "it turned out"). It is also explicit in his remark on the group's capacity to amplify these tiny measured currents. "Fortunately Fred Sigworth had just joined the laboratory. With his *experience in engineering,* he improved the electronic amplifiers to match the advances in recording conditions" (1991, 15). Science writer (and biochemistry Ph.D.) Karen Hopkin has documented further remarks by Neher, Sakmann, and collaborators on their achievement of the gigaseal (Hopkin 2010). Their "tinkering-first" attitude is unmistakable in those remarks. For example, Hopkins quotes Neher suggesting that experimental know-how led to his breakthrough: "you had to apply *a little bit* of suction in order to pull some membrane into the orifice of the pipette ... if you *did it the right way* it worked" (Hopkin 2010; my emphases). She quotes lab member Owen Hamill recalling "a weird period where we could no longer get gigaseals ... Then Bert [Sakmann] suggested that you have to blow before you suck" (Hopkin 2010). Blowing solution through the clean pipette tip as it approached the membrane apparently ejected any minute particles in the tip that weakened the seal. No theory guided that discovery; it had nothing to do with membrane polishing, Sakmann's expertise. Rather, this discovery was made "on the bench" by an experienced (and first-rate) laboratory tinker.

Armed with their now-reliable new tool, Neher, Sakmann, and collaborators quickly demonstrated experimentally that the macroscopic ionic Na^+ and K^+ currents in neurons measured in voltage clamp experiments going back to Hodgkin and Huxley's work were the sum of a huge number of microcurrents through individual channels specific to each ion. The latter were now reliably measurable by the gigaseal patch clamp. Either current could be induced through the voltage clamp stimulating electrode by changing macroscopic membrane current. During multiple current inductions, Na^+ or K^+ currents could be measured through the patch clamp, with the other type of channels blocked pharmacologically by antagonists. An average of all of those (thousands of) patch clamp recordings could then be computed and graphed. The graph of time with respect to ion microcurrents exactly matched that for membrane macrocurrents. The activities of Hodgkin and Huxley's speculative "voltage gates" in neuron membranes, and their role in generating action potentials, were now observable on the lab bench. Coupling these patch clamp discoveries with ones using an even older experimental tool, X-ray crystallography (which had been around for nearly a century by that time), quickly revealed channel structure. They were configured proteins with differently charged amino acids at specific locations. And the theory of ion channels and active transporters in neural conductance that we possess today was quickly fleshed out experimentally. There is an often-traced direct line of theory progress in neurobiology from Hodgkin and Huxley's Nobel Prize to Roderick MacKinnon's half-share of the Nobel Prize in Chemistry in 2003 for his work on the structure and mechanistic functioning of K^+ channels. That path runs directly through Neher, Sakmann and results obtained using their patch clamp.

And that was just the beginning of the patch clamp's contributions to neurobiology. As Salk Institute neurobiologist Charles Stevens, whose Yale lab had hosted Neher's 1975–1976 visit, remarked a decade ago, "everything that we're learned about the nervous system over the past 25 years we could not have done without patch camping. Erwin's discovery of the gigaseal made all the difference in the world" (quoted in Hopkin 2010). The next few years following the reliable establishment of the gigaseal bear out Stevens' assessment. Ingenious experimenters quickly discovered numerous ways the isolated patches of neuron membrane could be manipulated. In his Nobel Prize address, Neher refers to these further discoveries as "Unexpected Benefits" (1991, 15). They were "unexpected" because they were not predicted by any theory; they were discovered purely by chance or trial-and-error experimentation; nobody saw these coming. In the words of this paper, they were the result of extended laboratory tinkering. First, numerous variations on cell surface patching were found. Hamill et al. (1981) reported that a strong pulse of suction through the pipette would not only establish the gigaseal but would also lesion the sealed membrane. This made the cytoplasm of the cell continuous with the interior of the pipette and afforded experimenters a means to manipulate interior neuron function molecularly in real time. These so-called "whole cell recordings" via the patch clamp remain a laboratory standard in electrophysiology to this day.

Hamill et al. (1981) also reported that by applying suction to establish the gigaseal, then slowly lifting the pipette, the patch of membrane sealed inside the pipette could be detached from the cell. This "inside-out" patch-clamp variation exposed the cytoplasmic surface of the membrane and its channels or receptors to molecular manipulation via the solution in the nutrient bath. Finally, and most remarkably, the gigaseal could be established with the cell membrane, strong suction applied to lesion the membrane, as with the whole-cell recording technique, then the pipette lifted to rupture the cell membrane, only lifting slightly more slowly than with the inside-out technique to remove slightly more cell membrane on either side of the seal. The two detached strands of the membrane would anneal together. This "outside-out" patch clamp variation made the extracellular domain and its channel or receptor components accessible to molecular manipulations for the first time via the nutrient bath. *All* of the experimentally-confirmed theory we now possess about receptors, including metabotropic receptors and the variety of intra- and intercellular signaling their activation leads to, traces back to these innovations with basic patch clamp techniques. All these variations had been developed, refined, and put to use in numerous laboratories worldwide by the time Sakmann and Neher published their first comprehensive scientific review paper of the patch clamp technique and its principal results, in 1984.

Neher himself, in his Nobel Prize address one decade later, remarked on how transformative the patch clamp had already been in electrophysiology. He notes that the whole-cell recording variant quickly became "the method of choice for recording from most cell culture preparations" because of its range of experimental applications: "many cell types, particularly small cells of mammalian origin, became accessible to biophysical analysis for the first time" (1991, 17). These cells simply "would not tolerate multiple conventional impalements" that previous tools required (1991, 17). Patch clamp whole-cell recording, inside-out, and outside-out variants could also be used in combinations in detailed multiple-experiment designs, and suddenly "individual current types could be separated through control of solution composition on both sides of the membrane" (1991, 17). The patch clamp radically shifted experimental practices in laboratory neurobiology. It made the cells of real interest, including mammalian neurons, experimentally accessible, which technical limitations had precluded previously. And experiments changed drastically, almost overnight. Neher reports some details:

> This development shifted the emphasis of electrophysiological studies away from large-celled preparations, which usually were of invertebrate origin, towards mammalian and human cell types. In the first half of 1981, just before we first published a whole-cell characterization of a small mammalian cell (bovine adrenal chromaffin cells), only 5 out of 14 voltage-champ studies in the *Journal of Physiology* were performed on cells of mammalian origin. The first 1991 issue of the same journal alone contained 10 voltage-clamp studies on mammalian cells, none on invertebrates, and all using either the whole-cell or single-channel recording techniques.
>
> (1991, 17)

This shift constituted a real revolution in neurobiology, one reflected in the actions, not just the words of bench neurobiologists. As I emphasized in my (2016) concerning gene targeting techniques and optogenetics, the revolution in neurobiology stemming from the patch clamp was likewise built strictly on the development and ingenious use of this experiment tool, itself the product of laboratory tinkering. The theory-centric components of Kuhn's (1962) famous model—paradigms, anomalies, crisis science—are likewise not found in this history.

The most eye-opening and long-range influence of experiments with the patch clamp were ones through which experimenters began to unravel the vast networks of intracellular signaling pathways in active neurons. These investigations constituted the leading edge of the "molecular revolution" in neurobiology. The role of the patch clamp in this work began with early reports of "rundown" or "wash-out" when investigating calcium (Ca^{2+}) channels. We now know these channels to be subject to modulation by second messengers, G-proteins, and phosphorylation; but nearly 40 years ago none of this was known. Fenwick et al. first reported "a slow run-down" of Ca^{2+} currents observed when using whole-cell recordings, with "the speed of rundown … dependent on intracellular Ca^{2+} concentration" (1982, 595). Channel activity measured through the patch clamp disappeared rapidly, as a result of the perturbations initiated by rupturing the cell membranes with whole-cell recording and excised patch (inside-out, outside-out) techniques. Fenwick et al. speculated that the rundown "was apparently due to a progressive elimination of the channels available for activation" (1982, 595). Less than one decade later, in his Nobel Prize address, Neher could already assert that these puzzling results were "due to the loss of regulators, which at that time were unknown," through the ruptured membranes (1991, 19). But these initially puzzling results only spurred more work using these new experiment tools. As Neher claims, "subsequently, ingenious use of these tools by many laboratories has revealed a whole network of interactions between channels, second messengers, G-proteins, and other regulatory proteins" (1991, 19). But in order to reveal this network, electrophysiological recordings from these special channel-containing cells were not enough. Experimenters also needed "to control or change systematically the concentrations of second messengers" (1991, 19). And the patch clamp and its standard variants, with their capacities to expose different areas of the cell membrane and the cytoplasm to differing solutions in the pipette and the surrounding nutrient bath, made these experimental interventions possible.

The floodgates to increased knowledge of intracellular signaling had opened. In his Nobel address, Neher cites three publications that quickly followed Fenwick et al.'s (1982) initial report of rundown in Ca^{2+} channel-containing cells. These three papers show the patch clamp's expanding role in both molecular neurobiology and physiology generally. Fesenko et al. (1985) used the patch clamp to investigate "intracellular messengers" which couple activation of vertebrate retinal photoreceptive rod cell outer segments to single-channel activity. They found that the activity of second messenger cyclic guanine monophosphate (cGMP) "inside the inner membrane" was matched by increased cation conductance through the individual channels (1985, 310). Kameyama et al. (1986) found modulation of second messenger Ca^{2+} ion currents during the phosphorylation cycle in patch-clamped guinea pig heart cells. This work extended the use of patch clamping to investigate second messenger activities in a wider range of tissue types. And Penner et al.

(1988) used the patch clamp to investigate multiple second messenger pathways, including those involving Ca^{2+} and cyclic adenosine monophosphate (cAMP) in rat peritoneal mast cells, producing elevated intracellular Ca^{2+} concentrations released from intracellular storage sites. In the three-decades span since Neher cited those three papers in his Nobel Prize address, what we now know about these and other intracellular signaling pathways and their significance for neuronal function has increased by orders of magnitude. What is now presented in textbooks for undergraduates (see, e.g., Purves et al. 2017, chapters 7 and 8) would have astonished Neher and his fellow ground-breakers back in 1991. The patch clamp and its standard variants made all this progress possible. This tool continues to be used by electrophysiologists and molecular neurobiologists today, and sometimes still in the very forms that Neher and others developed more than 40 years ago. All this is impressive history for a tool whose development resisted four years of "systematic" attempts to achieve the gigaseal but yielded its promises to one lucky accident by an observant experimentalist, which was followed quickly by improvements found by a host of laboratory tinkers worldwide.

5 Answering the Call for "More Theory in Neuroscience"

I have used some historical details about the development of the metal microelectrode and the patch clamp to illuminate the double dependency of theory progress in neurobiology, not only on the development of new research tools but also the latter's dependence on atheoretical laboratory tinkering:

laboratory tinkering → new experiment tool development → theory progress

I end this chapter by developing two further points of interest to both philosophers and neuroscientists.

Nowadays we routinely hear calls for "more theory" in neuroscience, especially from cognitive, computational, and systems neuroscientists and their philosopher friends. Francis Crick was among the earliest callers for this. As far back as 1979, while still an admitted "novice" in neuroscience, Crick wrote an invited commentary on a series of essays published in *Scientific American* on then-state-of-the-art neuroscience, all written by leading neuroscientists. He remarked that while the articles "give a good general idea of the progress that has been made" in understanding the functioning, sensing, cognizing, emoting, and action-guiding brain,

what is conspicuously lacking is a broad framework of ideas within which to interpret all these different approaches. Biochemistry and genetics were in such a state until the revolution in molecular biology. It is not that most neurobiologists do not have some general concept of what is going on. The trouble is that the concept is not precisely formulated ...How then should *a general theory of the brain* be constructed?

(1979, 133; my emphasis)[6]

Crick's request for "more theory in neuroscience" was not unique to him. Neurophilosopher Patricia Churchland, in her book that initiated that field, likewise insisted that, at least concerning how ensembles of neurons work to generate complex behaviors and cognition, "there is no widely accepted theoretical framework, nor even a well-defined conception of what a theory to explain such things as sensorimotor control or perception or memory should look like" (1986, 403). And while she admitted "some sympathy" for neuroscientists who judged that "theorizing about brain function is ... slightly disreputable and anyhow a waste of time," she nevertheless offered a number of reasons for "the value of theory" (1986, 403–407). Chapter 10 of that book, nearly 80 of the book's 482 pages, presents three nascent "theories of brain function," each one "illustrat[ing] some important aspect of the problem of theory in neuroscience" (1986, 411). This same attitude carried over into her computational neuroscience primer published six years later and co-authored with prominent neuroscientist Terrence Sejnowski (Churchland and Sejnowski 1992). "'Data rich but theory poor' is a description frequently applied to neuroscience," they write; "in one obvious respect, this remains true, inasmuch as we do not yet know how to explain how brains see, learn, and take action" (1992, 16). The hope they express throughout that book is that computational modeling, coupled with continued experimentation into real brains by biochemists through neuropsychologists, will provide the most promising strategy for generating missing but needed theory.

Philosophers of neuroscience Ian Gold and Adina Roskies sounded this familiar lament in their survey chapter from more than a decade ago:

Neuroscience ... has very few broad theories. It might be said that the field is governed by a few global frameworks—a crude physicalism and perhaps computationalism—but these serve as fundamental or guiding assumptions rather than theories: They don't provide neuroscientists with predictive power in the way that physical theories do... Given its lack of theoretical richness, and the rather local character of the theories that do exist, neuroscience looks quite different from both physics and evolutionary biology.

(2008, 351)

And as recently as 2016 Churchland and Sejnowski still lament: "neuroscience is theory-poor" (2016, 667).

If it is a more and better theory that neuroscience needs or neuroscientists want, then the lesson from a metascience of tool development recommends how to get that. *Build new and better research tools!* Without obvious exception, the best, most well-confirmed theory in neuroscience has resulted from the development of new research tools and their ingenious uses on lab benches. As we saw in the previous section, the development of one specific research tool, the patch clamp, generated the "molecular wave," not just a theory but a world view that has dominated mainstream neurobiology for three decades.

A metascience of tool development in neurobiology yields an additional recommendation for those who want "more theory" in neuroscience. My basic framework for tool development experiments (Bickle 2016), coupled with the new emphasis stressed in this chapter on the place of laboratory tinkering, have all been derived retrospectively, from historical case studies. But its basic concepts and lessons can also be applied prospectively, to new tools under active initial development, or even to ones simply being envisioned or imagined now. Furthermore, the four case studies I have now analyzed provide exemplars for developing *revolutionary* new tools. What features does a new tool currently under development share with, e.g., those that drove the development of gene targeting techniques in behavioral neuroscience? Or those that drove the patch clamp toward achieving the gigaseal reliably? In what ways might the practical problems confronting developers of some envisioned new tool, to make it work, resemble those Hubel confronted and solved in his tinkerings that built the metal microelectrode and hydraulic microdriver? Might new tool developers gain insights from details of these historically successful cases and a metascientific analysis of their shared dynamics? Might grant proposal reviewers, convinced of the primary place of laboratory tinkering and new research tools for the best-confirmed instances of theory progress across all of neuroscience, look more favorably at proposals that emphasize the development of new research tools?[7] The abstract nature of my (2016) initial metascientific account of components shared across different instances of tool development grow increasingly detailed with each new case study to which they get applied.

Interestingly, some neuroscientists seem to be groping toward conclusions like these. Churchland and Sejnowski (2016), for example, couple their claim (cited above) about neuroscience still being "theory-poor" with a surprising conjunct: "at the level of neuronal networks, neuroscience is also decidedly data poor" (2016, 667). Very much in keeping with the lessons I am urging, they advocate explicitly for the BRAIN initiative—Brain Research through Advancing Innovative Neurotechnologies—as a promising solution to this dual theory-data poverty. Launched in the U.S. in 2013, the BRAIN Initiative is a multi-federal agency public-private collaboration "aimed at revolutionizing our understanding of the human brain ... by accelerating the development and application of innovative technologies" (https://www. braininitiative.nih.gov/). As Churchland and Sejnowski insist, the hope is that this Initiative will generate

> new tools to obtain the data ... new methods to analyze them ... inventing new technologies that will, it is hoped, foster the discovery of a unified set of principles that link all levels of nervous systems and thorough which brains perform their jobs.
>
> (2016, 667)

The direction of influence that the BRAIN Initiative stresses should be familiar to readers of this paper: new experiment tools → theory progress. Will BRAIN funders take heed of the lessons urged in this chapter, that 'atheoretical laboratory tinkering' drives new tool development, and put money toward proposals to do that?

6 Coda: Do Scientists Less Beholden to Theory Make the Best Laboratory Tinkers?

I close this chapter by raising a related question. Are the scientists who wind up inventing the research tools that revolutionize experiment-driven fields typically the ones less beholden to or enamored with theory in their day-to-day scientific activities? Does this attitude make them more amenable toward the laboratory tinkering that drives new tool development? And might this aspect of laboratory scientific practice become institutionalized in the ways we train scientists?

I return to the attitudes of one of this chapter's heroes. David Hubel was a laboratory junkie. After he had perfected the process for making and insulating tungsten microelectrodes, he recalls that he "spent the next few months recording everything in the anesthetized cat's nervous system, from spinal cord to cochlear nucleus to olfactory bulb, almost forgetting the original plan to record from awake, behaving animals" (1996, 303–304). This laboratory tinkering resulted in his getting "scooped" in publishing results using his new tool. Herbert Jasper of McGill University, who ironically had been Hubel's laboratory mentor when Hubel was a medical student, traveled to Walter Reed in 1957 to learn firsthand Hubel's tungsten electropolishing technique. He and his post-docs returned to McGill, started producing the electrodes, and were first to publish successful recordings from single neurons in awake animals (primates) engaged in a cognitive (learning) task. In his scientific autobiography, Hubel recalls his initial regret at his own dalliance: "I wished I hadn't taken so much time recording from so many parts of cats' brains" (1996, 304). But he also recalls soon coming to appreciate the time he spent tinkering with his new tool:

> The chance to *play around* at an early stage of one's training is a luxury denied to most beginning graduate students, who often start in on a specialized problem assigned by an advisor, before having a chance to try a few things for themselves.
>
> (1996, 304; my emphasis)[8]

In the same paragraph, Hubel also remarks, "It has always surprised me how few attempts are made to devise new methods—perhaps it is because one is generally rewarded not for inventing new methods but for the research which results from their use" (1996, 304). The lament of a tinker!

This attitude pervaded Hubel's entire approach to science. Speaking for himself and Wiesel, he remarks that "we felt like 15th century explorers, like Columbus sailing West *to see what he might find*" (1996, 312; my emphasis). The impact of theory on their landmark research was minimal:

> If we had any "hypothesis" it was the simple-minded idea that the brain, in particular the cerebral cortex, with all its ordered complexity, must be doing something biologically meaningful with the information that comes into it ... So we recorded cells to see what we might find.
>
> (1996, 312–313)

And he generalizes this last point beyond himself and Wiesel: "I suspect that much of science, especially biological science, is primarily exploratory in this sense" (1996, 313).

Hubel's account of science's "main pleasures" will be unfamiliar to theorists: "To me the main pleasures of doing science are in getting ideas for experiments, doing surgery, designing and making equipment, and above all the rare moments in which some apparently isolated facts click into place like a Chinese puzzle" (1981, 48). The first joy on Hubel's list is that of experimentalists, the second that of lab technicians, and the third and fourth those of the tinkers, both mechanical and intellectual.

The task of writing Hubel's obituary for *Neuron*, published a few days after his death in October 2013, fell to Margaret Livingstone, his second long-time research collaborator. She notes that he was "a giant in our field," but also "the guy in the lab who did the work that made him great, and there is surely some connection between the way he daily went about doing science and how successful he was" (2013, 735). She notes the "two characteristics" that were most important to his scientific success: "his mechanical inventiveness and his perseverance" (2013, 735).

She closes his obituary by remarking on the teaching Hubel undertook after ending his research career:

> When David did start teaching, he taught a Freshman Seminar at Harvard College that was extraordinary popular, with ten times as many students signing up each year as could be accommodated. He taught them things that he thought were important but were missing from most young people's upbringing today: how to solder, how to use power tools, how to suture skin, and how to wire up a simple circuit.
>
> (2013, 737)

I trust that Hubel's tinkering-first attitude about science-in-general is readily apparent in Livingstone's remarks!

Intuitively, Hubel's attitude about science seems fitting for someone destined to develop useful new experiment tools. The dedicated explorer-experimentalist will be attuned to the motivating problems for new tools (Bickle 2016), and the dedicated tinker will be someone with the patience and skills needed to build these new tools through ongoing trial-and-error. But is there evidence for a general lesson here, between those who've successfully built neuroscience's most revolutionary, influential experiment tools and the general approach to science Hubel articulated? If so, might this attitude be tracked, encouraged, and maybe even taught as part of basic neurobiological training? Only further metascientific work like that presented here can answer this question. But if the lessons I'm stressing about the importance and dynamics of tool development in neurobiology are correct, then neurobiology might stand to gain enormously from these investigations.

Notes

1 A detailed investigation of this connection must await future work.
2 Microns, μm, millionths of one meter. The necessary tip dimensions thus ranged from less than 4 one-hundred thousandths of an inch to less than 2 ten-thousandths of an inch.
3 By passing a 2- to 6-volt alternating current between the tungsten wire and a nearby carbon rod, with the wire inserted into a 27-gauge hypodermic needle, and its tip exposed and inserted into a saturated aqueous potassium nitrite solution. I draw all details in this paragraph from Hubel's (1957) paper.
4 In the terminology of my metascientific model of tool development experiments (Bickle 2016), these three publications present the metal microelectrode's *second-phase hook experiments*, which bring the tool and its usage potential to a wider range of scientists, and sometimes to the broader general public, beyond specialists in the field in which the tool is developed.
5 These numbers were obtained from PubMed Central (https://www.ncbi.nlm.nih.gov/pmc/), queried May 12, 2021.

6 Crick maintained this judgment to the end of his life. See one of his last publications before his death, co-authored with Christof Koch, where the pair propose "a framework" for a neurobiology of consciousness, emphasizing that a framework is not a theory, but rather just a "suggested point of view for an attack on a scientific problem" (2003, 119).

7 See, e.g., my discussion (Bickle 2019) of Mario Capecchi's remark about his experiences with an NIH panel on his initial funding request for developing techniques of gene targeting by homologous recombination, followed by subsequent remarks from the same panel a couple of years later after he had persisted in his research despite that panel's initial mistaken—and theory-grounded!—pessimistic judgment about its potential.

8 Hubel's wording here should remind the reader of one of Ian Hacking's (1983) most quoted remarks about the development of microscopes: "We should not underestimate ... the pretheoretical role of ... fooling around."

References

Atanasova, N. (2015). "Validating animal models." *Theoria: An International Journal for Theory, History and Foundations of Science 30*: 163–181.

Bickle, J. (2003). *Philosophy and Neuroscience: A Ruthlessly Reductive Account.* Dordrecht: Springer.

Bickle, J. (2015). "Marr and reductionism." *Topics in Cognitive Sciences (TOPICS)* 7: 299–311.

Bickle, J. (2016). "Revolutions in neuroscience: Tool development." *Frontiers in Systems Neuroscience 10*: 24. doi: 10.3389/fnsys.2016.00024.

Bickle, J. (2018). "From microscopes to optogenetics: Ian Hacking vindicated." *Philosophy of Science 85*: 1065–1077.

Bickle, J. (2019). "Linking mind to molecular pathways: The role of experiment tools." *Axiomathes: Where Science Meets Philosophy 29*(6): 577–597.

Bickle, J. (2020). "Laser lights and designer drugs: New techniques for descending levels of mechanisms in a 'single bound'?" *Topics in Cognitive Sciences (TopiCS) 12*: 1241–1256.

Burian, D. (2007). "On microRNA and need for explanatory experimentation in post-genomic molecular biology." *History and Philosophy of the Life Sciences 29*(3): 283–310.

Churchland, P.S. (1986). *Neurophilosophy: Toward a Unified Science of the Mind-Brain.* Cambridge: MIT Press.

Churchland, P.S. and Sejnowski, T.J. (1992). *The Computational Brain.* Cambridge: MIT Press.

Churchland, P.S. and Sejnowski, T.J. (2016). "Blending computational and experimental neuroscience." *Nature Reviews Neuroscience 17*(11): 567–568.

Crick, F.H. (1979). "Thinking about the brain." *Scientific American 241*(3) (September): 219–232.

Crick, F.H. and Koch, C. (2003). "A framework for consciousness." *Nature Neuroscience 6*: 119–126.

Desimone, R., Albright, T.D., Gross, C.G., and Bruce, C. (1984). "Stimulus-selective properties of inferior temporal neurons in the macaque." *Journal of Neuroscience 4*(8): 2051–2062.

Fenwick, E.M., Marty, A., and Neher, E. (1982). "Sodium and calcium currents in bovine chromaffin cells." *Journal of Physiology 331*: 595–635.

Fesenko, E.E., Kolesnikov, S.S., and Lyubarsky, A.L. (1985). "Induction of cyclic GMP in cationic conductance in plasma membrane of retinal rod outer segment." *Nature 313*: 310–313.

Franklin, L. (2005). "Explanatory experiments." *Philosophy of Science* (Proceedings) *72*: 888–889.

Funahashi, S., Chaffe, M.V. and Goldman-Rakic, P.S. (1993). "Prefrontal neuronal activity in rhesus monkeys performing a delayed anti-saccade task." *Nature 365*: 753–756.

Gold, I. and Roskies, A.L. (2008). "Philosophy of neuroscience." In M. Ruse (ed.), *The Oxford Handbook of Philosophy of Biology*. New York: Oxford University Press, 349–380.

Gross, C.G., Rocha-Miranda, C.E., and Bender, D.B. (1972). "Visual properties of neurons in inferotemporal cortex of the macaque." *Journal of Physiology 35*(1): 96–111.

Hacking, I. (1983). *Representing and Intervening*. Cambridge: Cambridge University Press.

Hamill, O.P, Marty, A., Neher, E., Sakmann, B., and Sigworth, FJ. (1981). "Improved patch clamp techniques for high-resolution current recording from cells and cell-free membrane patches." *Pflügers Archiv (European Journal of Physiology) 391*: 85–100.

Hodgkin, A.L and Huxley, A.F. (1952). "A quantitative description of membrane current and its application to conduction and excitation in nerve." *Journal of Physiology 117*: 500–544.

Hopkin, K. (2010). "It's electric." *The Scientist.* https://www.the-scientist.com/uncategorized/its-electric-43471.

Hubel, D.H. (1957). "Tungsten microelectrode for recording from single units." *Science 125*(3247): 349–550.

Hubel, D.H. (1981). "Evolution of ideas of the primary visual cortex, 1955–1978. A biased personal history." *Nobel Lecture.* https://www.nobelprize.org/nobel_prizes/medicine/laureates/1981/hubel-lecture.pdf.

Hubel, D.H. (1996). "David H. Hubel." In L. Squire (ed.), *The History of Neuroscience in Autobiography, vol. 1.* Washington, DC: Society for Neuroscience, 294–317.

Hubel, D.H. and Wiesel, T.N. (1959). "Receptive fields of single neurons in the cat's striate cortex." *Journal of Physiology 148*: 574–591.

Hubel, D.H. and Wiesel, T.N. (1962). "Receptive fields, binocular interaction, and functional architecture in the cat's striate cortex." *Journal of Physiology 160*: 106–154.

Hubel. D.H. and Wiesel, T.N. (1965). "Receptive fields and functional architecture in two non-striate visual areas (18 and 19) of the cat." *Journal of Neurophysiology 28*: 2290289.

Kameyama, M., Herscheler, J., Hofmann, F., and Trautwein, W. (1986). "Modulation of Ca current during the phosphorylation cycle of the guinea pig heart." *Pflügers Archiv (European Journal of Physiology) 407*: 123–128.

Kuhn, T. (1962). *The Structure of Scientific Revolutions*. Chicago, IL: University of Chicago Press.

Livingstone, M. (2013). "David H. Hubel, 1926–2013." *Neuron 80*: 735–737.

Mishkin, M., Ungerleider, L.G., and Macko, K.A. (1983). "Object vision and spatial vision: Two cortical pathways." *Trends in Neurosciences 6*: 414–417.

Neher, E. (1991). "Ion channels for communication between and within cells." *Nobel Lecture*. https://www.nobelprize.org/nobel_prizes/medicine/laureates/1991/neher-lecture.pdf.

Neher, E. and Sakmann, B. (1976). "Single-channel currents recorded from membrane of denervated frog muscle fibers." *Nature 260* (April 29): 799–802.

Neher, E., Sakmann, B., and Steinback, J.H. (1978). "The extracellular parch clamp: A method for resolving currents through individual open channels in biological membranes." *Pflügers Archiv (European Journal of Physiology) 375*: 219–228.

Penner, R., Matthews, G., and Neher, E., (1988). "Regulation of calcium influx by second messengers in rat mast cells." *Nature 334*: 499–504.

Purves, D., Augustine, G.J., Fitzpatrick, D., Hall, W.C., LaMantia, A.-S., Mooney, R.D., Platt, M.L., and White, L.E. (2017). *Neuroscience, 6th Ed.* New York: Oxford University Press.

Robins, S.K. (2016). "Optogenetics and the mechanism of false memory." *Synthese 193*: 1561–1583.

Robins, S.K. (2018). "Memory and optogenetic intervention: Separating the engram from the ecphory." *Philosophy of Science 85*(5): 1078–1089.

Romo, R., Hernández, A., Zainos, A., and Salinas, E. (1998). "Somatosensory discrimination based on cortical microstimulation." *Nature 392*: 387–390.

Sakmann, B. and Neher, E. (1984). "Patch clamp techniques for studying ionic channels in excitable membranes." *Annual Review of Physiology 46*: 455–472.

Salzmann, C.D., Murasugi, C.M., Britten, K.H., and Newsome, W.D. (1992). "Microstimulation in visual area MT: Effects on direction discrimination performance." *Journal of Neuroscience 12*(6): 2331–2355.

Sellars, W. (1965). "Scientific realism or irenic instrumentalism." In R.S. Cohen and Marx W. Wartofsky (eds.), *Boston Studies in the Philosophy of Science, vol. II*. New York: Humanities Press, 171–204.

Sigworth, F.J. and Neher, E. (1980). "Single Na^+ channel currents observed in cultured rat muscle cells." *Nature 287*: 447–449.

Silva, A.J., Landreth, A., and Bickle, J. (2014). *Engineering the Next Revolution in Neuroscience*. New York: Oxford University Press.

Sullivan, J.A. (2009). "The multiplicity of experimental protocols: A challenge to reductionist and non-reductionist models of the unity of neuroscience." *Synthese 167*: 511–539.

Sullivan, J.A. (2010). "Reconsidering 'spatial memory' and the Morris water maze." *Synthese 177*: 261–283.

Sullivan, J.A. (2018). "Optogenetics, pluralism and progress." *Philosophy of Science 85*(5): 1090–1101.

Van Essen, D.C., Anderson, C.H., and Felleman, D.J. (1992). "Information professing in the primate visual system: An integrated systems perspective." *Science 255*(5043): 419–423.

2 Tools, Experiments, and Theories

An Examination of the Role of Experiment Tools

Gregory Johnson

1 Introduction

John Bickle (2016, 2018, 2019) offers two frameworks for thinking about the role of experiment tools in neurobiology. First, he argues that "revolutions in neuroscience" do not proceed in a Kuhnian manner such that a dominant paradigm is replaced in response to an accumulation of anomalies. Rather, revolutions in this science begin with *motivating problems* that spur the development of new experiment tools, the importance of which is revealed in *initial-* and *second-phase hook experiments* (2016). The initial-phase hook experiments demonstrate the feasibility of the new tool. The second-phase hook experiments demonstrate its usefulness in a wider range of experimental contexts and bring it to the attention of a much larger audience—both scientific and more general.

Bickle extends this to a second framework, which is grounded in a critique of "theory-centrism" in the philosophy of neuroscience (2018, 2019). As Bickle has it, theory-centrism is the view that neuroscience needs theories—on the model of physics, early modern astronomy, or evolutionary biology—that will drive successful research efforts. One advocate of this view is Patricia Churchland. She writes,

> If neuroscience is to have a shot at explaining—really explaining—how the brain works, then it cannot be theory-shy. It must construct theories. It must have more than anatomy and pharmacology, more than physiology of individual neurons. It must have more than patterns of connectivity between neurons. What we need are small-scale models of subsystems and, above all, grand-scale theories of whole brain function.
>
> (1986, p. 406)

And then, more than two decades later, Ian Gold and Adina Roskies say,

> The question remains whether neuroscience is the sort of science that is doomed to be theory-poor, or whether this poverty is due to its relative immaturity as a science. ... The brain is an exceedingly

DOI: 10.4324/9781003251392-4

complex biological organ which has evolved to perform a variety of sophisticated tasks. It yields its secrets grudgingly. Nonetheless, there is no principled reason why we cannot expect that, in time, we will be able to formulate more general theories about the neural processing that underlies these diverse functions.

(2008, p. 353)

Bickle aims to dispel this view that theory should have a central position in our understanding of neuroscience. Rather, he argues that we should appreciate the central role of tool development and use. To the extent that theory has a role in contemporary neuroscience, it is "tertiary" in importance:

> Rather than being the crux point on which everything else depends, ... theory turns out to be doubly dependent, and hence of tertiary, not primary, importance. Our best confirmed theory is totally dependent on what our experiment tools allow us to manipulate. And those tools developed by way of solving engineering problems, not by applying theory.

(2019, p. 578)

This can be interpreted in two ways. On the one hand, when a theory is proposed, the theory depends on experiments and the tools used in those experiments for its confirmation. Hence, without those tools, the theory would fail to be confirmed. Arguably, though, dependence in this sense doesn't detract from a central role for theory in the scientific process. This sense of dependence, however, doesn't seem to be what Bickle has in mind. For instance, in one place, he writes,

> The molecular mechanisms of cognitive functions rank among contemporary neuroscience's greatest theoretical achievements. And yet this theory is tertiary in dependence. It comes directly from the development and ingenious experimental use of some novel experiment tools, to intervene into specific molecular processes in behaving mammals. And those tools come from a catch-as-catch-can, make-it-work, engineering-first attitude of the sort famously alluded to by Hacking (1983), in his "microscope" argument for the relative independence of "the life of experiment" from theory.

(2019, p. 594)

Here it seems that we are meant to understand that the temporal order, as well as the order of importance, is, as Bickle later lays it out, "engineering solutions → new experiment tools → better theory" (2019, p. 595). I will call this the *tools first* (or *anti-theory-centric*) *method* with the idea that, as Bickle stresses, the application of an experiment tool is, along with other factors, central to the investigation—but one of those other factors is *not* the testing of a theory.

Surprisingly, given the role that it has in his analysis, Bickle is studiously coy about what he means by *theory*. For the most part, rather than use this term, I will use *hypothesis*, defined here as *an explanation for a process or phenomenon that still requires confirmation*. By focusing on hypotheses, I am deliberately setting aside *theory* used in the sense of *understanding, knowledge of the discipline*, or *completed explanation*—or, as Churchland says, "this conglomeration of background assumptions, intuitions, and assorted preconceptions" (1986, p. 405). I will take it for granted that *theory* in this latter sense is pervasive at all stages of neurobiological investigations.[1]

Bickle's assertion that the tools first method is *always* used in contemporary neurobiology is a strong claim, and it will be our focus. In Sections 2 and 3, I will look at two cases. The first, gene targeting and investigations of the relationship between memory and long-term potentiation, is extensively discussed by Bickle (2016, 2019). I find, however, that a well-defined hypothesis does have a prominent role in these investigations. In short, a hypothesis was developed and then confirmed by experiments using gene targeting. The second case, however—an optogenetic investigation of neurons in the extended amygdala that were found to drive both anxiety and anxiety-reduction—illustrates the application of Bickle's tools first method.

The takeaway, then, is twofold. First, scientific method in contemporary neurobiology is more varied than Bickle suggests, and sometimes theory does have a central role. But, second, there are important investigations in neurobiology that proceed without a hypothesis or theory as the starting point (and without either coming into play at any point, for that matter). This is, in part, a consequence of, as Bickle argues, experiment tools that allow for ever more precise investigations of cellular and molecular processes. It is also a consequence of the explanatory goals in neurobiology, namely, the description of mechanisms. When these two consequences come together, there is no longer an apparent need for theories of the sort encountered in physics or evolutionary biology.

2 Gene Targeting and LTP

The first case involves two research tracks that intersected with productive results in the 1990s. Long-term potentiation (LTP) is a lasting increase in the efficacy of synaptic transmission following a sufficiently strong stimulation from the pre-synaptic neuron. This phenomenon was first reported by Terje Lømo in 1966 and then in more detail by Lømo and Tim Bliss in 1973 (Lømo 1966; Bliss & Lømo 1973). The idea that changes in the efficacy of synapses would be the neural basis for learning and memory had been proposed before Bliss and Lømo's work (Hebb 1949; Gardner-Medwin 1969), but even in the 1990s, the idea that LTP—in particular, LTP at the CA3-CA1 synapses in the hippocampus—was the basis for at least some types of learning and memory was still a hypothesis.

Richard Morris added some confidence to the hypothesis by demonstrating that a pharmacological intervention targeted at NMDA receptors impaired spatial learning (Morris et al. 1986; Morris 1989). DL-2-amino-5-phosphonopentanoic acid (AP5) prevents NMDA receptors from allowing Ca^{2+} ions into the post-synaptic neuron, and, from *in vitro* studies of hippocampal slices, AP5 was known to prevent LTP (Harris et al. 1984). Morris infused AP5 into the ventricular system of rats and then tested their performance on the Morris water maze. In this test of spatial memory, rats or mice, swimming in a pool of opaque liquid, explore until they find a submerged platform. After training, they remember the location of the platform quite well using cues from outside the pool to orient themselves to its location—e.g., objects naturally occupying the room (filing cabinets, posters on the wall, etc.) or images placed around the room so that they can be seen from the pool. Morris found, however, that rats that had received the AP5 infusions were impaired at learning the location of the platform, although they were not impaired on a test of visual discrimination learning, which does not depend on hippocampal functioning. These results support "the hypothesis that the underlying neural mechanisms of LTP are activated during and required for certain kinds of learning" (Morris & Kennedy 1992, p. 511). But, as Morris noted, the AP5's disruption of the NMDA receptors' function could have effects elsewhere in the hippocampus that are unrelated to LTP, and those other effects could be responsible for the spatial memory impairment (Morris 1989, p. 3053).[2]

The second research track was the development of targeted gene replacement as a tool for investigating the effects that specific genes and the proteins that they encode have on behavior. When this technique is used, as the name suggests, the gene for a single protein is replaced with a non-functional copy. This was done, first, to fruit flies by Seymour Benzer and his colleagues in the 1970s, and in the mid-1980s, Mario Capecchi successfully knocked out developmental genes in mice. (See Bickle 2016, 2019 for a fuller description of the development of this tool in the 1980s.) This brings us to the intersection of targeted gene replacement and the relationship between LTP and spatial memory. Bickle writes,

> Taken together, the predicted general applicability of Capecchi's gene targeting techniques to mammalian nervous tissue, and the experimental demand to block LTP without disrupting other aspects of synaptic function in order to test the alluring LTP → (rodent spatial) learning and memory hypothesis, constituted the *motivating*

problem for the application of gene targeting techniques in mammalian behavioral neuroscience.

(2016, p. 4)

In the early 1990s, in response to this motivating problem, Alcino Silva and Susumu Tonegawa used gene targeting for the first time in neurobiology to prevent LTP in mice and to investigate the LTP → spatial memory hypothesis (Silva et al. 1992a, 1992b). They replaced the gene for the α-form of calcium-calmodulin-dependent kinase II (α-CaMKII), a protein that was believed at the time to have a role in LTP and is now known to be needed for the insertion of new AMPA receptors in the post-synaptic cell's membrane, one of the early steps that increases the efficacy of transmission at the synapse. They found that this prevented LTP in hippocampal neurons *in vitro* (1992b) and impaired spatial learning in the Morris water maze (1992a). The α-CaMKII deficient mice were not impaired, however, on a test of non-spatial memory.

Silva et al. report that their results "considerably strengthen the contention that the synaptic changes exhibited in LTP are the basis for spatial memory" (1992a, p. 206). But elsewhere, when discussing this use of targeted gene replacement, Tonegawa points out,

> In 1992, this work led to the report of the first knockout mice in neuroscience. It was shown that deletion of the α-CaMKII gene causes a deficit in LTP at Schaffer collateral-CA1 synapses and an impairment of spatial learning. Even before publication, however, we were aware of the limitations of this approach in conventional knockout mice. These limitations were primarily because the gene of interest is deleted in the entire animal throughout the animal's life. Although no obvious developmental defects were observed in the α-CaMKII knockout mice, more subtle defects could not be excluded. Furthermore, the universal absence of the protein in question (in this case, α-CaMKII) certainly did not permit the establishment of a causal relationship between CA1 LTP and spatial learning.
>
> (2001; see also Tsien et al. 1996, p. 1327)

So, while Silva et al. showed that gene targeting could be used in neurobiological investigations and their study added some degree of confirmation to the LTP → spatial memory hypothesis, their results encountered much the same problem as did Morris's. Like Morris, Silva and his colleagues disrupted one component in the process that gives rise to LTP and, at the same time, this intervention impaired spatial learning. But, in both cases, the intervention was broad enough to raise questions about whether it was the absence of LTP or the impairment of some other process that was responsible for the poor performance on the spatial memory task. Four years later, however, further work on the gene targeting technique by Joe Tsien—who was also working in Tonegawa's lab—made it possible to draw a stronger conclusion.

Silva et al. had introduced the non-functional copy of the α-CaMKII gene into embryonic stem cells that were then injected into fertilized mouse embryos. The embryos were implanted in the uteruses of surrogate females, and some of the mice that were born contained the mutant gene. Mating those mice with wild types and then mating mice that were heterozygous for the mutant gene eventually yielded mice that were homozygous for the mutant gene. This ensured that these mice lacked α-CaMKII in CA1 neurons in the hippocampus. But these mice also lacked this protein at all stages of development and in all brain areas where it would normally be expressed: throughout the hippocampus, in the cortex, septum, striatum, and amygdala.

Shortly after Silva et al.'s study was published, Tsien used the same embryonic stem cell method to create two lines of mice. One line expressed an enzyme derived from the bacteriophage P1 only in pyramidal cells in the hippocampus's CA1 region. This enzyme, Cre recombinase, targets specific sequences of DNA, 34 base pair "loxP" sites, and it will excise a sequence of DNA that is flanked by these 34 base pair sequences. (Or, in a procedure that was, at this point, not yet developed, Cre recombinase can flip the orientation of a gene so that, depending on its original orientation, it either will be transcribed or won't be transcribed.) In the other mouse line, loxP sites flanked the NMDAR1 gene, a gene that encodes an essential subunit of the NMDA receptor. But besides the inclusion of the loxP sites, these mice had normal genomes and developed normally with a functioning NMDR1 gene. Mating mice from these two lines produced offspring in which the Cre recombinase would excise the NMDR1 gene in CA1 neurons, but nowhere else (since Cre recombinase wasn't expressed in any other neurons). And, since Cre recombinase only begins to be expressed several weeks after birth, the loss of the NMDR1 gene did not interfere with prenatal or perinatal development.

Tsien and his colleagues found that the mice that lacked the NMDAR1 gene exhibited impaired spatial learning on the Morris water maze without an impairment to non-spatial learning, and, *in vitro*, stimulating CA3 axons did not induce LTP in CA1 neurons. Tsien et al. conclude: "these results provide strong support for the hypothesis that NMDAR-mediated LTP in the CA1 region is crucially involved in the formation of certain types of memory" (1996, p. 1328). And a little later they add:

> Previous studies examined the correlation between spatial memory and the site of hippocampal LTP (i.e., CA1, CA3, and dentate gyrus) by using a variety of conventional knockout mice. ... Our new evidence, while still correlational, is much stronger than that in the earlier reports because we have singled out the CA1 synapses as a site of plasticity impairment.

> (1996, p. 1335)

That said, the issue here is not whether this hypothesis has been suffi- ciently confirmed or by whom. Rather it is that, in these studies, the re- searchers are clearly seeking to confirm a hypothesis. Morris even lays it out in textbook fashion when he says that "the hypothesis makes the im- portant and testable prediction that AP5 should impair a subset of those learning tasks that are impaired by hippocampal lesions but should be without effect on tasks unaffected by such damage. The present series of experiments tests this prediction" (1989, p. 3041). Each team of in- vestigators, then, is judicious about the degree of confirmation provided by their own results and even more so about the degree of confirmation provided by the investigation that preceded theirs.

The LTP → spatial memory hypothesis was dependent on gene tar- geting for its eventual confirmation, but, temporally, the hypothesis pre- ceded the application of the tool, and verifying the hypothesis was the goal of these investigations. Hence, the investigations did not employ the tools first method, which is based on the absence of a well-defined hy- pothesis.[3] This, however, takes nothing away from gene targeting being a revolutionary new tool, which, at least on Bickle's terms, it has been. It changed the types of investigations that could be undertaken, and its use has become pervasive across cellular and molecular neuroscience (2016, p. 2). Arguably, it has a greater claim to triggering a revolution for the field than the second tool Bickle (2016) discusses, optogenetics, since optogenetics depends on the manipulation of genes.

3 Optogenetics

The second "neuroscientific revolution" that Bickle (2016) describes is the development and subsequent use of optogenetics. This tool, which was initially developed in the early 2000s by Karl Deisseroth, Edward Boyden, and colleagues working at Stanford University, uses light to control the activation or inactivation of neurons (Boyden et al. 2005). This is done by taking genes for light-activated proteins from algae, archaebacteria, and other microbial organisms and expressing them in the neurons of interest. For instance, the frequently used ion channel channelrhodopsin-2 occurs naturally in the green alga *C. re- inhardtii*. When it is expressed in the neural membrane and exposed to blue light, channelrhodopsin-2 allows positively charged ions to enter the cell, which causes an excitatory response. Conversely, halor- hodopsin, which is found in the single-celled archaeon *N. pharaonis*, pumps negatively charged chloride ions into the cell when it is ex- posed to yellow or orange light. This hyperpolarizing current inhibits the cell. Once the light-sensitive protein is expressed in neurons, an optical fiber that has been implanted in the animal's brain over the area of interest is used to deliver a specific wavelength of light. Thus, neurons can be activated or inhibited while still allowing the animal to move freely.

Bickle describes the motivating problem that spurred the development of optogenetics this way:

> The motivating problem for optogenetics stemmed from the causal-mechanistic explanatory goals of mainstream neurobiology. To test hypotheses about the causal role played by specific neurons to produce behaviors routinely taken as indicators of particular cognitive functions in mammalian models, experimenters need the capacity reliably to intervene into the hypothesized mechanisms *in vivo*—to activate or inhibit them in the behaving organism, as directly and as efficiently as possible. ... If successful, neurobiology would then have a great new experimental interventionist tool to explore causal-mechanistic hypotheses relating activity in specific neurons to behaviors—including behaviors routinely taken to indicate the occurrence of particular cognitive functions. This was optogenetics' motivating problem.
>
> (2016, pp. 10–11)

This captures the central issue, but we can give a less hypothesis-centric characterization of the problem. Here is how Boyden puts it:

> As I interviewed for PhD programs in neuroscience in spring 1999, I asked the scientists I met on each stop the same question: what tools should a physical sciences-trained investigator develop, to help understand the brain?
>
> One fact that emerged from those conversations was that there are many different kinds of neuron in the brain, which possess different morphologies, molecular compositions, and wiring patterns, and which undergo different changes in disease states. New neuron types, and new properties of existing neuron types, are being discovered all the time. ... In order to determine how different kinds of neuron in the brain work together to implement brain functions, and to assess the roles that specific sets of neurons play within neural circuits, it would ideally be possible to drive or quiet the activity of defined neurons embedded within an intact neural network. By driving the activity of a specific set of neurons, it would be possible to determine what behaviors, neural computations, or pathologies those neurons were able to cause. And by silencing the activity of a specific set of neurons, it would be possible to determine what brain functions, or pathologies, those neurons were necessary for.
>
> (2011, p. 2)

This is, of course, related to Bickle's characterization of the motivating problem, but here we begin, not with "causal-mechanistic hypotheses," but with the nature of the neuronal milieu. When distinguished by structure, function, the genes they express, or how they are arranged and project to other neurons, the types of neurons packed into each brain area are extremely diverse. Lesioning, pharmacological interventions, and electrical stimulation and recording are useful tools, but they lack the specificity to intervene on only a narrowly defined set of neurons. Thus, the need for optogenetics, which allows for control of neurons that are identified by genetic markers (which is related to their function and structural features), location, and where their axons project.

Whereas before we saw gene targeting deployed to confirm the hypothesis that LTP underlies spatial memory, we will now turn to a study that is not investigating a hypothesis. This is not how all investigations using optogenetics proceed, but the study is a fair exemplar of the tools first method in neurobiology.

3.1 Optogenetics and Divergent Motivational States

The dopamine pathways in the brain are composed of dopamine-releasing neurons in the midbrain's ventral tegmental area (VTA) and substantia nigra that project to the prefrontal cortex, nucleus accumbens, and striatum. Electrical stimulation, pharmacological interventions, and lesioning have shown that these neurons have a role in reward-seeking and motivated behaviors (e.g., Olds & Milner 1954; Ungerstedt, 1971; Crow 1972; Wise et al. 1978). Not surprisingly, however, given that dopaminergic and non-dopaminergic neurons are intermingled in the VTA and have these diverse projections, the increased specificity of cell-type targeting afforded by optogenetics has been embraced. Some of this work has been done by Garret Stuber, who, not long after the very first *in vivo* studies using optogenetics were performed, began investigating the effects that dopaminergic neurons have on neurons outside of the VTA and on behavior (Tsai et al. 2009; Stuber et al. 2010; Adamantidis et al. 2011). He then investigated, again using optogenetics along with other tools, the function of non-dopaminergic neurons in the VTA that synapse on dopamine-releasing neurons (van Zessen et al. 2012). Then, stepping further back from the dopaminergic neurons, he began investigating the functions of neurons in other parts of the brain—the lateral habenula, the bed nucleus of the stria terminalis, and the lateral hypothalamus—that project directly or indirectly to the VTA (Stamatakis & Stuber 2012; Jennings et al. 2013; Stamatakis et al. 2016). This has yielded an increasingly detailed picture of the functional and structural features of the neurons that provide inputs to the VTA-based dopamine system. (For reviews of some of this work see Deisseroth 2014; Stamatakis et al. 2014.)

In the study that investigated the functional properties of neurons in the bed nucleus of the stria terminalis that project to the VTA, Joshua Jennings, Stuber, and colleagues found that a small number of neurons can drive *and* prevent behavior that reflects anxiety in mice (Jennings et al. 2013). They introduce the study this way:

> The extended amygdala, including the bed nucleus of the stria terminalis (BNST), modulates fear and anxiety, but also projects to the ventral tegmental area (VTA), a region implicated in reward and aversion, thus providing a candidate neural substrate for integrating diverse emotional states. However, the precise functional connectivity between distinct BNST projection neurons and their postsynaptic targets in the VTA, as well as the role of this circuit in controlling motivational states, have not been described.

(2013, p. 224)

There is no question that they are starting with a thorough understanding—such as was available—of these brain areas. Their goal, however, is not hypothesis-testing but rather to describe "the precise functional connectivity" of these neurons and how these circuits control motivation and behavior.

To carry out this investigation, they began with two genetically modified mouse lines. In the first, Cre recombinase was expressed only in neurons that release the neurotransmitter glutamate. The adeno-associated virus was then used to deliver the channelrhodopsin-2 gene to neurons in the ventral BNST (vBNST). Most of the viral DNA had been removed from each copy of the virus and replaced with the gene for channelrhodopsin-2 inverted between loxP sites. When this viral construct was injected into the vBNST, it infected, harmlessly, all neurons there. Expression of the channelrhodopsin-2 gene, however, was dependent on Cre recombinase flipping the gene to the correct orientation so that it could be transcribed. Thus, only the excitatory glutamate-releasing neurons ended up with the light-sensitive ion channels. And since the viral construct was only injected into the vBNST, the expression of channelrhodopsin-2 was limited to that area of the brain. In the other mouse line, the mice expressed Cre recombinase only in neurons that release the neurotransmitter γ-aminobutyric acid (GABA). Using the same viral construct, channelrhodopsin-2 was expressed only in inhibitory GABA-releasing neurons in the vBNST in these mice.

After injecting the virus, Jennings et al. let four to six weeks elapse so that channelrhodopsin-2 would be expressed, not only in and around the neurons' cell bodies but also in the presynaptic terminals that reach into the VTA. The optical fiber for photostimulating the vBNST neurons with blue light was then implanted in the VTA, thus ensuring that, while vBNST → VTA neurons would be photostimulated at their distal axons, neurons in the vBNST that project elsewhere would not be.[4] The result was that the neurons that could be optogenetically manipulated were selected on the basis of the neurotransmitter that they release—glutamate or GABA—the location of their cell bodies, and where their axons project, all without any apparent adverse effects on the mice.

Once the mice were prepared, Jennings et al. used several tests to investigate the functions of these neurons in freely moving mice. First, they combined optogenetic control of the neurons with recording from a microelectrode array implanted in the vBNST. So that they could distinguish the neurons in the vBNST that project to the VTA from other neurons in the vBNST, they photostimulated the presynaptic terminals in the VTA to generate action potentials that propagated up the neurons' axons (i.e., from the pre-synaptic terminals to the cell bodies). Detection of a spike less than 20 ms after the first light pulse was delivered indicated that the neuron being recorded was either a glutamatergic or GABAergic vBNST → VTA neuron. With the ability to record the activity of these neurons, Jennings et al. submitted the mice to an unpredictable foot-shock procedure: mice received about 20 foot-shocks over a 20-minute period while also being exposed to two constant contextual cues, light from a house lamp and white noise. During this period—and excluding the moments when the mice received the foot-shocks—they found that, compared to an earlier baseline period, there was increased activation of the glutamatergic vBNST → VTA neurons. Conversely, the GABAergic vBNST → VTA neurons showed a reduction in activity during the 20-minute period. This established that the glutamatergic neurons respond during an aversive event while the activity of the GABA-ergic neurons is suppressed during such an event.

In the remaining parts of the study, photostimulation was delivered during the experiments. In the first two, mice could choose to receive or avoid photostimulation of the vBNST → VTA neurons either by staying on one side of an arena or by nose poking. Mice in which the glutamatergic neurons would be stimulated avoided photostimulation, while the mice in which the GABAergic neurons would be stimulated sought it out. Next, and interestingly, in an experiment with mice that had been food-deprived, constant photostimulation of the vBNST → VTA glutamatergic neurons caused a reduction in nose poking that would deliver a food reward. In the final experiments, each group of mice was submitted to one of two tests that are frequently used to assess anxiety in rodents, the open field test, and the elevated plus maze. In the first, following 20 minutes of constant photostimulation of the glutamatergic vBNST → VTA neurons, mice spent significantly more time in the corners of the open field arena—a 25 × 25 cm chamber—and less time in the center compared to controls, behavior that indicates a heightened level of anxiety. Meanwhile, mice that received constant photostimulation of the GABAergic neurons spent more time, compared to control mice, exploring the open arms (as opposed to the enclosed arms) of an elevated plus-shaped maze, indicating reduced levels of anxiety.

The takeaway is straightforward. Activation of the glutamatergic vBNST → VTA neurons enhances anxiety, while activation of the GABA-ergic vBNST → VTA neurons suppresses it. There is more to say about the neurons that are targeted by these vBNST → VTA neurons, but, even without that detail, we can see that these different types of neurons—from the same brain area and projecting to the same brain area—cause very different types of motivation and behavior.[5] Jennings et al. conclude: "Although the canonical view of BNST function proposes a dominant role of this structure in promoting anxiety states, the cellular and functional complexity described here illustrates that particular BNST circuit elements orchestrate divergent aspects of emotional and motivational processing" (2013, p. 228). Granting that "the canonical view" is theory is some loose sense, their goal was to investigate and describe these neural circuits and that is what they accomplished. Moreover, a few years after the study was completed, Stuber said this about their aims:

> One thing that we began to think about more as we were finishing this study was that these are ways that we can manipulate different cell populations, but these are still very broad-spectrum cell targeting strategies. We are still, essentially, targeting all glutamatergic neurons or all GABAergic neurons within this structure. And so, after our 2013 paper, we began to search for other genes—which may be enriched in these structures, such as the BNST—that could serve, potentially, as genetic handles or entry points [and] would allow us to tap in and modulate and study more precise cell types.
>
> (2016)

This led them to investigate the functional properties and connectivity of the subpopulation of GABAergic neurons in the BNST that express the gene for the neuropeptide nociceptin (Rodriguez-Romaguera et al. 2020). While it may be that Stuber and his team have expectations or thoughts about what their experiments will reveal, their interest appears to sidestep theory or hypotheses. Instead, they are seeking out more and more details of these neural mechanisms.

4 Conclusion

Scientific method in contemporary neurobiology is varied. Hypotheses may be formulated and tested, but they need not be. Ian Hacking (1983) discusses this point, and it is instructive to see how far he is willing to take it. He begins by quoting the 19th-century chemist Justus von Liebig who wrote,

> Experiment is only an aid to thought, like a calculation: the thought must always and necessarily precede it if it is to have any meaning.

An empirical mode of research, in the usual sense of the term, does not exist. An experiment not preceded by theory, i.e., by an idea, bears the same relation to scientific research as a child's rattle does to music.

> (*Über Francis Bacon von Verulam und die Methode der Naturforschung*, 1863; in Hacking 1983, p. 153)

Hacking, then, explains that there is a weak and a strong version of Liebig's statement about the role of theory. The weak version, which Hacking finds uncontroversial, is simply that

> you must have some ideas about nature and your apparatus before you conduct an experiment. A completely mindless tampering with nature, with no understanding or ability to interpret the result, would teach almost nothing.
>
> (1983, p. 153)[6]

The strong version of Liebig's statement, meanwhile, has it that "your experiment is significant only if you are testing a theory about the phenomena under scrutiny" (1983, p. 154), and this Hacking believes to be false. Of course, sometimes it is true that we precede that way, but "one can conduct an experiment simply out of curiosity to see what will happen" (1983, p. 154). The strong versus the weak reading of Liebig's statement is the distinction that we have encountered. Morris, Silva, Tonegawa, Tsien, and their colleagues were testing a theory (or a hypothesis, at least) about LTP and spatial memory. Jennings, Stuber, and their colleagues—while having "some ideas about nature and [their] apparatus"—were experimenting to see what they would find.

But while Hacking allows that experiments can be productively carried out without being tests of a theory, he then adds that theory will eventually be needed to make sense of the results (1983, pp. 158, 164–165). One of his examples is Brownian motion. Although Robert Brown was not the first to notice the phenomenon, he observed and carefully recorded the motions of pollen in water in 1827. But, Hacking reports, "for long it came to nothing" (1983 p. 158). It took Einstein's molecular theory of heat—which was itself confirmed in a series of experiments by Jean Perrin—to explain Brown's observations.

This is where we break from Hacking. He is not concerned to make every experiment look like a test of a theory, but in the end, he maintains that "plenty of phenomena attract great excitement but then have to lie fallow because no one can see what they mean, how they connect with anything else, or how they can be put to some use" (1983, p. 158). He then concludes, "Thus I make no claim that experimental work could exist independently of theory" (1983, p. 158). Similarly, Churchland worries that "by shunning theory, one runs the risk that the data-gathering may be random and the data gathered, trivial" (1986, p. 404). Hacking may be right when the examples come from physics, and Churchland is writing in the 1980s, before the development of the tools discussed here and before the mechanistic turn in the philosophy of biology, a point to which we will turn in a moment. Their worries, in any case, appear not to apply to Jennings et al.'s results. We may wish to know more about the projections of dopaminergic neurons in the VTA, their effects on behavior, and the inputs that they receive, but there is no real difficulty with making sense of the results.

Part of the reason for this is because explanations in cellular and molecular neurobiology are mechanistic. Carl Craver, for one, is clear on this point. Referring to "early twenty-first-century physiological sciences, such as neuroscience," he writes, "In such fields, the language of mechanism is literally ubiquitous, and most scientists continue to demand that adequate explanations reveal the hidden mechanisms by which things work" (2013, p. 134). As is well known, this involves identifying the parts that compose the system, both their structures and functions, and how those parts are organized. William Bechtel puts it this way:

> On my analysis, *a mechanism is an organized system of component parts and component operations. The mechanism's components and their organization produce its behavior, thereby instantiating a phenomenon* (Bechtel & Abrahamsen, 2005; ...). According to this view, a mechanism is a system operating in nature, and a mechanistic explanation is an epistemic product. To arrive at a mechanistic explanation, scientists must represent (sometimes verbally, but often visually in diagrams) the component parts and their operations and the ways in which they are organized.
>
> (2005, pp. 314–315, italics in the original)

Seeking mechanistic explanations does not, however, by itself lead to the tools first method. To the contrary, as Craver points out, these are "hidden mechanisms," and if we had little or no access to them, then theorizing would be a prominent part of trying to understand them. But, even though the components and operations of the brain are heterogeneous, fragile, and relatively inaccessible, experiment tools that have been developed for investigating the brain are, as we have seen, providing access to cellular and sub-cellular mechanisms.[7] Gene targeting (as well as the viral delivery of genes) and optogenetics are two prominent examples, but there are many others. One that bears mentioning because it is, in a way, the complement to optogenetics is calcium imaging, which uses proteins that can absorb and emit light (delivered to neurons by the same methods that are used for light-sensitive ion channels) to image neurons firing individual action potentials.

While this is only a subset of the experiment tools used in contemporary neurobiology, it illustrates their scope nicely. Proteins can be removed or added to specific types of neurons with gene targeting or with viral gene delivery. At the cellular level, precise types of neurons in specific locations can be activated or inhibited with optogenetics. How these interventions effect behavior can then be tracked. Calcium imaging, meanwhile, allows the activity of individual neurons to be tracked when animals are given a behavioral task. Consequently, when the goal is descriptions of 'organized systems of component parts and component operations' and when the tools exist to identify those parts, their operations, and how they are organized, then, rather than expecting the development of theories that must be submitted to experimental tests, we should expect neuroscientific practice to be a process of exploring and, piece by piece, adding detail to mechanistic explanations.

Acknowledgments

This chapter has benefited from many discussions of John Bickle's work on tool development at Mississippi State University and at the 2018 and 2019 Philosophy and Neuroscience at the Gulf annual meetings. I would also like to thank John Bickle for his comments on a draft of this chapter.

Notes

1 I am not claiming that *theory* in the sense of *a hypothesis* (or *a collection of hypotheses*) can be cleanly distinguished from any of the other senses of *theory* or that we should always want to make such a distinction. I am only claiming that the distinction will be useful here.

Bickle, for his part, uses *theory* in different ways. When he invokes and rejects "theory-centrism," he is adopting Churchland, Gold, and Roskies' call for theory in the sense of proposed explanations that direct experimental investigations and are confirmed or disconfirmed by those investigations. But he also uses *theory* in the sense of well-confirmed and mainly completed explanations—for instance, when he says,

> neuroscience, I claim (Bickle 2015, 2016, 2018), has lots of good, well-confirmed theory; ... the mechanisms of neuronal conductance and transmission at chemical synapses, receptor and ion channel function, mechanisms of synaptic plasticity, including its molecular-genetic and epigenetic mechanisms, details of anatomical circuitries linking neurons to other neurons, and ultimately to sensory receptors and muscle tissue.
>
> (2019, p. 580).

Then, in his description of the development of gene targeting and optogenetics, he is at pains to show that these tools were developed by "catch-as-catch can laboratory tinkering" (2019, p. 594) not by the considered application of theory—that is, not by the application of well-confirmed scientific explanations (2018, pp. 1071–1074; 2019, pp. 591–594).

2 Silva et al., in the introduction to their own study, make the point plainly:

Although LTP has been studied as a mechanism responsible for some types of learning and memory, the actual evidence for this hypothesis is not extensive. The main support for LTP as a memory mechanism is the observation that pharmacological agents that block hippocampal glutamate receptors of the N-methyl-D-aspartate (NMDA) class and thus prevent the induction of LTP also impair spatial learning in rodents (Morris et al. 1991). The problem with this evidence is that blocking NMDA receptors disrupts synaptic function and thus potentially interferes with the in vivo computational ability of hippocampal circuits. Perhaps the failure of learning results not from the deficit in LTP but simply from some other incorrect operation of hippocampal circuits that lack NMDA receptor function.

(1992b, p. 201)

3 Bickle's analysis is different. He focuses on the theory, or lack thereof, that was used by Capecchi to develop gene targeting in mice (2019, pp. 591–594). That, however, switches the focus from the theory that is stated in the motivating problem, and which clearly concerned these investigators, to theory in a different context.

4 Control animals were from the same two lines of mice. Each received the injection of the viral construct and the optical fiber was implanted in its VTA. But, for these mice, the viral construct did not contain the gene for channelrhodopsin-2, and so their vBNST → VTA neurons could not be activated by light.

5 For the curious, using immunohistochemical staining, photostimulation, and patch-clamp recording in brain slices, Jennings et al. found that the vBNST → VTA neurons "formed functional synapses primarily onto non-dopaminergic and medially located dopaminergic neurons." They then add, "these data provide a circuit blueprint by which vBNST subcircuits interact with VTA-reward circuitry" (2013, pp. 225–226).

6 Although, he later adds,

Indeed even the weak version is not beyond doubt. The physicist George Darwin used to say that every once in a while one should do a completely crazy experiment, like blowing the trumpet to the tulips every morning for a month. Probably nothing will happen, but if something did happen, that would be a stupendous discovery.

(1983, p. 154)

7 Bickle, in another context, has made this same connection between new experiment tools that began to be developed in the 1980s and 1990s and mechanistic explanations (2015; see especially Section 4).

References

Adamantidis, A. R., Tsai, H.-C., Boutrel, B., Zhang, F., Stuber, G. D., Budygin, E. A., Touriño, C., Bonci, A., Deisseroth, K., & de Lecea, L. (2011). Optogenetic interrogation of dopaminergic modulation of the multiple phases of reward-seeking behavior. *Journal of Neuroscience, 31*(30), 10829–10835.

Bechtel, W. (2005). The challenge of characterizing operations in the mechanisms underlying behavior. *Journal of the Experimental Analysis of Behavior, 84*(3), 313–325.

Bechtel, W., & Abrahamsen, A. (2005). Explanation: A mechanist alternative. *Studies in History and Philosophy of Biological and Biomedical Sciences, 36*, 421–441.

Bickle, J. (2015). Marr and reductionism. *Topics in Cognitive Science, 7*(2), 299–311.

Bickle, J. (2016). Revolutions in neuroscience: Tool development. *Frontiers in Systems Neuroscience, 10*, 1–13.

Bickle, J. (2018). From microscopes to optogenetics: Ian Hacking vindicated. *Philosophy of Science, 85*(5), 1065–1077.

Bickle, J. (2019). Linking mind to molecular pathways: The role of experiment tools. *Axiomathes, 29*(6), 577–597.

Bliss, T. V. P., & Lømo, T. (1973). Long-lasting potentiation of synaptic transmission in the dentate area of the anaesthetized rabbit following stimulation of the perforant path. *The Journal of Physiology, 232*(2), 331–356.

Boyden, E. S. (2011). A history of optogenetics: The development of tools for controlling brain circuits with light. *F1000 Biology Reports, 3*(11), 1–12.

Boyden, E. S., Zhang, F., Bamberg, E., Nagel, G., & Deisseroth, K. (2005). Millisecond-timescale, genetically targeted optical control of neural activity. *Nature Neuroscience, 8*(9), 1263–1268.

Churchland, P. S. (1986). *Neurophilosophy: Toward a unified science of the mind-brain.* Cambridge: MIT Press.

Craver, C. F. (2013). Functions and mechanisms: A perspectivalist view. In P. Huneman (Ed.), *Functions: Selection and mechanisms* (pp. 133–158). Dordrecht: Springer.

Crow, T. J. (1972). A map of the rat mesencephalon for electrical self-stimulation. *Brain Research, 36*(2), 265–273.

Deisseroth, K. (2014). Circuit dynamics of adaptive and maladaptive behaviour. *Nature, 505*(7483), 309–317.

Gardner-Medwin, A. R. (1969). Modifiable synapses necessary for learning. *Nature, 223*(5209), 916–919.

Gold, I., & Roskies, A. L. (2008). Philosophy of neuroscience. In M. Ruse (Ed.), *Oxford handbook of philosophy of biology* (pp. 349–380). Oxford: Oxford University Press.

Hacking, I. (1983). *Representing and intervening: Introductory topics in the philosophy of natural science.* Cambridge: Cambridge University Press.

Harris, E. W., Ganong, A. H., & Cotman, C. W. (1984). Long-term potentiation in the hippocampus involves activation of N-methyl-D-aspartate receptors. *Brain Research, 323*(1), 132–137.

Hebb, D. O. (1949). *The organization of behavior: A neuropsychological theory.* New York: Wiley.

Jennings, J. H., Sparta, D. R., Stamatakis, A. M., Ung, R. L., Pleil, K. E., Kash, T. L., & Stuber, G. D. (2013). Distinct extended amygdala circuits for divergent motivational states. *Nature, 496*(7444), 224–228.

Lømo, T. (1966). Frequency potentiation of excitatory synaptic activity in the dentate area of the hippocampal formation. *Acta Physiologica Scandinavica, 68*(S277), 128.

Morris, R. G. M. (1989). Synaptic plasticity and learning: Selective impairment of learning rats and blockade of long-term potentiation *in vivo* by the

N-methyl-D-aspartate receptor antagonist AP5. *Journal of Neuroscience,* 9(9), 3040–3057.

Morris, R. G. M., Anderson, E., Lynch, G. S., & Baudry, M. (1986). Selective impairment of learning and blockade of long-term potentiation by an N-methyl-D-aspartate receptor antagonist, AP5. *Nature, 319*(6056), 774–776.

Morris, R. G. M., Davis, S., & Butcher, S. P. (1991). Hippocampal synaptic plasticity and N-methyl-D-aspartate receptors: A role in information storage? In M. Baudry & J. L. Davis (Eds.), *Long-term potentiation: A debate of current issues* (pp. 267–300). Cambridge: MIT Press.

Morris, R. G. M., & Kennedy, M. B. (1992). The Pierian Spring. *Current Biology, 2*(10), 511–514.Olds, J., & Milner, P. (1954). Positive reinforcement produced by electrical stimulation of septal area and other regions of rat brain. *Journal of Comparative and Physiological Psychology, 47*(6), 419–427.

Rodriguez-Romaguera, J., Ung, R. L., Nomura, H., Otis, J. M., Basiri, M. L., Namboodiri, V. M. K., Zhu, X., Robinson, J. E., Munkhof, H. E. van den, McHenry, J. A., Eckman, L. E. H., Kosyk, O., Jhou, T. C., Kash, T. L., Bruchas, M. R., & Stuber, G. D. (2020). Prepronociceptin-expressing neurons in the extended amygdala encode and promote rapid arousal responses to motivationally salient stimuli. *Cell Reports, 33*(6), 108362.

Silva, A. J., Paylor, R., Wehner, J. M., & Tonegawa, S. (1992a). Impaired spatial learning in alpha-calcium-calmodulin kinase II mutant mice. *Science, 257*(5067), 206–211.

Silva, A. J., Stevens, C. F., Tonegawa, S., & Wang, Y. (1992b). Deficient hippocampal long-term potentiation in alpha-calcium-calmodulin kinase II mutant mice. *Science, 257*(5067), 201–206.

Stamatakis, A. M., & Stuber, G. D. (2012). Activation of lateral habenula inputs to the ventral midbrain promotes behavioral avoidance. *Nature Neuroscience, 15*(8), 1105–1107.

Stamatakis, A. M., Sparta, D. R., Jennings, J. H., McElligott, Z. A., Decot, H., & Stuber, G. D. (2014). Amygdala and bed nucleus of the stria terminalis circuitry: Implications for addiction-related behaviors. *Neuropharmacology, 76,* 320–328.

Stamatakis, A. M., Van Swieten, M., Basiri, M. L., Blair, G. A., Kantak, P., & Stuber, G. D. (2016). Lateral hypothalamic area glutamatergic neurons and their projections to the lateral habenula regulate feeding and reward. *Journal of Neuroscience, 36*(2), 302–311.

Stuber, G. D. (2016, September 28). *Functional and molecular dissection of a neural circuit for anxiety* [Conference presentation]. DECODE Summit, Palo Alto, CA. https://youtu.be/lj4_54w91wI.

Stuber, G. D., Hnasko, T. S., Britt, J. P., Edwards, R. H., & Bonci, A. (2010). Dopaminergic terminals in the nucleus accumbens but not the dorsal striatum corelease glutamate. *Journal of Neuroscience, 30*(24), 8229–8233.

Tonegawa, S. (2001). Roles of hippocampal NMDA receptors in learning and memory. *Riken BSI News, 12.* https://bsi.riken.jp/bsi-news/bsinews12/no12/issue1e.html.

Tsai, H.-C., Zhang, F., Adamantidis, A., Stuber, G. D., Bonci, A., de Lecea, L., & Deisseroth, K. (2009). Phasic firing in dopaminergic neurons is sufficient for behavioral conditioning. *Science, 324*(5930), 1080–1084.

Tsien, J. Z., Huerta, P. T., & Tonegawa, S. (1996). The essential role of hippo-campal CA1 NMDA receptor–dependent synaptic plasticity in spatial memory. *Cell, 87*(7), 1327–1338.

Ungerstedt, U. (1971). Adipsia and aphagia after 6-hydroxydopamine induced degeneration of the nigro-striatal dopamine system. *Acta Physiologica Scandinavica, 82*(S367), 95–122.

van Zessen, R., Phillips, J. L., Budygin, E. A., & Stuber, G. D. (2012). Activation of VTA GABA neurons disrupts reward consumption. *Neuron, 73*(6), 1184–1194.

Wise, R. A., Spindler, J., deWit, H., & Gerberg, G. J. (1978). Neuroleptic-induced "anhedonia" in rats: Pimozide blocks reward quality of food. *Science, 201*(4352), 262–264.

3 Science in Practice in Neuroscience

Cincinnati Water Maze in the Making

Nina A. Atanasova, Michael T. Williams and Charles V. Vorhees

1 Introduction

Historically, philosophy of science was largely preoccupied with questions regarding the nature of scientific theories, what makes one theory better than another, and what implications scientific theories have for traditional philosophical questions. Philosophers conceptualized scientific change in terms of theory change. Theory was considered a finished product independent from its social and institutional context. However, the process of theory in the making has yet to be carefully studied in philosophy of science.

In our view, an integrated approach viewing science as a human practice embedded in a historical and institutional context should be adopted for the study of multiple relevant factors involved in the making of theories. This approach requires zooming out of the narrow view of science which reduces it to its theories and looking at the bigger picture of science as a practice, which generates theories along with technological, medical, and social innovations motivated by societal needs and available funding. Here we present a case study from contemporary experimental neuroscience which focuses on the routine practices of grant-funded research and tool development which drive the research process in biomedical science. We propose an account of science in which theories serve as interpretative devices of experimental data. This result contradicts some philosophical accounts of science that tend to reduce it to its theories. By *theory,* we mean abstract models and narratives which postulate comprehensive ontologies for the explanation of target phenomena and the mechanisms that produce them.

Our approach recognizes the multiple functions of theories such as prediction, explanation, and modeling, which have been extensively analyzed in philosophy of science. While we recognize the importance of all these functions, we show that the role theory plays in contemporary neuroscience is as a device for interpretation of data generated by exploring focused hypotheses about specific interventions, for example, lesions of the hippocampus and their corresponding deficits in spatial

DOI: 10.4324/9781003251392-5

navigation. Contemporary neuroscience is data-driven. Scientific innovation consists in the development and consolidation of ensembles of experimental tools and techniques. It depends largely on the availability of funding and relevant technology.

Our goal is to present a case study which utilizes an integrated methodology in which philosophers and scientists reflect together on the practice of science. The authors are a philosopher and two neuroscientists in whose lab the philosopher worked while a graduate student. Although the majority of the narrative is a first-person recount of the two scientists, we use a third-person structure in order to ease the flow of the text.

In what follows, we provide a brief characterization of two traditional philosophical views of science which we challenge. We then turn to the philosophy of science-in-practice. Consistent with the turn to the philosophy of science-in-practice, philosophers of neuroscience have focused their attention on experimentation and tool development (Bickle 2006; Sullivan 2009; Silva et al. 2014; Atanasova 2015). This motivated our choice to trace the invention, development, and the continuous refinements of an experimental tool in neuroscience, the Cincinnati water maze (CWM). The case demonstrates the significance of the turn to the philosophy of science-in-practice by exemplifying the notion of research repertoires advanced by Leonelli and Ankeny (2015) and Ankeny and Leonelli (2016). We show how factors such as availability of funding, technology, and collaborations determine many rational choices in research practice. Finally, we introduce the notion of theories as interpretative devices to capture the role of theory in contemporary neuroscience.

1.1 Postpositivist Views of Science and Scientific Change

Early-20th-century philosophy of science was dominated by logical positivism which viewed empirical science as the most rigorous source of knowledge. Scientific knowledge, according to logical positivism, is based on empirical observations of the natural world that result in law-like generalizations. Scientific explanations consist of identifying generalizations from which the observed phenomena could be logically derived. Theories, in this view, do not serve explanatory functions, they are merely useful prediction devices. The success of science, according to logical positivism, is measured by the success of its predictions.

By mid-20th century, many of the core beliefs of logical positivism were challenged. Postpositivism took two forms: scientific realism and scientific relativism. Scientific realists (e.g., Putnam 1976; Boyd 1980) challenged the claim of positivism that scientific theories are merely prediction devices. If they are so successful in predicting events, scientific realists noted, theories must be getting something right about the unobservable world. Scientific theories tell us truths about the world even if we cannot directly observe all entities and processes they postulate. This inspired many to treat scientific theories as explanatory devices with comparable significance for both science and philosophy. Thus, the borders between theoretical science and metaphysics were blurred (Chakravartty 2007).

Scientific relativists (e.g., Kuhn 1970; Feyerabend 1988/1975), on the other hand, criticized both positivists and realists for their conceptualization of science as a rational activity detached from the lives of the human beings who practice it. They focused on science as a social activity and studied human interactions among scientists instead of the relationship between theories and the world. Nevertheless, theories play a central role in this account of science.

Inspired by the notion of the theory-ladenness of experiment and observation (Hanson 1965), Kuhn and Feyerabend claimed that the practice of science is defined by the theories adopted by different scientific communities. Theories, from this view, function as local ontologies which define the worldviews of the communities which adopt them. Thus, scientific disagreement is attributed to incompatible worldviews characteristic of rival communities. Since the proponents of this view believe that there is no objective way to determine that one ontology is better than another, all ontologies and corresponding theories are equally legitimate. Therefore, scientific change, according to relativists, consists in switching from one worldview to another. It is a radical replacement of one theory with another.

Both kinds of postpositivist approaches have rendered valuable insights. However, taken to an extreme, both present a distorted image of science. On one end of the spectrum, naïve scientific realists have a dogmatic attitude toward science as a flawless source of ultimate knowledge about the world. On the other end, radical relativists leave no room for science as a specialized source of knowledge. This divide culminated in the infamous Science Wars of the 1990s which drove a wedge between intellectuals from the humanities and social sciences on one side and natural scientists on the other (Gross and Levitt 1994; Gross et al. 1996; Ross 1996). Philosophy of science has since carved space for a middle ground. A number of philosophers of science now look both at the theories generated in science and at the interactions between scientists. Philosophy of science has turned to studying science-in-practice.

1.2 The Philosophy of Science-in-Practice

Postpositivist philosophy of science was preoccupied with scientific theories. While we take issue with naïve realism which assumes, often uncritically, the epistemic authority of science, we nevertheless assume that there are facts of the matter regarding the way the world is. However, judging which theory is better than another, in our view, depends on judgments about the validity of the methods used to generate that theory.

It matters, for example, how scientists come to know the mechanism of long-term potentiation in order for discussions about its role in memory-formation to be justified. If the phenomenon of long-term potentiation is not reproducible across laboratories and experimental conditions, if it is not reliably associated with behaviors indicative of memory-formation, we would not be able to make sense of the discussions about its causal role in the process (Dringenberg 2020). This is why it is important to look behind the scenes of knowledge production to understand the practice that makes it possible. Studying the practice of science is thus as important as studying its products, the theories. This realization is at the core of the turn to the philosophy of science-in-practice.

1.2.1 The Society for Philosophy of Science in Practice

The philosophy of science-in-practice traces its roots to 20th-century philosophy of experiment (Hacking 1983). However, it was not until the mid-2000s that the approach matured as a distinct methodology of philosophy of science. It was institutionalized with the initiation of the Society for Philosophy of Science in Practice (SPSP), founded in 2006 by Rachel Ankeny, Mieke Boon, Marcel Boumans, Hasok Chang, and Henk de Regt. SPSP held its founding meeting at the biennial meeting of the Philosophy of Science Association in Vancouver. The idea for SPSP was conceived of the previous year at the conference "Philosophical Perspectives on Scientific Understanding" in Amsterdam. According to SPSP's mission statement:

> Philosophy of science has traditionally focused on the relation between scientific theories and the world, at the risk of disregarding scientific practice. In social studies and technology, the predominant tendency has been to pay attention to scientific practice and its relation to theories, sometimes willfully disregarding the world except as a product of social construction. Both approaches have their merits, but they each offer only a limited view, neglecting some essential aspects of science. We advocate a philosophy of scientific practice, based on an analytic framework that takes into consideration theory, practice, and the world simultaneously.
>
> (SPSP Mission Statement)

The society has grown and given rise to a trend surpassing the framework of postpositivism. Prominent leaders of the society, Rachel Ankeny and Sabina Leonelli, introduced the notion of *research repertoire* to account for the collaborative practices in the contemporary life sciences. They define research repertoire as follows:

> ...a distinctive and shared ensemble of elements that make it practically possible for individuals to cooperate, including norms for

what counts as acceptable behaviours and practices together with infrastructures, procedures and resources that make it possible to implement such norms.

(Leonelli and Ankeny 2015, p. 701)

...well-aligned assemblages of skills, behaviors, and material, social, and epistemic components that groups may use to practice certain kinds of science, and whose enactment affects the methods and results of research, including how groups practice and manage research and train newcomers.

(Ankeny and Leonelli 2016, p. 20)

Our case study exemplifies the enactment of one such repertoire in behavioral neuroscience. It shows the superiority of this account of science over the, still influential, notion of scientific paradigm first advanced by Thomas Kuhn and Paul Feyerabend in the 1960s–1970s.

1.2.2 Post-Kuhnian Philosophy of Science

The notion of repertoire was inspired by the realization of the limitations of postpositivist philosophy of science. It was introduced as an alternative to Kuhn's (1970 [1962]) notion of a paradigm. Acknowledging Kuhn's equivocal use, we take *paradigm* to refer to the idea that a scientific community is defined in terms of a shared ontology, shared ways of formulating hypotheses, and standardized experimental methodologies. The knowledge claims formulated by such a community are context-dependent, bound by the corresponding ontological assumptions. This often precludes members from one community to have meaningful exchanges with members of other scientific communities. This dissonance ultimately precludes the integration of scientific knowledge generated by different communities. Recent recounts of this concern include Sullivan (2009), Longino (2014), and Hochstein (2016).

However, the philosophy of science-in-practice has brought about post-Kuhnian alternatives to the stage. Ankeny and Leonelli's notion of scientific repertoire captures the interactions of local epistemic communities belonging to a single institution as well as large consortia which may be spread out into a global network of collaborations.

1.2.3 Philosophy of Neuroscience in Practice

In this new line of philosophical studies of science, a number of philosophers of science have engaged with analysis of current experimental practices in neuroscience (Atanasova 2015; Bickle 2016; Robins 2016; Sullivan 2016). With this research came the recognition of the central role that tool development and innovation play in neuroscience.

Neuroscientific practice is experiment-driven. Theory often catches up after critical data are generated and are in need of synthesis and interpretation. Experiments are often inspired by the available technology rather than inspiring the design of novel technologies themselves. Many decisions regarding what experiments to design and run are based on pragmatic considerations (personnel, facilities, and funding).

Tool development and improvement thus need to take center stage in the philosophy of neuroscience. The case study we offer is meant to do justice to the epistemic and pragmatic problems through which tool development progresses. The case study exemplifies the fundamental role of the calibration strategy identified by Atanasova (2015). The story about the development and refinement of the CWM we tell below is a narrative about its calibration as a tool for the study of cognitive functions and deficits in rats.

This case study exemplifies the dynamic interplay between tool development, experiment, and theory. We aim to show that even though theoretical considerations and background assumptions are implicit in experimental design, this is not to say that comprehensive theories necessarily guide experiments. Theoretical constructs such as "learning" and "memory" are often very loosely defined and are rather fluid concepts. They serve as placeholders in experimental hypotheses and are under continuous reinterpretation and refinement in light of experimental results. As such they function like experimental tools (Feest 2010). We thus maintain that while comprehensive theories about learning and memory do get articulated, they often follow rather than precede the experiments which support them.

2 The Cincinnati Water Maze in the Making

The CWM is an apparatus used for testing rat egocentric (based on internal bodily cues) learning and memory when performed in darkness and requiring learning a sequence of turns to navigate to a goal (see Figures 1a and b). In the beginning, the CWM was used to study a mixture of egocentric and allocentric (based on external cues) learning and navigation when rats were run under standard room lighting but has since been modified as a test of egocentric memory complementary to the widely utilized MWM which tests allocentric learning. The CWM was introduced by Vorhees (1987) and has evolved continuously in the Vorhees/Williams Lab at Cincinnati Children's Research Foundation ever since. The maze consists of a series of interconnected T-shaped cul-de-sacs through which a rat navigates from a fixed start to an invariant goal. The maze is partly submerged in water and the task is for rats to find by trial and error the escape platform. The motivational factor in this task is the natural aversion of rats to water. The CWM was inspired by a simpler maze, the Biel water maze (BWM).

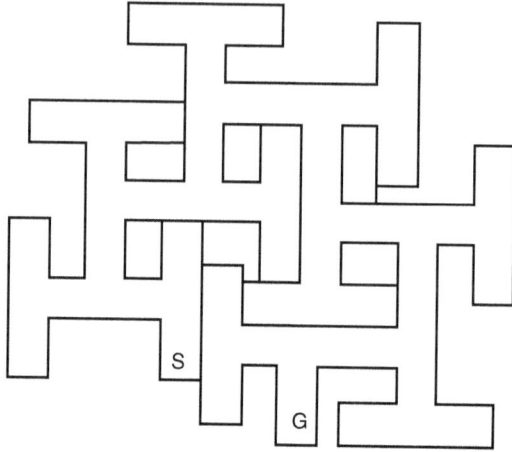

Figure 1a Drawing of Cincinnati water maze featuring the training path which begins at S (start) and ends at G (goal). The two points are reversed during reversal tests.

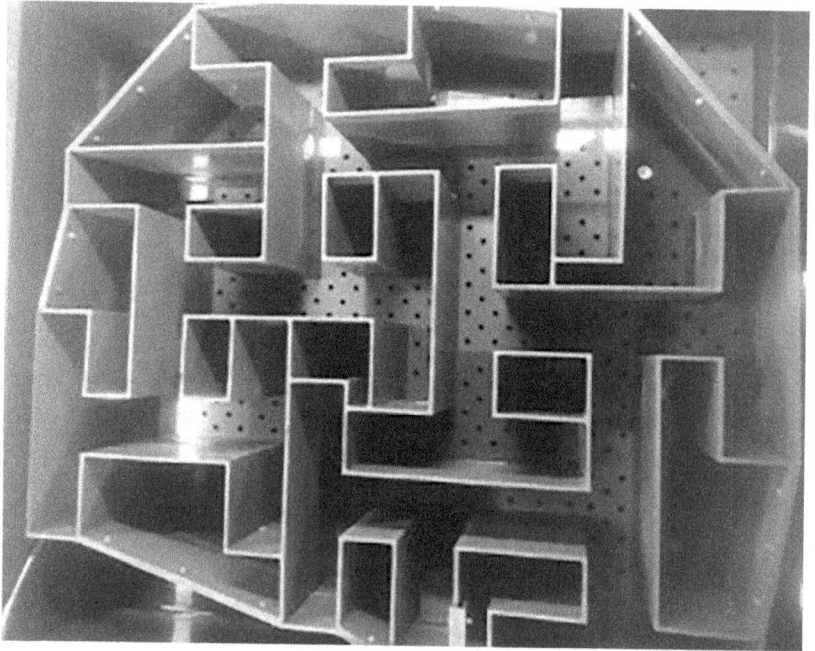

Figure 1b Photograph of Cincinnati water maze.

2.1 The Biel Water Maze

The BWM was introduced by William Biel (1940). The apparatus was used to explore developmental changes in the ability of young rats to learn a complex task. Rats were trained to navigate by swimming through a maze to reach an escape ladder. The maze consisted of a long straight channel along one side used for preliminary training and a series of five shorter T-shaped cul-de-sacs. Rats were placed in the starting position and tested until they located the goal at the end of the long arm where there was a ladder which afforded escape from the water. Rats were given training trials for 2.5 days. Rats received one trial in the straight arm in the morning and four maze training trials in the afternoon. The next day they received five more training trials. There were 24 maze trials divided among two test sessions each day, one in the morning and one in the afternoon. The first maze trial was in the morning after the last training day and consisted of one trial and two trials in the afternoon, followed by two morning and two afternoon trials for the next five days ending with a single trial on the last day. Trials ended when the rat found the escape ladder, but if it did not find it within ten minutes, it was removed. Biel recorded the number of errors (not specified what counted as an error), trials to reach criterion (criterion not specified), and latency to reach the goal.

The maze was later used by Polidora and colleagues in a series of experiments testing rat cognition. Polidora et al. (1963) aimed to "devise a learning task, simple enough for rapid mastery by rats, but difficult enough for reliable detection of relatively small differences in learning ability" (pp. 817–818). They tested rats for five days. Rats were given five pre-test trials in the straight channel on the first day. For the next three days, rats were given seven trials per day in the maze. On the fifth day, they were given five post-test trials in the straight channel. Rats were given ten minutes of rest between trials. Polidora and colleagues recorded transit time and errors (whole-body entries into a blind alley).

A few years later, the apparatus was utilized in a series of experiments exploring behavioral and biochemical consequences of exposure to several neurotoxins, after either pre- or postnatal exposure, by Richard Butcher's Lab at Cincinnati Children's Research Foundation throughout the 1970s. Butcher et al. (1970) used different procedures in which, in addition to the training in the straight channel and the original start-to-goal path in the maze, tested rats in a path which reversed the start and the goal points of the maze after a number of trials in the original, forward, path. Rats were given five trials in the straight channel on the first day of the experiment. For the next two days, rats were given five trials a day. Over the last two days, rats were tested on the reverse path for five trials a day. Rats were removed from the maze if they did not find the goal within ten minutes. Time and errors (whole body entries into blind alleys) were recorded.

In 1976, Dr. Vorhees joined Dr. Butcher's lab. While running experiments using the BWM, Vorhees noticed that rats, treated in various ways (experimental groups), tended to perform worse on the reverse path compared with control groups, even though there were no differences on the forward path. This prompted him to investigate why this happened. After numerous observations of how rats went through the maze and made decisions, he noticed that if a rat was in the forward path, it was forced to make a decision only at the end of a channel when it encountered a perpendicular wall, where it had to turn right or left. This was an inherent feature of the design of the maze. However, if the rat was in the reverse path and swam until encountering a wall, it was always a dead-end cul-de-sac, such that no matter whether it turned right or left, it reached another dead-end. To advance through the maze, the rat had to backtrack and take a side channel or anticipate the dead-end and turn before it reached the end of a channel. Vorhees conjectured that learning this anticipatory turn might be the reason why it was more difficult for rats to solve the task in the reverse path. He hypothesized that this more difficult aspect of the reverse path might be more sensitive to subtle differences between treatments. If so, treatments might show more pronounced effects if the maze was made more complicated and had more anticipatory turns.

2.2 Introduction of the Cincinnati Water Maze

By 1987, Vorhees was the principal investigator of the lab. He set out to explore his hypothesis that a more complex maze would increase the sensitivity of the test. This is when he designed the CWM (Vorhees 1987). The new maze was made of nine T-shaped channels, as opposed to five plus the long arm in the BWM. The channels were wider than the BWM to accommodate adult rats and the long arm was eliminated. Vorhees compared the sensitivity of the two maze designs to cognitive deficits occurring in rats after prenatal exposure to phenytoin. The choice of drug was made on the basis of the well-established neurotoxicity of the compound. He tested four groups of rats, one control and three with exposure to different doses of the drug. The results showed dose-dependent cognitive impairments in both mazes. However, the differences in performance between groups were significantly larger in the CWM.

This approach to establishing the validity of a behavioral test in neurobiology is analyzed in Atanasova (2015) where she refers to it as *calibration*. Behavioral tests such as the CWM are typically used in combination with other tests such as locomotor ability, anxiety, and vision. These tests are known as test batteries. For each test in the battery, the rest serve as calibration devices. Some of them are meant to establish prerequisite abilities for the test of main interest and others are used for detection and elimination of artifacts of the procedure. When a test is established within this larger context, it gets validated as an animal model of some human ability, disorder, or other research-worthy condition. Further, when a new experimental design, or tool, is introduced, neuroscientists calibrate it by testing it against factors that are known to produce certain effects under circumstances similar to the test conditions. For example, when a new animal model of depression is introduced, it is run with antidepressants that are known to be effective in the treatment of the symptoms of depression. Once it is established that antidepressants have effects that correspond to the modeled mood disorder, the animal model is used to assess novel compounds for effectiveness as antidepressants.

Similarly, Vorhees took a compound, phenytoin, known to produce cognitive impairments and a tool, the BWM, which was established as a valid test of cognitive impairments and redesigned it to make it more useful. The validity of the test refers to the capacity of the tool to accurately detect positive control agents known to be detrimental, but also to accurately identify negative control agents as not toxic (Vorhees 1987, p. 239). The BWM was successful at detecting the effects of known neurotoxins. Vorhees took the new tool, the CWM, and tested it against an established positive control compound. The new tool detected the same effects better than the old one, and in later experiments, it detected effects which the old apparatus did not detect. This allowed Vorhees to conclude that the new tool was more sensitive than the old one.

2.3 Trials and Errors

Michael Williams joined the lab in 1997. The CWM was continuously used to study the cognitive deficits resulting from exposure to various drugs and neurotoxins. Consistent with the calibration strategy, Vorhees and Williams used test batteries. Among the tests they commonly employed was the MWM introduced by Richard Morris (1981). The test is the most widely utilized spatial learning and memory test in neurobiology. The MWM consists of a large circular tank filled with water with a submerged escape platform (see Figures 2a–c). Animals are trained to navigate to the platform using distal cues on the walls of the testing room and away from the edge of the tank. There are numerous versions of the installation and control conditions under which the test is run (Vorhees and Williams 2006). In the Vorhees/Williams lab, the MWM is used as a test complementary to the CWM in the sense that the MWM is used to test allocentric navigation and the CWM – egocentric navigation.

The two instruments share a number of similarities. For example, both detect cognitive deficits. However, while the CWM detects deficits

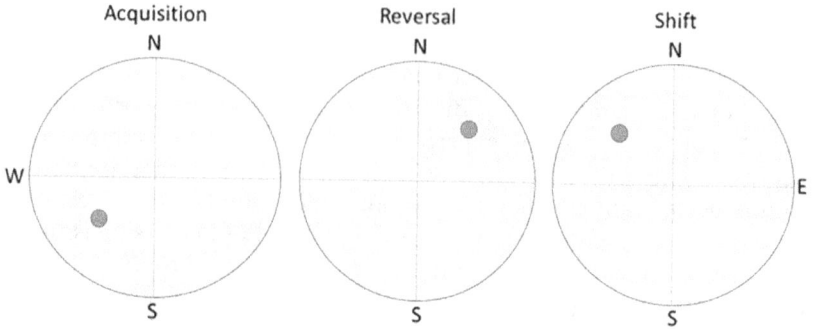

Figure 2a Drawing of Morris water maze featuring different positions of the escape platform during different training and testing phases.

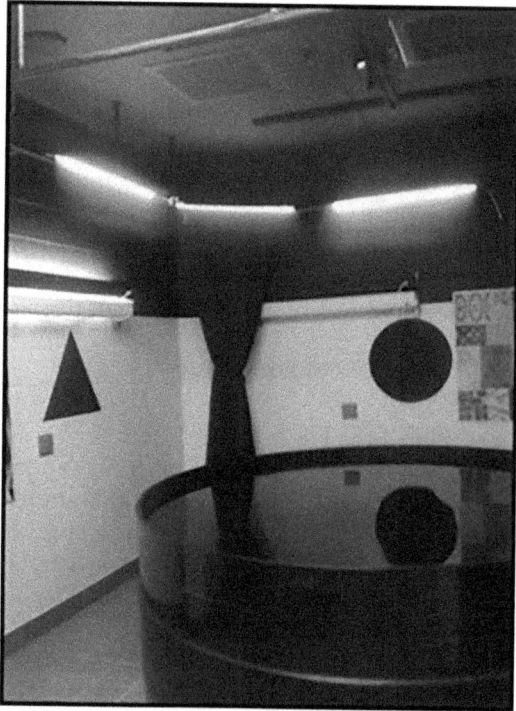

Figure 2b Photograph of Morris water maze.

in sequential/egocentric learning, the MWM detects deficits in spatial navigation. Running multiple experiments in both mazes, Vorhees and Williams noticed that after some treatments the performance in both tasks was disrupted (Morford et al. 2002; Williams et al. 2003), but

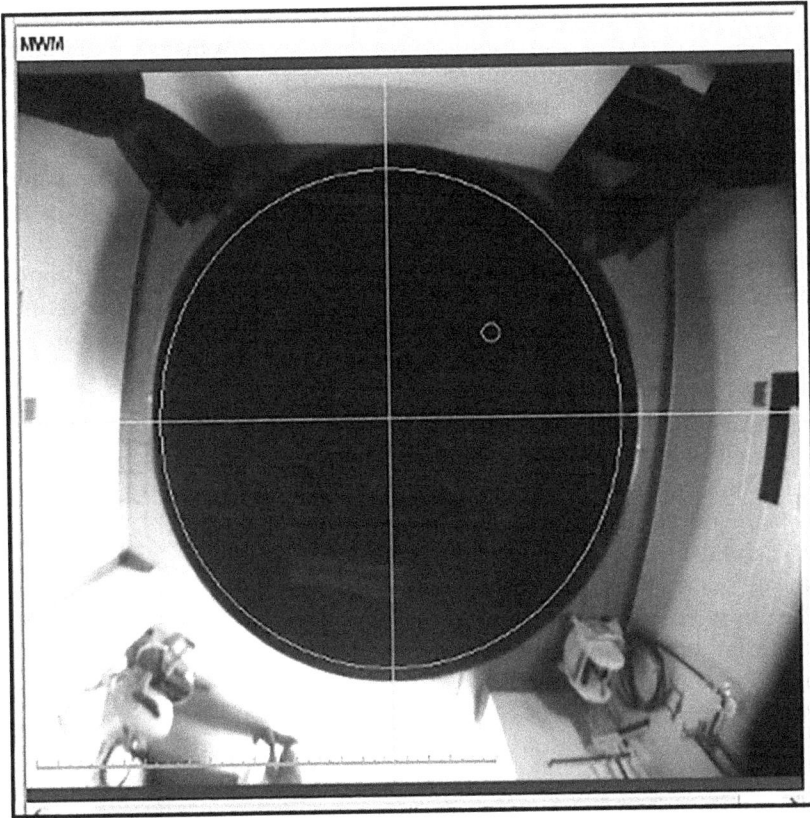

Figure 2c Screenshot of a bird's-eye view of Morris water maze through a recording camera.

after other treatments, the performance in one but not the other was impaired (Williams et al. 2002, 2003). Vorhees and Williams realized that such data pointed to a corresponding difference in the brain areas and the neurotransmitters that were involved in solving the two tasks. This inspired theoretical questions, but the maze would undergo several modifications in response to calibration issues before they could be addressed.

Vorhees and Williams discussed what makes the CWM unique and what brain regions were involved in solving it. They knew that distal cues are important for spatial memory, but the room that housed the CWM had no prominent cues but had many standard room features (such as air intake ducts and electrical outlets on the wall). Williams wondered, "Are the rats using background spatial cues as well as proximal cues in the CWM?" The task had presumably been solved on the basis of egocentric route-based proximal cues. So, they explored ways to eliminate spatial cues and the first thing they tried was hoods to cover the rats' eyes so that they could not see distal cues. Whishaw and Maas-winkel (1998) made hoods to obstruct rats' vision using a large circular platform maze where they first found food visually, then had to re-find it blindfolded.

Inspired by this publication, a student in the Vorhees/Williams lab, Tracy Blankemeyer, made rat hoods. However, when the rats were tested in the maze and the hoods got wet, they pried the hoods off, then searched for the goal. Efforts to get the rats accustomed to the hoods also failed by having the rats wear them for a week prior to maze testing. The rats did adjust to the hoods and left them on but when put in the maze, they again pried them off.

Therefore, Vorhees and Williams considered surgically blinding the rats but found this objectionable. Neither thought they could sew the eyelids shut even though this is a published procedure. They settled on a more humane solution: they turned off the lights but provided a red light because rat vision is reported to be deficient at the red end of the visible spectrum. The maze was harder than under white light, but the rats still solved the task rapidly. This suggested that there was enough light that the rats were still able to see room cues. At that time, it was known that a single landmark can be sufficient to solve an MWM. Therefore, Vorhees and Williams thought rats might be using even minimal red light as an orientation beacon to navigate to the goal.

This led to the decision to use infrared light. In this setup, rats performed worse than under red light, but they still appeared to orient to some unidentified light source. It turned out that the light leaking underneath and around the door was sufficient for the rats to orient. A hint that it was the door came out of experiments a graduate student, Nicole Herring, did. She found that rats treated with methamphetamine had CWM deficits (Herring et al. 2008). However, when she attempted to replicate the results, the effect was smaller. Something had changed. After inspection, it was determined that in the second experiment the door was not closing fully, providing more light than in the first experiment.

Therefore, trim was installed around the door and the closer was fixed so no light could get in the room. The principal investigators stood in the room making sure after dark adaptation that nothing could be seen. When experimenters entered the room to test a rat, they carried a red-light flashlight to see enough to place rats in and out of the maze without interfering with the dark adaptation of rats waiting to be tested. The difficulty rats had in solving the task under complete darkness meant that they were no longer using visual cues for navigation. Performance was monitored using an infrared-sensitive camera mounted above the maze connected to a monitor in an adjacent room where the experimenter scored performance. The tool was now calibrated to detect the effects which the investigators studied. In this process, there was little theoretical speculation about what the effects of the experimental procedures would imply for the nature of egocentric learning and memory, although tacit knowledge about the behaviors of rats under experimental conditions informed procedural changes. Some of the findings were accidental others were predicted.

Another inadvertent discovery was the importance of training. This came about when Vorhees and Williams helped another lab to set up a CWM by providing them with drawings for the maze. Later, the lab called Vorhees stating that the CWM was not working and that all rats failed to learn even when tested under normal light. The other lab had only asked for drawings, not test procedures. Vorhees had not provided information on the straight channel trials under the assumption they would later ask for procedures, but they never did. Hence, their rats did not learn that escape was possible and because the CWM even in the light is complex, and rats gave up searching without ever finding the escape. The tool was not properly calibrated, not all procedures for its proper use were followed. This is when Vorhees appreciated that the straight channel was essential to teach rats about escape. Without this knowledge, the rats became frustrated and would give up and tread water until removed. Hence, it became clear that minimal training was required for rats to solve a maze as difficult as the CWM. Until then, running the rats through the straight channel, just like Biel did, was considered an assessment of the rats' swimming capacities before they went into the maze, not a learning experience with positive transfer of training to the maze. It was meant to establish that rats were proficient swimmers and motivated to escape the water, and ensure they had no motoric impairment if they were in the treated group. This procedure accounted for the possibility that a treatment affecting swim speed could confound the interpretation of group differences obtained in the maze. Because the straight channel was used in the lab to obtain performance (swim speed) information, it was not initially appreciated that it was an essential part of the procedure. Employing the test for this purpose is part of the calibration strategy, but it became clear that it was a necessary component of the experimental setup. This shows that tacit procedural knowledge can make a difference in the way research develops without the employment of a theory about the process which underlies the studied behaviors. The causal connection between this element of the procedure and the observed behavior was articulated after the fact. It was not a hypothesis that was tested purposefully.

An even more recent change in the maze design was the introduction of a tenth T cul-de-sac. Williams noticed something that Vorhees overlooked. In Vorhees' drawing, one wall was slightly out of alignment limiting the maze to nine cul-de-sacs. However, once the alignment was corrected, there was room for an additional T. Recent data from the new design show that the change made a difference in maze difficulty and it now requires more trials for rats to become proficient. The rats' optimal performance in the ten-T version for the equivalent number of testing days is not as good as in the nine-T version.

More changes were introduced in response to calibration problems. For example, initially, only the errors in the arms of a T at the end of a cul-de-sac were counted. Now stem and T-errors are counted in recognition of the fact that all turns not leading to the goal are errors whenever a rat deviates from a direct path to the end regardless of whether it goes the full distance to the end of a right or left arm of a T. Moreover, counting only the end of cul-de-sac errors was not capturing valuable information about mistakes rats made. As rats learn, one of the intermediate steps they go through is recognizing when they make a wrong turn and swim down the stem of a T. Once the rats have visited that dead-end T several times, thereafter when they turn in down that stem, they recognize that they have been there before. The rat then stops short and reverses course. Counting only T-arm errors missed these intermediate errors. Adding stem errors further increased the sensitivity of the test. The change in error counting occurred at a lab meeting when it became clear that group differences were larger on some occasions depending on how different experimenters counted errors. They needed to calibrate experimenters as well as definitions of errors more precisely. This is not trivial because when rats begin to learn the maze, they progressively inhibit errors. At first, rats go all the way to the end of a T and turn right and left, and sometimes go back and forth before exiting. Later, rats hesitate partway down the stem before turning around. These 'intermediate' mistakes were being missed. The lab considered whether arm errors were in a sense more severe than stem errors. To find out, the next experiment counted both types of errors. Analysis of the data provided no support for the idea that arm errors represent a more severe deficit than stem or arm + stem errors in revealing group differences. Therefore, all errors are now treated the same.

In addition to errors, experimenters track the time it takes for a rat to find the platform (latency). However, there is a per-trial time limit of five minutes designed to prevent fatigue. This aspect of the test procedure also evolved. Initially, the time limit was 12 minutes. Rats were given two trials per day as before. However, rats that did not find the goal after 12 minutes would get exhausted. This caused rats to become tired faster on trial-2. The first approach to this problem was to give rats reaching the 12-minute limit, a one-hour rest. Later, the trial limit was reduced to ten minutes and the rest after a trial-1 failure was shortened to 30 minutes. Over a period of several years, the limit was gradually reduced from 10 to 6, and finally five minutes.

Some of the adjustments were also made in response to peer criticism. Critics pointed out that the resting time between trials might not be enough and, if insufficient, would compromise performance on trial-2 of each day. In response, Vorhees and Williams tested performance with rest intervals up to 30 minutes after a trial-1 failure to reach the goal and found it made little difference unless the trial time limit was shorter than five minutes. Therefore, five minutes was empirically determined and became standard practice. The data from these refinement experiments were not published separately because they were not sufficient by themselves to be worthy of a paper even though they were essential in the evolution of the method and are found within papers published across many years.

2.4 *The CWM in Practice*

The apparatus has become a standard tool for testing egocentric route-based learning and memory. It is an integral part of the test battery used in the Vorhees/Williams lab to measure behavioral responses to drugs, environmental agents, or gene mutations that cause neurological and cognitive dysfunction. The use of the CWM has followed three paths in its development, all of which are independent in their goals but intersect and reinforce the ultimate success of the task.

2.4.1 *Grant-Funded Research*

A recent project in the Vorhees/Williams lab is a study of the cognitive effects of proton exposure. It is a research question which arises in the context of cancer treatment. The motivation is to find what treatments minimize lasting cognitive side-effects from the treatment of brain tumors. Oncologists know that people treated for brain tumors by X-ray or proton radiation often have long-term cognitive problems. The questions they are addressing in normal rats include: "Do protons produce fewer or different long-term cognitive effects than X-rays, and do different dose, dose-fractions, and dose-rates produce fewer deficits than others?" The hypothesis is, since protons kill tumors more effectively, maybe they also produce less collateral damage to surrounding tissue than X-rays. Vorhees and Williams, working with oncologists, radiation biologists, and medical physicists, developed an experimental plan to test this hypothesis.

The way this works in practice is that the lab has tests of different cognitive functions. They then use this toolset in different settings to answer different experimental questions. In this case, by exposing rats to protons and testing them in the CWM, MWM, and other tests in their armamentarium, they can provide more comprehensive answers to the questions of interest. The experiments are meant to test a focused hypothesis about the cognitive effects of proton exposure. The researchers do not evoke an overarching theory of cognition. They operationalize cognitive deficits as deficits in behaviors observed under the experimental setup in response to a specific intervention. The toolkit is the crucial factor in this process.

When the lab sets out to study a drug, environmental agent, or gene mutation, they start by looking at the effect of the variable with the tools that they know since they know the brain regions that mediate each test. This provides first-pass information not only on what brain regions are affected but also provides clues to which neurotransmitters and receptors are likely affected. Once they generate preliminary data, they write grant proposals to supply the means for further study of the effects of the treatments.

2.4.2 Basic Research

Despite the fact that the majority of the choices made for the projects carried on in the lab depend on grant funding, Vorhees and Williams are driven by the quest for knowledge. For example, once Vorhees and Williams eliminated distal cues that rats could use for navigation in the CWM, they inferred that the rats' ability to use the hippocampus for spatial navigation in that task was discounted. This assumption was justified because the role of the hippocampus in spatial learning was well established. The next issue became to find out what part of the brain was used in solving the CWM. There were data published showing that the striatum is involved in path integration which is an overlapping ability with egocentric navigation. The next step, thus, was to lesion the striatum without affecting motor behavior and see if this created deficits in CWM learning.

When Amanda Braun entered the lab as a graduate student, she tested the role of striatal dopamine on CWM learning. Her experiments produced data showing that rats with dopaminergic striatal lesions performed much worse in the CWM than sham controls. However, to test the specificity of the effect, the rats were also tested in the MWM. Learning in the MWM was also impaired but less than in the CWM (Braun et al. 2012). Next, Braun lesioned subregions of the striatum to get a more specific idea of what regions were more important than others. She did four experiments, one for each regional lesion. She lesioned the dorsal striatum, the dorsal medial and dorsal lateral striatum, ventral striatum (n. accumbens), or prefrontal cortex.

The data supported the idea Vorhees and Williams had hypothesized. In these experiments, Braun again ran the rats in the CWM and MWM. Entire dorsal striatal dopaminergic lesions produced effects on learning in both mazes (Braun et al. 2012). This supported the notion that the two regions are interconnected. So, it was not an absolute difference between the two but the effect in the CWM was greater. When she lesioned the medial vs. lateral dorsal striatum, she was able to differentiate between effects in the CWM vs. MWM (Braun et al. 2015). Hence, with the entire dorsal striatum lesioned there were effects in both mazes whereas lesions in subregions produced smaller or no effects on the MWM. They also found that n. accumbens lesions impaired CWM learning, but prefrontal cortex dopamine lesions did not. This research was not extramurally funded and yet it made a difference in how they thought about the CWM compared with the MWM and other tests of learning and memory. It changed their approach to searching for other structure-function cognitive relationships.

Braun's experiments addressed concerns of other researchers about the CWM as a unique tool. In the beginning, Vorhees and Williams' peers would ask: "What does it mean? What are you measuring? Yes, you get a difference among groups but what is the basis of the difference?" The initial lack of answers to these questions shows that the early CWM experiments were not inspired by a preconceived theory about what unobservable processes were producing the observed behaviors. Braun's results identified the principal brain regions involved in CWM learning. Since the lesions were specific for dopamine, these studies implicated dopamine as a key neurotransmitter in mediating CWM learning. Now a claim about the causal connection between affected brain regions and behaviors was articulated. This eliminated many criticisms because the results were empirically derived.

One of the projects Vorhees and Williams are considering is testing the hippocampus' involvement in CWM learning by lesioning the hippocampus and running rats through both mazes since the MWM is known to depend on the hippocampus and NMDA receptors but the involvement of the latter for the CWM is not known. There are NMDA receptors in the striatum too, but whether glutamate mediates egocentric navigation circuits between the striatum and hippocampus is poorly understood. These experiments would help elucidate the relationship between these forms of learning and memory. However, time and money limit what can be done. Graduate students and postdocs have the luxury to run experiments to test hypotheses based on curiosity and are less constrained by the specific aims done for a funded grant. Principal investigators need to fulfill the aims of the grant and explore other ideas, time and resources permitting.

2.4.3 Making Tools Better

The development of the maze was empirical, incremental, and based on focused hypotheses at each step. It was motivated by trying to make improvements in the utility of the apparatus to detect differences hypothesized to be caused by different interventions. In other words, this was a process of progressive calibration of the CWM. Method improvements came along because experimenters needed something more than the method provided at any given time; a tool that would do a better job than in the past. Most changes resulted in the CWM working better based on experimenter reasoning that was tested experimentally. When a new idea suggested an improvement and the improved procedure worked, the question became: Why does it work better? At this stage, the apparatus inspired theoretical questions.

For example, Williams came up with a way to test the role of distal cues (Vorhees and Williams 2014). The idea was to test one group of rats in the dark and switch them to the light and another group in the light and switch them to the dark. The results showed that when rats started in the light and were switched to the dark, they made large numbers of errors even though they knew the path to the goal. But if the rats started in the dark, then were switched to the light, they had no disruption in learning. Having learned the maze in the dark the rats knew the way without distal cues and adding these cues had little effect. The rats may have made a cognitive map or formed a rule of how to solve the maze. These are theoretical hypotheses. Rats learning under light learned faster and made fewer errors, but rats used distal and proximal cues to find their way. Once distal cues were eliminated, they did not have enough proximal cue information to find the goal and had to do extensive relearning that proved highly disruptive. This was informative. It showed that once rats developed an internal map, they were able to use it regardless of vision-based cues. But for rats that used vision, when it was eliminated, they had too few internal cues to fall back on because their default solution relied more on the use of distal rather than internal cues. When put in the dark, the rats were initially lost and made many errors. The hippocampal spatial maps the rats developed no longer worked and they were forced to switch to striatum-based learning. Hence, rats have two navigational systems and when encountering a new situation, rely on the system that is most efficient under the conditions they confront. Generally, this is spatial rather than egocentric navigation. This is an example of how the CWM started to generate theoretical insights. However, exploring theoretical hypotheses is still constrained by the dynamic interplay between tool building and experimental design.

Most tests in the Vorhees/Williams lab are improved incrementally as experimental work progresses. During a renovation, they were able to build a larger, eight-foot diameter, MWM. The reasoning was derived from what they had learned with the CWM: if the task is made more difficult, perhaps it will be more sensitive to treatment effects. If their hypothesis is correct, they would be able to detect treatment effects that were previously not detected in a smaller diameter MWM, and they did. Treatments that had not shown differences in six and seven-foot MWMs showed significant effects in the eight-foot version. This was another improvement that grew out of their experience in developing the CWM. Note that the hypothesis they tested was not derived from a theory. It was a hypothesis about how the experimental tool would interact with animal behavior. This shows how new theoretical hypotheses are inspired by the new possibilities afforded by improved tools.

The CWM is sensitive to perturbations of the striatum. And so, if a treatment, whether pharmacological, lesion, or genetic, affects the striatum, the CWM generally detects it. The procedures are still being refined. One idea Vorhees and Williams are exploring is reversal learning; a well-established phenomenon in learning theory. In classic T-mazes, it is well known that after initial learning to one reinforced arm, switching to the other (reversal) is easier or harder depending on the strength of the initial learning. Over-training tends to make reversal learning easier (the overlearning reversal effect). In the MWM, reversal learning is approximated by moving the hidden platform to the opposite quadrant once the first position is learned. What is reversal learning in the CWM? Williams and Vorhees reasoned it would be a mirror image of the maze. Would it be harder for rats to learn the mirror image after reaching asymptotic performance on the original version because they would have retroactive interference? Or would it be easier because of positive transfer of training and the prior learning would help them solve the mirror image faster as in the overlearning reversal effect? They built a mirror image maze and ran the experiments. As it turned out, the transfer was positive. The negative interference the rats experience is outweighed by the positive transference they get from knowing the general features of the maze. This is an example of how, at this stage of the tool development and utilization, theoretical questions inspire technological innovation.

The experimental goal of learning how a novel cognitive task could be solved went hand in hand with the goal of making the apparatus more sensitive. A lot of the refinements never make it into the scientific literature. At the most, they are referenced as 'we have shown previously that ..., say 5 min between trials was sufficient to not compromise trial-2 performance.' Changes are described the first time they are published, but after that, it is treated as standard. It disappears into the past. These incremental steps are found periodically in review articles, such as Vorhees and Williams (2006, 2014, 2015, 2016), but can be hard to detect in data-based articles.

3 Reflections on Research Practices in Neuroscience

The case of the invention and development of the CWM exemplifies general trends in neuroscience which generalize to most biomedical sciences. We have identified three fundamental drivers of scientific innovation: resources, collaborations, and theory-building.

3.1 Resources: Funding and Tool Availability

The CWM case exemplifies the significance of factors such as funding and experimental equipment. The development of tools such as the

CWM is a lengthy process. It took the Vorhees/Williams lab decades to calibrate their equipment to work in ways that improved utility. Because the test has been continuously refined, they are now in a position to look at the data in a new experiment testing a new variable to determine if the data do or do not fit predictions for a given test article. In such cases, they can hypothesize what will be found and if the data are not consistent with prediction, they can revise their hypothesis confident in the knowledge that the CWM provided accurate data. This is the know-how they acquired through the continuous use of the apparatus over time.

It is not irrational to choose to perform some experiments and not others because of available funding. For example, an insufficient number of experimental subjects (be they humans or nonhuman animals) because of insufficient funding, would jeopardize the statistical significance of the results articulated in a study. Avoiding mistakes is another reason for limiting the experimental design choices to a core set of tools that the experimenter knows well. This is not to say that one should never introduce new tools in the toolkit. It is, however, important to recognize when a certain tool-making endeavor needs to be abandoned. Sometimes a lab cannot get some equipment to generate useful data. In such cases, experimenters tend to "cut their losses," abandon a method that does not seem productive, and try another one given the limits on money, time, and personnel.

3.2 The Role of Collaboration

The specialization of labs using different tools and experimental techniques would leave unbridgeable gaps and lead to incommensurable theoretical commitments across the research communities trained in a certain lab if Kuhn were correct about the rigidity of the worldviews he ascribed to scientists. Contemporary neuroscience proves this ascription unjustified. Ankeny and Leonelli's scientific repertoires capture what happens much better. Some labs have solved problems others have encountered. A single lab cannot install all equipment needed in the field.

To calibrate their results, scientists often reach out to colleagues in other labs that have different tools in their toolboxes. This is why collaboration, rather than competition, is crucial. The venues for establishing collaborations are, not surprisingly, the professional conferences where neuroscientists "trade experience."

On the large scale of present-day grant-funded research, collaborations between multiple laboratories are crucial for innovation. Different labs have different equipment and expertise, some of which can be expensive and difficult for every lab to set up and maintain. The CWM is one such tool. It is mostly used by the Vorhees/Williams lab because of fabrication costs and space requirements. The MWM is widely used because all one needs is a room, a circular water tank, and a platform.

Moreover, many MWM tanks are drained and put in storage until needed again. For many labs, it is impractical to build a large, complex, permanently installed maze such as the CWM. However, having the CWM in their toolbox, the Vorhees/Williams lab can answer questions that labs without such a striatally based test cannot. There are no other tests that measure egocentric learning and memory as well as the CWM.

Conversely, when other questions need to be addressed and Vorhees and Williams do not have the equipment for it, they send their rats to other laboratories. The decisions regarding tool utilization are constrained by the availability of resources and the stage of the research. If the studies in the collaborating laboratories "were to find something new," Vorhees and Williams typically try to get the equipment set up in their lab so they can continue. Alternatively, they may collaborate on an ongoing basis with the other lab and apply jointly for grant support.

What hypotheses are explored depends on the available funding, equipment/expertise, and collaboration between laboratories. For example, the Vorhees/Williams lab developed a genetically modified rat using CRISPR/Cas9 genome editing to delete exon 3 of the latrophilin-3 gene associated with some cases of Attention Deficit Hyperactivity Disorder (ADHD) (Regan et al. 2019). The LPHN-3 knock-out rat is hyperactive, hyper-reactive to sudden stimuli, and has cognitive deficits, but they have no direct way of testing attention and impulsivity. Therefore, they sent these rats to Dr. Helen Sable at the University of Memphis who uses operant conditioning to test attributes Vorhees and Williams could not. Her data affirm that these rats are less attentive and more impulsive than wildtype littermates.

Ankeny and Leonelli's notion of research repertoires captures the collaborative practice of contemporary neuroscience. What the CWM case shows is how laboratories develop specialized skills and techniques that they contribute to larger-scale research in collaborative projects. The research practice of neuroscience is driven by the availability of funding, institutional infrastructure, and interactions between researchers.

3.3 Theory-Building: Theories as Interpretative Devices

Where did theory go? The influence of postpositivism is still strong in the contemporary philosophy of science. Some versions of the Kuhnian notion of paradigm lurk behind the concerns about the equivocal use of terminology and theoretical constructs by different research teams in neuroscience (Sullivan 2016), the claims about irreconcilable pluralism in the study of behavior (Longino 2013), and irreconcilable codependence of psychology and neuroscience (Hochstein 2016). However, when analyzed in detail, the practice of neuroscience displays the incremental change of experimental practices and theoretical narrations rather than "big paradigm shifts." Neuroscience is characterized by an interplay of tool development, experiment, and theory articulation. A single experiment often leaves many unanswered questions. If a given hypothesis seems to explain a certain effect, then there is the question of whether it should be tested further to establish that it is indicative of a general phenomenon. Unfortunate as it is, in neuroscientific practice, this question is often left unaddressed, many times due to pragmatic considerations of tool availability or funding. Therefore, opportunities to articulate comprehensive theories of the phenomena of interest are often unexplored. This shows that the end goal of experimental neuroscience is not always the articulation of theories.

Twentieth-century philosophy of science developed largely as a reflection of theoretical physics. It led to the view that the rest of the scientific disciplines would eventually achieve the maturity of physics, if not turn into physics themselves. This presupposed that the goal of science was to produce theories about the natural world. On this view, experiment plays only a supporting role to theory. Experiments are of interest only as long as they produce evidence for one theory over another. Tool development was not on the radar of philosophy of science until recently, particularly with the boom of biomedical technology which enabled experiments unthinkable 20 years ago.

In contemporary neuroscience, it is uncommon for researchers to be guided by abstract theory in experimental practice. If neuroscientists mention theories or when they announce that they are going to give a "theoretical talk," what they mean is something along the lines of: "We need to think more broadly. We need to figure out how to fit all these pieces of information together in a coherent hypothesis." Unlike theory-driven physics, neuroscience typically articulates theories after a significant number of diverse experimental data have accumulated and the data need to be synthesized and made sense of within a theoretical framework. In other words, the role of a theory is to interpret conglomerations of data resulting from the testing of multiple focused hypotheses. For example, the theory of cognitive maps in the hippocampus grew out of electrophysiological experiments with recording electrodes put into the awake rat hippocampus. It was combined with later experiments where the relationship with the hippocampus was found using hippocampal lesions to disrupt radial-arm maze learning. Then came Morris' invention of the MWM that made assessing spatial learning clearer. Many more electrophysiological experiments mapping "place cells" in the hippocampus were performed, followed by many experiments showing how hippocampal place cells map onto entorhinal grid cells and other experiments that found head direction cells. These and other experiments eventually culminated in a theory of the hippocampus-entorhinal cortex of memory formation, consolidation, and retrieval. This is the theory for which John O'Keefe, Edvard Moser, and May-Britt Moser won the 2014 Nobel Prize for the discovery of "cells that constitute a positioning system in the brain" which is the basis of memory. In this case, theory followed rather than preceded the experiment.

In a sense, neuroscience is still working within an area of black boxes. A lot is known about the brain and about how it functions. Neuroscientists often ask: " What is the mechanism underlying a particular observed change?" In reality it could be many different things. Neuroscience proceeds through experimental testing of focused hypotheses about the effects of specific interventions under specific conditions until a bigger picture of what happens is gradually assembled. This is when articulating a comprehensive theory of the studied phenomena comes into play.

This is how our case study unfolds. The CWM was originally used to study spatial memory and navigation similarly to the MWM. Allocentric and egocentric navigation were recognized as distinct behaviors but there was no assumption that they had distinct neural mechanisms. When Vorhees and Williams started to observe systematic differences in the performance of rats in the two mazes under identical interventions, they started to ask questions about the underlying causes of the differences. They published their results, but peer reviews asked the question about what CWM results meant. Vorhees and Williams sought an explanation. This meant asking theoretical questions about how to interpret data. Initially, they guessed they were studying path integration. However, a colleague pointed out that this could not be since path integration is manifested in taking shortcuts in navigating a familiar terrain and this was not possible in the CWM. Hence, they hypothesized that they were studying route-based egocentric navigation. This was what prompted the modifications of the maze that eventually led to using an infrared camera to test the rats in darkness. Once the maze was standardized, they were able to use it in the search for the underlying mechanism of egocentric navigation.

Vorhees and Williams did not have a preconceived model of that mechanism. There was not a theory to guide their efforts. To the extent that they were operating under the assumption that observable behaviors (e.g., navigation) attributed to a cognitive capacity (e.g., memory) have underlying neural patterns, there was a theoretical assumption. This assumption, however, characterizes neuroscience as a research endeavor. It is not a theory that the CWM could test. Vorhees and Williams articulated a theory to explain route-based egocentric navigation, which had not been thoroughly investigated at the time. Their experiments gradually identified the striatum as the predominant region involved in egocentric navigation in the CWM. The next step was to identify the neurotransmitters involved. Experiments showed that dopamine is one of them but there may be others. All along Vorhees and Williams have been testing focused hypotheses about the effects of specific interventions on specific brain areas during egocentric navigation. These steps are taking them closer to a comprehensive theory of the mechanism of egocentric navigation, but this is still a theory in the making. Such is the case with many research domains in neuroscience. This is why we contend that the philosophy of neuroscience is best served by studying experiment and tool development along with the theories they generate.

4 Conclusion

We presented a case study of the invention and calibration of a tool in experimental neuroscience, the Cincinnati water maze. Our results show that making choices regarding what experiments to pursue more often than not relies on pragmatic considerations of funding, equipment, and collaborations. Our analysis is consistent with the notion of scientific repertoire and challenges approaches to philosophy of science which focus on the study of scientific theories rather than scientific practice. The case we presented is exemplary of the tendency in contemporary neuroscience for theories to be articulated for the purposes of interpretation of disparate experimental data that need to be integrated into a cohesive framework. Theory in this case functions as an interpretative device.

References

Ankeny, R. A. and S. Leonelli (2016). "Repertoires: A post-Kuhnian perspective on scientific change and collaborative research". *Studies in History and Philosophy of Science, 60*: 18–28.

Atanasova, N. (2015). "Validating animal Models". *THEORIA: An International Journal for Theory, History and Foundations of Science, 30*(2): 163–181.

Bickle, J. (2006). "Reducing mind to molecular pathways: Explicating the reductionism implicit in current cellular and molecular neuroscience". *Synthese, 151*(3): 411–434.

Bickle, J. (2016). "From microscopes to optogenetics: Ian Hacking vindicated." *Philosophy of Science, 85*(5): 1065–1077.

Biel, W. (1940). "Early age differences in maze performance in the albino rat." *The Journal of Genetic Psychology, 56*: 439–453.

Boyd, R. (1980). "Scientific realism and naturalistic epistemology." *PSA: Proceedings of the Biennial Meeting of the Philosophy of Science Association, 2*: 613–662.

Braun, A. A., D. L. Graham, T. L. Schaefer, C. V. Vorhees and M. T. Williams (2012). "Dorsal striatal dopamine depletion impairs both allocentric and egocentric navigation in rats." *Neurobiology of Learning and Memory, 97*: 402–408.

Braun, A. A., R. M. Amos-Kroohs, A. Guetierez, K. H. Lundgren, K. B. Seroogy, M. R. Skelton, C. V. Vorhees and M. T. Williams (2015). "Dopamine depletion in either the dorsomedial or dorsolateral striatum impairs egocentric Cincinnati water maze performance while sparing allocentric Morris water maze learning." *Neurobiology of Learning and Memory, 0*: 55–63.

Butcher, R., C. Vorhees and H. Berry (1970). "A learning impairment associated with induced phenylketonuria." *Life Sciences*, 9, Part I: 1261–1268.

Chakravartty, A. (2007). *A metaphysics for scientific realism. Knowing the unobservable*. Cambridge: Cambridge University Press.

Dringenberg, H. C. (2020). The history of long-term potentiation as a memory mechanism: Controversies, confirmation, and some lessons to remember. *Hippocampus, 30*: 987–1012.

Feest, U. (2010). "Concepts as tools in the experimental generation of knowledge in cognitive neuropsychology." *Spontaneous Generations: A Journal for the History and Philosophy of Science, 4*(1): 173–190.

Feyerabend, P. (1988/1975). *Against method*. London and New York: Verso.

Gross, P. R. and N. Levitt (1994). *Higher superstition: The academic left and its quarrels with science*. Baltimore, MD: Johns Hopkins University Press.

Gross, P. R., N. Levitt, and M. W. Lewis (eds.) (1996). *The flight from science and reason*. New York: New York Academy of Sciences.

Hacking, I. (1983). *Representing and intervening: Introductory topics in the philosophy of natural science*. Cambridge and New York: Cambridge University Press.

Hanson, N. R. (1965). *Patterns of discovery*. Cambridge: Cambridge University Press.

Herring, N. R., T. L. Schaefer, G. A. Gudelsky, C. V. Vorhees and M. T. Williams (2008). "Effects of (+)-methamphetamine on path integration learning, novel object recognition, and neurotoxicity in rats." *Psychopharmacology, 199*(4): 637–650.

Hochstein, E. (2016). Giving up on convergence and autonomy: Why the theories of psychology and neuroscience are codependent as well as irreconcilable. *Studies in History and Philosophy of Science, 56*, 135–144.

Kuhn, T. (1970). *The structure of scientific revolutions*. Chicago, IL: University of Chicago Press. First published 1962.

Leonelli, S. and Ankeny, R. A. (2015). "Repertoires: How to transform a project into a research community". *Bioscience, 65*(7): 701–708.

Longino, H. E. (2013). *Studying human behavior: How scientists investigate aggression and sexuality*. Chicago, IL: University of Chicago Press.

Morford, L. L., S. L. Wood, G. A. Gudelsky, M. T. Williams and C. V. Vorhees (2002). "Impaired spatial and sequential learning in rats treated neonatally with d-fenfluramine." *European Journal of Neuroscience, 16* (3), 491–500.

Morris, R. G. M. (1981). "Spatial localization does not require the presence of local cues". *Learning and Motivation, 12*: 239–260.

Polidora, V. J., D. E. Boggs and H. A. Waisman (1963). "A behavioral deficit associated with phenylketonuria in rats." *Proceedings of the Society for Biology and Medicine, 113*: 817–820.

Putnam, H. (1976). "X* – What is 'realism'?" *Proceedings of the Aristotelian Society, 76*(1): 177–194.

Regan, S. L., J. R Hufgard, E. M. Pitzer, C. Sugimoto, Y. Hu, M. T. Williams and C. V. Vorhees (2019). "Knockout of latrophilin-3 in Sprague-Dawley rats causes hyperactivity, hyper-reactivity, under-response to amphetamine, and disrupted dopamine markers." *Neurobiology of Disease, 130*: 104494.

Robins, S. K. (2016). "Memory and optogenetic intervention: Separating the engram from the ecphory". *Philosophy of Science, 85*(5): 1078–1089.

Ross, A. (ed.) (1996). *Science wars*. Durham, NC: Duke University Press.

Silva, A. J. and J. Bickle (2009). The science of research and the search for molecular mechanisms of cognitive functions. In J. Bickle (Ed.), *The Oxford handbook of philosophy and neuroscience* (pp. 91–126). Oxford: Oxford University Press.

Silva, A., A. Landreth and J. Bickle (2014). *Engineering the next revolution in neuroscience*. New York: Oxford University Press.

Sullivan, J. A. (2009). "The multiplicity of experimental protocols: A challenge to reductionist and non-reductionist models of the unity of neuroscience." *Synthese, 167*: 511–539.

Sullivan, J. A. (2010). "Reconsidering 'spatial memory' and the Morris water maze." *Synthese, 177*: 261–283.

Sullivan, J. A. (2016). "Optogenetics, pluralism, and progress." *Philosophy of Science, 85*(5): 1090–1101.

Vorhees, C. V. (1987). "Maze learning in rats: A comparison of performance in two mazes in progeny prenatally exposed to different doses of phenytoin." *Neurotoxicology and Teratology, 9*: 235–241.

Vorhees, C. V. and M. T. Williams. (2006). "Morris water maze: Procedures for assessing spatial and related forms of learning and memory." *Nature Protocols, 1*(2): 848–858.

Vorhees, C. V. and M. T. Williams (2014). "Assessing spatial learning and memory in rodents." *ILAR Journal, 55*(2): 310–332.

Vorhees, C. V. and M. T. Williams (2015). "Reprint of 'Value of water mazes for assessing spatial and egocentric learning and memory in rodent basic research and regulatory studies.'" *Neurotoxicology and Teratology, 52*: 93–108.

Vorhees, C. V. and M. T. Williams (2016). "Cincinnati water maze: A review of the development, methods, and evidence as a test of egocentric learning and memory." *Neurotoxicology and Teratology, 57*: 1–19.

Whishaw, I. Q. and H. Maaswinkel (1998). "Rats with fimbria-fornix lesions are impaired in path integration: A role for the hippocampus in 'sense of direction'". *The Journal of Neuroscience, 18*(8): 3050–3058.

Williams, M. T., L. L. Morford, A. E. McCrea, S. L. Wood and C. V. Vorhees (2002). "Administration of D, L-fenfluramine to rats produces learning deficits in the Cincinnati water maze but not in the Morris water maze: relationship to adrenal cortical output." *Neurotoxicology and Teratology, 24*: 783–796.

Williams, M. T., L. L. Morford, S. L. Wood, S. L. Rock, A. E. McCrea, M. Fukumura, T. L. Wallace, H. W. Broening, M. S. Moran and C. V. Vorhees (2003). "Developmental 3,4-methylenedioxymethamphetamine (MDMA)-induced learning deficits are not related to undernutrition or litter effects: Novel use of litter size to control for MDMA-induced growth decrements." *Brain Research, 968*(1), 89–101.

4 Where Molecular Science Meets Perfumery

A Behind-the-Scenes Look at SCAPE Microscopy and Its Theoretical Impact on Current Olfaction

Ann-Sophie Barwich and Lu Xu

1 Introduction: A Cognitive Approach to Tool Use

Imagine studying an entire brain in action, live stream in all its complex interactive signaling, down to the single-cell level. You are able to image an entire nervous system or large intact tissue sections reacting to a stimulus. So, you may spritz an odor at a fruit fly or look at muscle contractions in larvae to see what cells react and when. This must sound like a dream to any neuroscientist studying structure function interactions in the central nervous system and beyond. This dream turned into reality with the invention of a new tool by the Hillman lab at Columbia: SCAPE (Swept, Confocally-Aligned Planar Excitation microscopy), a tool for three-dimensional, rapid live-stream imaging of small living, freely moving organisms (e.g., C. elegans, drosophila) and large intact brain tissues of bigger animals (as: in mice). Despite the relative recency of its invention, SCAPE has already provided groundbreaking insights into the workings of the mammalian and insect nervous and motor system (Bouchard et al. 2015; Vaadia et al. 2019; Xu et al. 2020), one of which will be the topic of this chapter.

Science in general, and neuroscience in particular, is driven by new tools and technologies. Philosophical analysis of science has engaged with various historical episodes, meticulously reconstructing the impact of technologies on the trajectory of a field and its models. Yet, a clear understanding of the epistemic role of tools in the research process still remains at large. Of course, the general significance of tools in experimental science is indisputable: research tools support observation and inference-making, enlarge data production and accelerate data analysis, and shape the communal standards with which materials and models are selected as paradigmatic cases to explain phenomena of interest. Meanwhile, another—and perhaps less obvious—function of tools in science is their explicitly *cognitive* dimension.

DOI: 10.4324/9781003251392-6

Previous cognitive theories of science, meaning cognitive approaches that target the mental mechanisms and environmental affordances making scientific reasoning possible, have been principally applied to scientific models and theories (Giere 1988; Churchland 1996; Thagard 2012), not the specific nature of tools. In recent years, Bickle (2016, 2019, 2020, this volume) has shown with historical examples that engineering and tinkering with tools has been a central *driver of theories* throughout the history of neuroscience. Such an account pointing toward the cognitive role of tools in neuroscience further invites a contemporary perspective to complement and expand upon our understanding of scientific tool use in action.

This chapter offers the rare opportunity of going behind the scenes at the frontiers of science to get a better look at the pragmatic and cognitive dimensions of tool use and development. Specifically, it provides a first-hand account of how SCAPE arguably revolutionizes current research on the brain by revealing how this tool was made to fit its experimental potential, and notably one with tremendous theoretical implications.

The authors are well positioned to undertake this challenge. Between 2015 and 2018, Barwich was the resident philosopher in the Firestein lab at Columbia University (Barwich 2020a), where Xu was the lead scientist in the process of adopting the new tool of SCAPE to tackle mixture coding in the nose (Xu et al. 2020). The results of these experiments would turn out to be remarkable: Xu et al.'s study, published in *Science*, uncovered a previously unknown molecular mechanism in the sensory periphery of olfaction.

In what follows, we present a combined narrative of tool development and its broader philosophical implications to better understand scientific reasoning at the laboratory bench. This chapter integrates philosophical analysis with contemporary scientific history to engage with the fundamental question of how scientists use new experimental tools to access yet unknown features of research materials. Specifically, we want to understand how tools can perform a cognitive function that opens new theoretical perspectives for scientists in their experimental investigations. What characterizes the cognitive function of scientific tool use in action? Specifically, how do tools structure scientific reasoning by providing the observational and conceptual scaffolds that create or stimulate the ability to conceive new perspectives on research objects or processes? How does tool use afford the conceptual reconfiguration of a research topic? In short, we want to understand how tools unlock conceptual possibilities that were previously difficult to imagine.

SCAPE is an excellent example to show how tool innovations can provide scientists with new *cognitive scaffolds* in the advancement of scientific theorizing. Traditionally, the cognitive structure of tools in research practice has been considered mostly in terms of their theory-ladenness, meaning their construction and application embody *existing theoretical assumptions* that shape what we see and learn to understand with their use (e.g., van Fraassen 1980, 2008; Barwich 2017). According to this view, tools primarily *assist and supplement* scientific thinking. Here, we want to highlight that research tools also embody a crucially *constitutive* part of that thinking process, so much so that tools occupy an essential causal role in the mental mechanisms of scientific reasoning. In other words, tools do not merely embody existing theoretical knowledge. Instead, tools are *active drivers* of new models and theories by accommodating and, moreover, *extending the cognitive process* of scientists.

We present our analysis in three steps. First, we introduce the scientific challenges and developments in recent research on odor coding, involving the receptors and the stimulus (Section 2). This will help to situate the significance of the SCAPE study for general readers and highlight the theoretical impact of its results. Then the SCAPE study takes center stage (Section 3). Here, we blend the scientific study and its published results with Xu's own experience on getting the experiments to work in the first place. In other words, we get a glimpse of how the sausage was made! These details present the backdrop against which we clarify the theoretical impact of the SCAPE study for theories of odor coding (Section 4). We conclude with a (*brief*) philosophical reflection on the cognitive dimensions of tool use (Section 5). Specifically, we draw on theories of distributed cognition in recent cognitive science to suggest that tools are a constitutive and active part of the reasoning process by which scientists generate new exploratory and explanatory concepts.

2 The Scientific Challenge: A Code in the Nose

Crucial to any new technology's success is identifying the right kind of problem, specifically a situation more difficult to probe with previous tools. SCAPE had found its perfect match in the mechanisms of odor coding at the sensory periphery.

2.1 At the Periphery: The Olfactory Receptors

Why olfaction? Odor coding at the receptor level has been notoriously difficult to investigate. Notably, the olfactory receptors were discovered only 30 years ago (Buck and Axel 1991). This discovery transformed the field of olfaction rapidly by catapulting it into mainstream neurobiology and genetics, almost overnight (Firestein 2005; Firestein, Mombaerts, and Greer 2014; Barwich 2020a, 2020b). The recognition of significance reached far beyond olfaction and led to the 2004 Nobel Prize in Physiology or Medicine for Buck (2005) and Axel (2005).

The reason for the great impact of the receptor discovery is twofold. On the one hand, the olfactory receptors provided the key causal elements connecting the distal stimulus of odorants (airborne odoriferous chemicals) with activity patterns in the brain. On the other hand, these receptors were identified as the largest and genetically most diverse members of the superfamily of G-protein coupled receptors (GPCRs). GPCRs are a fundamental entity in the inventory of biochemical research concerning a wide variety of biological processes, such as vision, the regulation of immune responses, the detection of neurotransmitters in the brain, and now also the encoding of chemical information as smells (Snogerup-Linse 2012; Barwich and Bschir 2017). Indeed, olfactory GPCRs proved a promising group of genes for future studies on general structure-function behavior in the GPCR superfamily (Barwich 2015a).

What makes the study of odor coding at the periphery so challenging? One central difficulty early on was the expression of odor receptors in tissues other than olfactory sensory neurons.[1] This hindered the ability of functional studies to test whether these receptors really constitute olfactory receptors, that is, that they responded to odorants instead of some other stimuli. Prior to the successful heterologous expression of odor receptors in other tissues (Dey et al., 2011; Mainland et al. 2015; Matsunami 2016), a study led by Haiqing Zhao in the Firestein lab (Zhao et al. 1998) established the functional role of this newly discovered GPCR family as unmistakably olfactory in nature. Briefly, this study introduced a selected olfactory receptor gene (the rat receptor OR-I7) via a viral vector into nasal epithelium tissue, resulting in a significant overexpression of that receptor in epithelium tissue, and thus allowing for the study of its foundational response and stimulus-response range.

However, this study could not yield insight into the principles of the molecular detection mechanism. The problem here is that GPCRs are generally quite difficult to stabilize. Besides, to this day there is no successful X-ray crystallography structure of the mammalian olfactory receptors—further exacerbating structure-function studies. (Although an X-ray crystallography structure has recently been obtained for an olfactory receptor of the genetically notably different insect receptors; see Butterwick et al. 2018).[2]

The breakthrough arrived with a functional study by Bettina Malnic in the Buck lab, which revealed that odorants are recognized combinatorially by the receptors (Malnic et al. 1999). "Combinatorial coding" means that one odorant is detected by different receptors, and one receptor can interact with different odorants. Notwithstanding, understanding of receptor-odorant interactions has experienced only limited progress since (Barwich 2020a). The reason for this stagnation resided in the ongoing experimental inaccessibility of odor receptors. But the situation started to change in recent years (detailed review in Kurian et al. 2021). Central to this change was the application of SCAPE to odor coding in the mammalian epithelium, specifically to the coding mechanism of mixtures (i.e., odor blends involving two or more odorants).

Mixture coding in olfaction had hitherto posed seemingly insurmountable experimental hurdles, so much so that the investigation of mixtures was considered impracticable and unfeasible. Frankly, it remains experimentally very tricky to examine the responses of individual receptors—or sensory neurons (with one neuron expressing one receptor gene; Mombaerts et al. 1996)[3]—even to single odorants. Indeed, most olfactory receptors have not yet been de-orphanized (meaning: their response range to odorants and repertoire remains unknown).[4] So how could you possibly measure and compare thousands and thousands of cells responding to multiple odors at once? You'd need a tool that can document the population behavior of these numerous cells while also allowing for detailed single-cell analysis.

This is what the invention of SCAPE microscopy afforded, and with surprising experimental results. Now, to explain why the results of the SCAPE study in olfaction were so surprising and remarkable, we first must do a quick detour to give some details about the nature of the stimulus and its perception.

2.2 In the Air: The Olfactory Table of Elements

If you tried counting odors, how many could you name? One peculiar feature of your sense of smell is that, once you start paying attention to it, the number of different scents seems almost endless. There are numerous flowers with different fragrances, an array of food odors, and every human or even every object has its own unique smell. We may not always be able to give names to these various olfactory impressions, but we can discriminate between them fairly well. At the same time, we clearly are able to group many of these odors into general qualities, such as being a green, a floral, a meaty, or a woody scent. How is that possible?

Imagine you want to invent a machine that can detect the slightest change of features or concentration in an ever-changing and chemically complex environment. This machine would need to be fast, adaptive, sensitive, and widely tuned. Your nose is precisely such an instrument.

Odors are numerous indeed, and their molecular basis is intriguingly complex. Odorants come from a variety of sources and are of immense structural diversity. Calculating the number of chemicals that can cause different odor impressions will not necessarily lead to a final estimate, though. An optimistic number was that *Humans Can Discriminate More than 1 Trillion Olfactory Stimuli* after a study of the same title by the team headed by Andreas Keller and Leslie Vosshall at Rockefeller University, published in *Science* in 2014 (Bushdid et al. 2014). While this staggering number has been disputed (Gerkin and Crasto 2015; Meister 2015), it remains unquestioned that the range of olfactory stimuli is mindbogglingly vast and covers at least several hundred thousand of different molecules.

(Besides, this further illustrates why the de-orphanization of olfactory receptors presents quite the laborious challenge.)

Compared to the (still growing) periodic table of elements in chemistry, the biological table of olfactory elements appears limited at first glance. Only molecules containing atoms of hydrogen, carbon, nitrogen, oxygen, and sulfur elicit odor sensations. Your nose does not seem to care much about other elements. Additionally, which of these molecules really are odorous depends on the receptors, not the chemistry of the stimulus in isolation because:

> it is nearly impossible to predict whether a given molecule will be odorous and what its odor quality might be from the chemical structure alone. Although all odor molecules are typically organic compounds of low molecular weight, they may be aliphatic or aromatic, may be saturated or unsaturated, and may have any of several polar functional groups. However, there are many molecules that conform to those characteristics, which are nonetheless odorless, to humans and other animals.
>
> (Poivet et al. 2018, 1)

Even within this seemingly restricted palette, the structural varieties and combinatorial possibilities are countless. While being constantly surrounded by hundreds of such odorants, your nose allows you to filter specific odor notes and detect differences resonating with minimal variances of elements in your surroundings. It does so with remarkable precision. A difference in one atom of two otherwise perfectly similar molecules can make your perception of their odor quality vary entirely. Consider nonanoic acid, a molecule smelling of cheese that has the chemical formula $CH_3(CH_2)_7COOH$. By adding only one methyl group, we end up with decanoic acid, $CH_3(CH_2)_8COOH$, which you will perceive distinctly different as rancid smelling. Similar cases where minor structural variations, even of just a single atom, result in drastic odor differences are abundant.

As early as 1895, olfactory scientists like the French scholar Frédéric Passy had noted that the sensitivity of the human nose is far greater than that for spectral analysis.[5] Or, in the more contemporary words of the neuroscientist Stuart Firestein: "Your nose is arguably the most accurate and sensitive chemosensor on the face of the planet!"[6]

The central scientific challenge in olfaction remains to explain just how the nose, in tandem with the brain, 'makes scents' of this multitude of volatile molecules. Scientists today still ask: is there any physical order to perceptual odor space? Is it even meaningful to assume a physical order? If it existed, how would such an order correspond to perceptual qualities?

Unlike the visual or auditory system, the physical stimulus of smell has not yet been reduced to a small number of measurable causal attributes.

This is not a result of the seemingly subjective nature of smells but is due to the molecular complexity of the olfactory stimulus. Consider the stimulus in vision or audition. As wavelengths, colors, or sounds come spatially ordered in a continuous linear scale. By contrast, the molecular basis of smells does not comply with such a linear arrangement. There is not one but multiple features that determine the quality of an odorant (Keller and Vosshall 2016). The concept of the chemical similarity between odorants encompasses a multitude of parameters, including, stereochemistry (a molecule's geometrical arrangement), molecular weight, functional groups, polarity, acidity/basicity, and many more (Ohloff, Pickenhagen, and Kraft 2012). This multidimensionality of physical features, encompassing approximately 5,000 molecular parameters, hinders a straightforward answer to our initial question of how perceptual odor space is connected to its physical stimulus space. To date, no general rule has been discovered that links a definite set of molecular features to a specific smell (Rossiter 1996; Sell 2006; Barwich 2015b, 2020a; Poivet et al. 2016, 2018).

Perhaps, the sensible way around this problem is not to focus primarily on the principles of organic chemistry but on the sensory system that translates these features into smells. To get to the link between molecules and odor, one might need to start with the system that extracts sensory information from the stimulus. It turns out the scientific answer to this challenge is far from obvious or even close to being settled.

3 Behind the Scenes: Notes of a Scientist

Investigations into the mechanism of mixture perception were considered to pose a challenge of experimental complexity primarily. However, the SCAPE study revealed that the challenge of understanding mixture coding at the sensory periphery is one of showing previously unconceived causal principles.

3.1 Introducing SCAPE to the Mix

Xu et al. (2020) found a molecular explanation for a peculiar and widespread phenomenon about mixture perception in olfaction. Perfumers have long known that odors do not behave additively in mixtures. A comparison with the visual system helps to clarify this issue. Color vision acts additively, which means that we can calculate colors by adding and subtracting ranges of electromagnetic wavelengths, translating into colors in the visible spectrum of light. Take the color pink. Pink has no associated wavelength but constitutes a brain's computational feature, namely: "pink is white light minus green." In contrast, olfactory mixtures as perceptual wholes are not the sum of their (chemical) parts. Additively in olfaction would imply we should be able to calculate what the sum of components will smell like by putting together its individual compounds. However, that is not the case.

Smell mixtures behave irregularly, often unpredictably. Perfumers working on a formula routinely note that, at times, they may put a tiny amount of a compound into a complex chemical blend, which then instantly alters the quality of that entire mix (e.g., Laudamiel in Barwich 2020a). Conversely, the opposite case is also known to occur. Perfumers can add significant amounts of a compound into a blend without resulting in any observable change in the overall scent quality of the mix. This phenomenon has also been well documented in several psychophysical studies (e.g., Cain 1974; Laing et al. 1984; Kay et al. 2005), referred to as *enhancement* and *suppression* effects. Odor notes appear enhanced or suppressed when blended into a mixture.

Such irregularity in complex mixture perception was assumed to constitute either an effect of blending different chemicals into a mixture or result from a higher-level mechanism in the neural computation of odor images. Meanwhile, there may be a third, hitherto unconceived alternative suggesting an unknown mechanism at the receptor level in the sensory periphery (instead of "higher-level" downstream computation). This mechanism came to the fore with the experiments in Xu et al. (2020).

This is where the technological affordances of SCAPE microscopy come into play.

SCAPE microscopy is a novel imaging technique developed by the Hillman lab. SCAPE is a form of light-sheet microscopy which uses a single, stationary objective lens at the sample. It can capture a sizeable 3D field of view (>1.2 mm × 1.2 mm × 400 μm) with cellular resolution at over 10 volumes per second (Figure 1). SCAPE forms a 3D image by illuminating the sample with an oblique light sheet, capturing fluorescence light excited by this sheet back through the same high numerical aperture (NA) objective. A single-axis galvanometer in the system both sweeps the light sheet from side to side at the sample and de-scans the returning light to form a stationary oblique intermediate image plane. This plane is then rotated using a set of two additional objective lenses (O2 and O3) and focused onto a fast sCMOS camera. Compared with other point-scanning based volumetric imaging methods, such as confocal or spinning disk confocal microscopy, the light-sheet based SCAPE approach dramatically increases the volumetric imaging speed and FOV [field of view] with lower photobleaching and phototoxicity while keeping similar spatial resolution in biological samples. (Further details in Bouchard et al. 2015; Hillmann et al. 2019; Voleti et al. 2019.)

In its current installment (SCAPE is being constantly improved), SCAPE microscopy allows studying the behavior of intact cells in timescales less than 0.1 s with a resolution high enough to analyze single-cell activation of the full brain or large-scale neuronal circuits with different animal models. This procedure creates several terabytes of data.

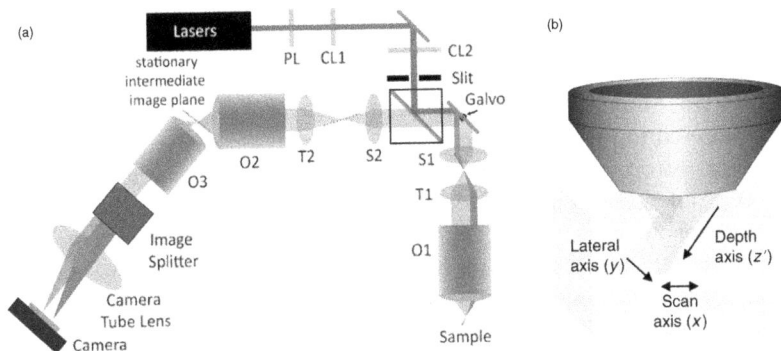

Figure 1 The SCAPE Microscopy System. (a) Schematic of the SCAPE layout. (b) Close-up of the O1 objective. An oblique light sheet images through the O1 stationary objective lens and scans the sample laterally in the x-direction to form a 3D image (Adapted from Voleti et al. 2019).

The application of SCAPE microscopy to the study of mixtures in olfaction sounded intuitive from the start, Firestein remarked (quoted in Barwich 2020a, 192): "The obvious thing to do with this would be blends or mixtures to see the code." SCAPE allowed us to observe two things simultaneously in intact tissue and in real-time: the reaction of individual cells to stimuli on the one hand and the behavior of entire cell populations on the other. In other words, Xu was able to expose a whole and intact section of epithelium tissue to one or more odors to observe which and how many different cells were activated in response to a specific stimulus.

So far reads the official story. Meanwhile, the idea to use SCAPE microscopy to explore the molecular nature of mixture coding in olfaction had some pragmatic, and also some romantic, origins. Hillman and Firestein were colleagues in the Biology Department at Columbia University. (Hillman's lab was originally on the fourth floor of the Shapiro building before moving to the new Zimmermann Institute (ZI); the Firestein lab remains on the tenth floor of the Fairchild building on the main Manhattan Campus to this day.) Meanwhile, there also existed another connection: Xu, back then doing her graduate research on smell receptors in the Firestein lab, is married to Wenze Li, a graduate student of Hillman and working on the further development of SCAPE:

It was 2015 when I first learned about SCAPE microscopy (the year that the Hillman lab published their first SCAPE paper). Wenze and I were walking our dog Muffin when he decided to show off his recent progress in the lab: a video showing a 3D Zebrafish heart beating. The contour of the heart was clearly outlined by the heart cells (which were labeled with some sort of fluorescence); as the heart contracts and relaxes, I could also see individual blood cells travel through the ventricle and atriums. Wenze told me that this was imaged with a 3D imaging technique called SCAPE.

At the moment, I was frustrated by the difficulty that I have encountered in my own research: the olfactory sensory neuron dissociation protocol (which I have been using for the past three years with no problem) no longer works, and this was the main method of my study at the moment. Briefly, what the protocol does is to first strip off the olfactory epithelium from the nasal turbinates of the mouse, digest with enzymes, then collect olfactory sensory neurons from the supernatant and place them on a piece of coverslip pre-coated with concavcalin A – this coverslip will later be used for calcium imaging. Normally I would get several hundred of neurons on each coverslip. But during that time, I was only getting ~50 cells per coverslip – a pathetic cell density, and I couldn't figure out why because my colleagues (Erwan Poivet and Narmin Tahirova) were using the same protocol and same reagents and they were getting a normal number of cells.

This was the original momentum of me seeking an alternative solution of imaging the olfactory sensory neurons. The cell dissociation protocol was not perfect anyway: first, during the dissociation process, the axons are severed from the olfactory bulb and the cilia are also damaged by the enzymes. Second, the efficacy is low. Even with a good cell density, we could only get ~200–400 neurons per field of view, among which only 5%–10% would respond to a particular monomolecular odor stimulus. The population will be further narrowed down if we want to study a receptor/neuron responding to multiple odors. Finally, the dissociation process is extremely time-consuming. If we start at 9:30 am, the cells would be ready for imaging at ~4 pm, during which we only have a 40min break for lunch, and there is no way to know if the dissociation is successful until the last step. Also, the cells can only be imaged the same day – if you leave them in a cell incubator, many of them will still be alive the following day but no longer functional.

As a lazy person,[7] I always wanted to take a shortcut. The easiest thing to come up with is to simply peel off the thin layer of the olfactory epithelium and image it directly. It seems to be straightforward, but in practice, it's difficult to mount the epithelium on a coverslip securely. And even though the epithelium is only ~100 um thick, its surface is curved, making it difficult to visualize many individual neurons in a single focal plane (imagine the difference of a flat piece of paper and a piece of crumpled paper).

The invention of SCAPE has brought new hope to this (almost) dead end. It's capability of imaging non-transparent tissue in 3D was exactly what I needed. How to harness this novel technique is yet another story.

(ps. Several months later, I finally figured out why the dissociation protocol was not working: we made a new batch of concavcalin A from a different manufacturer, and somehow it takes longer to dry out on the coverslip completely. If it's not dry, it will be washed off by the culture media along with all the neurons attached to it. I used to prepare the coverslip in the morning of the experiment day, which was fine for the old stock but not enough time for the new stock. Meanwhile, Erwan and Narmin had prepared the coverslip one night before, and that's why they never had the problem!)

These were the roots of the SCAPE study. But back to its experimental details: Xu used genetically engineered mice to track active cells with a fluorescent glow. In consultation with the master perfumer Christophe Laudamiel, she decided on two mixtures, each mixture consisting of three different compounds: (a) acetophenone, benzyl acetate, and citral, and (b) dorisyl, dartanol, and isoraldeine. The central criterion for choosing these components was that they were chemically and perceptually dissimilar. Additionally, the hypothesis was that the combination of these odorants would yield a configural odor image—configural meaning that the mixtures produced a quality different from their elemental components. Furthermore, odor set 1 was tested in equal concentration; odor set 2 in unequal concentration.

3.2 Challenges: Choosing the Chemical Stimulus and Testing Cell Responses

Scientific papers tend to present their findings without hiccups. Behind the scenes, the story reads differently. Indeed, Xu dealt with several challenges already at the stage of choosing the chemical stimulus, specifically the stimulus sets:

3.2.1 Choice of Odor Set 1

Stuart [Firestein] originally wanted me to test if "one odor can inhibit another odor," which sounds extremely counter-intuitive. I expected this kind of event to be extremely rare if it happens at all. Therefore, I want to use "potent" odors that activate a broad repertoire of neurons for me to analyze. It's easy to think of acetophenone and citral, as they are odors frequently used in olfactory studies and are known to activate a lot of cells. Fortunately, they also fit the criteria of being chemically and perceptually dissimilar. This is important because I was not looking for special cases of antagonism that would normally happen between a chemical and its derivative, but rather interactions that happen at a more general level.

To increase the complexity of odor interaction, I decided to introduce a third component, but not a fourth, because it increases the possible combinations from 7 (A, B, C, AB, AC, BC, ABC) to 15, which will be too complicated to test. It is yet difficult to find a third odor that is as potent as acetophenone and citral. Isoamyl acetate is a close one, and we finally replaced it with benzyl acetate, which has similar odor quality but is more frequently used in perfumery, according to Christophe [Laudamiel].

3.2.2 Choice of Odor Set 2

While I aimed to test chemically and perceptually unrelated odors with odor set 1, odor set 2 was selected to test the interaction between chemically unrelated but perceptually related odors. This reflects some cases in naturally occurring odors where perceptually similar odors produce harmonic odor perception, such as rose oxide and beta-damascone in rose. In fact, odor set 2 (named the "woody accord") is designed by perfumers to produce such harmonic smell at a particular concentration ratio. Interestingly, we have observed more inhibition in odor set 2 than odor set 1, indicating an underlying logic of doing subtraction (eliminating unwanted notes) rather than addition (adding extra notes) in perfumery.

With the stimulus selection in place, and over the course of several trying years, Xu repeatedly tested how the cells responded to each compound when administered individually, in pairs, and then in the tripartite mix (Figure 2):

The biggest challenge to me was to confirm that the modulation effects that I saw were real, not artifacts. It's relatively easy to answer qualitative questions ("Is this neuron activated by this odorant") as all you have to answer is yes or no. However, when it comes to quantitative questions ("how much a response is enhanced/inhibited"), the difficulty of answering increases exponentially (I'll explain why in the following paragraphs). I was constantly stuck in the "doubt – verification – confidence – doubt" cycle during the entire process of this project, and each round of self-questioning resulted in the optimization of some details.

A key technical challenge in Xu's experiments concerned sample mounting:

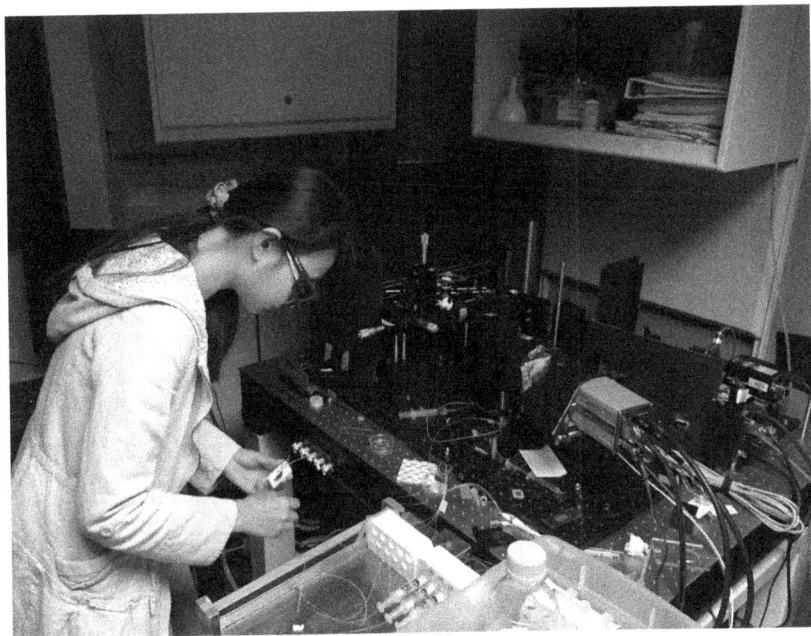

Figure 2 Lu Xu working with the SCAPE 1.0 system during the pilot experiments.

Rather than creating the SCAPE protocol from scratch, what I did was to use the old cell dissociation protocol as a starting point and gradually shaped it to the way I wanted (which ended up being quite different). In our very first experiment, I prepared the OE [olfactory epithelium] sample by cutting off the whole olfactory turbinates using a pair of fine scissors – this was actually an intermediate step during cell dissociation. The next steps were to peel off epithelium from the turbinates and cut it into pieces – I then placed it into a perfusion chamber with the epithelium side facing up. Perfusion is a standard thing to do in physiology in order to maintain the homeostasis of the extracellular environment, and I simply adopted the recipe of Ringer's solution we used to perfuse the dissociated neurons. Next, I tried to deliver odor stimulus by injecting odor solutions using an automatic syringe injector, which didn't work out because the sudden change of flow rate would cause the sample to float around. Given our field of view was only ~600 um × 400 um × 300 um at the moment, a displacement less than 1mm would make the sample disappear from the screen. Therefore, in the following experiments, we had to transport the Agilent isocratic pump from our lab to the Hillman lab using a small cart and used that for stable perfusion and odor delivery. This lasted until the Hillman lab moved to the ZI, and we purchased a new pump.

Nevertheless, the sample is still not stable enough in the chamber. At first, I thought of using a smaller chamber such as the sample is more confined in place, but then I realized it's actually easier if I don't cut the turbinates at all and leave them attached to the mouse head. This way all I have to do is to cut the mouse head sagitally and remove the septum to expose the OE. What's even better about this prep is that if I cover the mouse hemi-head with a coverslip, a narrow space will be naturally formed between the coverslip and the turbinates, which allows a very small volume of liquid to flow in through the nostril and out through the throat thanks to capillary action. Essentially, this is a re-construction of the nasal cavity by replacing the septum with a transparent coverslip, which allows us to observe the OE from the medial side. To implement this idea, we have designed our own perfusion chamber which resembles the shape of a mouse head. In the final prep, the mouse hemi-head is placed facing down to the coverslip on the bottom of the chamber, with an inverted objective acquiring the image from underneath (as shown in figure 1 of our published paper, and figure 3 in this chapter). During subsequent experiments, we further optimized sample mounting by applying a blue light-cured dental gel to fix the sample to the chamber. As a result, the displacement of the sample is now less than 10um at all three dimensions during a one-hour imaging session.

Naturally, challenges did not end here, and Xu further focused on the measures of response stability and the design of odor stimulation sequence:

Several key factors can significantly affect the interpretation of results: rundown, variation, and photobleaching. Rundown means when stimulated repetitively, the response magnitude of a cell will gradually decrease. Variation means the response to the same stimulus can fluctuate within a certain range. Photobleaching means the fluorescent signal gets dimmer under constant excitation light. Due to these factors, it is difficult to directly compare the response magnitude of two stimuli even if they are given subsequently. However, thanks to the pioneer work of Zita [Peterlin] et al. in our lab,[8] we already knew that the rundown of odor response is approximately linear, and the natural variation of odor response is about 10% (Peterlin et al. 2008). This result has been confirmed with SCAPE in our control experiment. In a simplified case [details of findings in sections 3.4 and 3.5], to measure the effect of a potential modulator B on odor A, the odor stimuli will be given as A – A + B – A, and compare A + B with mean (A); if A + B is larger than A, the

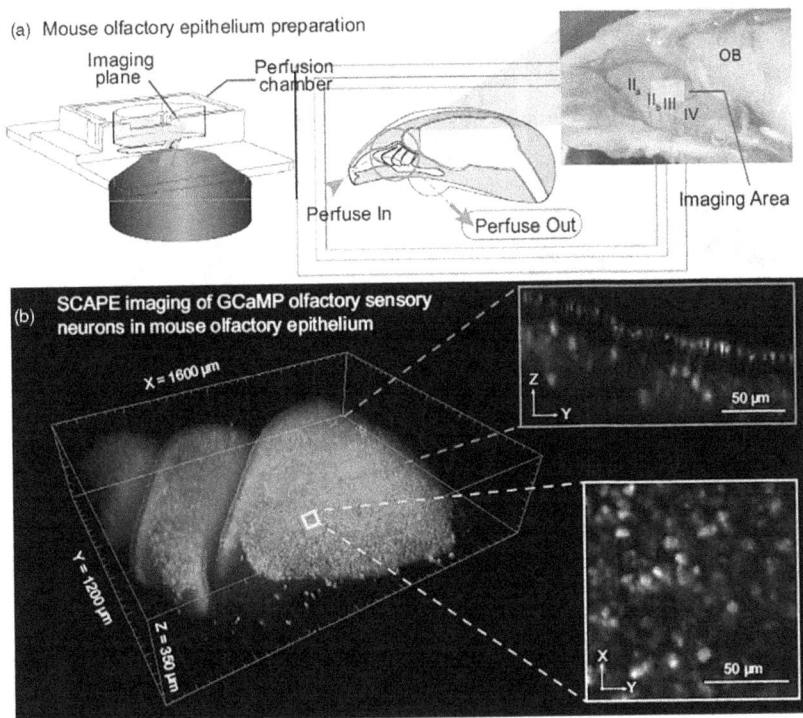

Figure 3 SCAPE microscopy of intact mouse olfactory epithelium capturing odor-evoked GCaMP activity with single OSN resolution. (a) The exposed olfactory turbinates were mounted in a 3D-printed perfusion chamber and imaged using SCAPE microscopy in an inverted configuration. Perfusion solutions flow through the inlet at the nostril and the outlet at the throat (bold arrows), the field of view covers the turbinate IIb and III, and some of the neighboring turbinate. (b) 3D volumetric rendering of SCAPE data acquired on the intact olfactory epithelium showing baseline GCaMP6f signals in a field of view of 1,170 × 1,000 × 235 (y-x-z, μm). Enlarged side and top views of the acquired volume are shown in the rectangle and square boxes accompanied with dotted lines respectively, demonstrating data acquisition with single-neuron resolution. GCaMP signals were extracted from 10,000's cells to evaluate their individual responses to odor mixes revealing both enhancement and suppression of odor responses by other odors at the sensory level (Xu et al. 2020).

response to B alone will be subtracted to avoid false interpretation of enhancement. In addition, we have set an inhibition/enhancement threshold over 30% to account for the variation of odor responses. These efforts may cause under-estimation of enhancement and inhibition but are critical to ensure the overall interpretation of results (Figure 4).

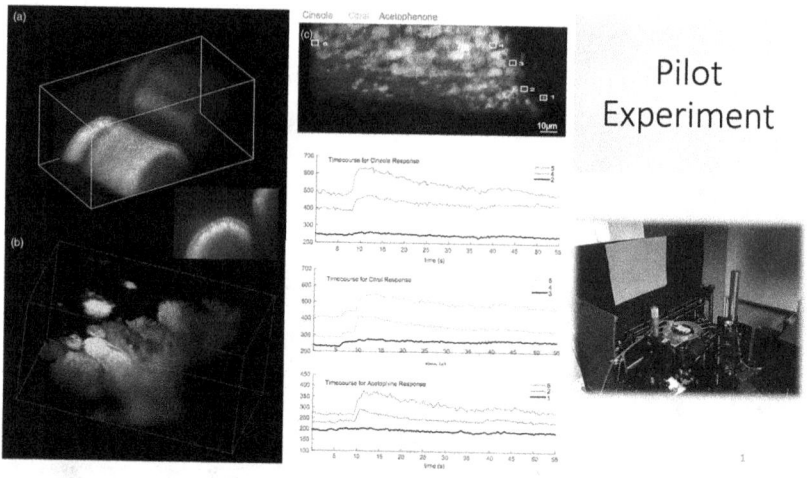

Figure 4 Evolution of the SCAPE technique. A comparison is made between data (3D images of mouse olfactory epithelium) acquired in 2015 and 2019, respectively. Note the improvement in both fields of view and resolution of the image.

Each challenge was tackled by iterative adjustments, thus resulting in an iterative improvement of the experimental procedure supporting data validity, as well as the *conceptual refinement* of the experimental design substantiating the possible scope of data interpretation.

Fine adjustments have also been made to minimize rundown by maintaining the tissue in a healthier state, including carboxgenation of the Ringer solution, adjustment of the Ringer recipe, improvement of dissection procedure, and optimization of the time interval between odor stimuli.

The control of photobleaching as well as further optimization of image quality was achieved mostly by Wenze and his colleagues. During the constant evolution of the SCAPE setup, the photobleaching effect has been decreased to a minimal level while the resolution and field of view has been greatly improved.

Obtaining stable measures and solid experimental results were not yet the end point. A final challenge involved data analysis, to which we come next.

3.3 Data Analysis

Another notable aspect in the making of the SCAPE study is its attention to data analysis of cell behavior. Xu analyzed a vast sweep of ~10,000 olfactory receptor cells via genetic tools that target calcium-dependent activity (GCaMP6f mice). That's humongous data to analyze and a plethora of individual cells for which one must identify and interpret their activity range and strength. Xu had to modify and work on the algorithm to accomplish this task. Data analysis took place in several steps:

3.3.1 Preprocessing

The raw SCAPE data are spool files and need a specific script to load into the workspace of Matlab. Since the specimen was scanned with an oblique light-sheet, each 3D volume needs to be de-skewed to the original scale. This part has been taken care of primarily by Wenze and his lab-mates.

3.3.2 Image Registration

After optimization of sample mounting, the drift of the sample during the experiment was minimal and easily corrected with various imaging processing packages. However, the tissue also underwent deformation at the scale of μm, which needed to be registered non-rigidly. Since the diameter of each neuron is only 5–10 um, the goal was to limit displacement at the submicron scale. Due to the lack of apparent "landmarks" at this scale, registration with commonly used methods (such as Matlab build-in functions or FIJI packages) did not yield satisfactory results.

To address this issue, I adopted the Non-Rigid Motion Correction (NoRMCorre) algorithm developed by Pnevmatikakis et al. (2017) and custom-modified it to perform deformable registration specifically for our own dataset. Since tissue drift and motion artifact within each 75 s trial was negligible, I took a single 3D volume (averaged from ten volumes during the resting state) from each trial and registered them to the template, which was also an averaged 3D volume from the reference trial. The displacement field was then applied to all the volumes in each trial. This modification has significantly reduced the calculation amount from the original frame-by-frame update scheme. One drawback of this algorithm is that it sometimes results in "outlier" output; to address this problem, I created a graphical use interface (GUI) to manually correct the registration when necessary.

The overall registration results generated by the custom NoRM-Corre scripts were satisfactory. However, manually validating image sub-patches was labor-intensive. To overcome this bottleneck, I switched to the Advanced Normalization Tools (ANTs) (Avants, Tustison, and Song 2009), an Insight Toolkit (ITK)-based open-source toolkit for image registration as well as segmentation, template-building, and many other functionalities. ANTs utilize a strategy termed Symmetric image Normalization (SyN) for deformable image registration. After fine-tuning, the performance of SyN was comparable with that of NormCorre, sometimes slightly better at resolving localized deformation. Although the SyN-based registration was still time-consuming (30–60 min per image pair), it did not require supervision and, therefore, can be automatically processed in batch through a custom bash script, which significantly accelerated the registration process.

3.3.3 Denoising and Demixing of Calcium Signals

OSNs [olfactory sensory neurons] are densely packed in the intact olfactory epithelium. Therefore, it is critical to eliminate the noise from neighboring cells when analyzing a given OSN. This was achieved through the application of Constrained Nonnegative Matrix Factorization (CNMF), a framework that implements denoising, deconvolution, and demixing of calcium imaging data simultaneously (Pnevmatikakis et al. 2016). CNMF is capable of processing both 2D and 3D data, yet the 3D version is computationally much more expensive. For this reason, Xu split the 3D image series into multiple non-overlapping 2D stacks and processed them with 2D CNMF. Now, the CNMF algorithm has undergone a series of updates since the publication of our paper, as well as many other computational tools, and it's possible to analyze our data with 3D CNMF in the future.

3.3.4 Data Sorting

The CNMF algorithm (as well as other demixing algorithms) inevitably picks up numerous non-neuronal components and spontaneously activated neurons during analysis. For about 10,000 extracted time courses in each experiment, only ~3,000 are from odor-responsive neurons suitable for further processing, the rest being motion-induced baseline fluctuation, spontaneous activity, or unhealthy neurons that stopped responding during the experiment.

Conventionally, time courses from dissociated neurons were screened manually. It's easier in practice than it sounds to screen several hundreds of neurons, as odor response curves share a clear temporal pattern that can be easily captured by trained eyes. However, when the number increases to 10,000, it becomes a different story. To accelerate the data sorting process, I designed a 2D convolutional neural network to perform the initial screening of the CNMF-extracted time-courses and spatial loci. Essentially, I trained a network to learn the way I would pick out the "good" (acceptable) or 'bad' (rejected) neurons with ~90% of accuracy. The screening results were then manually validated with a custom-designed GUI to ensure data fidelity.

To recap, the specific requirements in the application of SCAPE required several types of adjustment, including tissue preparation (e.g., sample mounting) and data analysis (e.g., material deformation). These adjustments likewise influenced the empirical grounding and validity of the resulting model interpretation (i.e., greater ecological validity due to perfusion chamber). Processing vast amounts of data, it soon became undeniable that the experimental results were striking indeed.

4 The Findings

The patterns of cell populations showed remarkable and widespread differences in their responses to the mixtures and their components in isolation. Specifically, up to 38% of cells responding to a mix differed compared to scans of the collection of cells responding to the individual odorants in such mixture. More importantly, Xu found two different and striking effects across receptor cell populations.

4.1 Effect One: Inhibitory Modulation

The first effect may have mirrored some expectations of olfactory researchers concerning the nature of mixture coding. Yet it presented a vital observation by confirming inhibition effects in odor coding at the sensory periphery. Exposure to mixtures showed reduced activity across epithelium cells (Figure 5, left), meaning that, overall, the number of cells responding to the tripartite mixture was not equal to the sum of the cells responding to its individual components. At first, this effect seemed less surprising because of the combinatorial nature of odor coding. Some odorants in a mixture may simply overlap in their activation of receptor cells. Still, this explanation was hypothetical. Also, what was not expected was the sheer amount of inhibition.

Was this observed effect just a sign of combinatorial overlap, or is there more to the story? Here, the ability to observe and compare the activity of individual cells with SCAPE cast a new light on what was really going on. Notably, some cells were responding to individual compounds and also to binary mixtures. However, these cells remained inactive when exposed to the tripartite blend. A closer look at cell responses to the tripartite and binary mix indicated that Isoraldeine (asterisk; Figure 5, left) served as the primary inhibitor instead of Dartanol (triangle; Figure 5, left). Moreover, Xu saw that some individual cells in the tripartite mix remained silent but showed responses to at least one of the two binary combinations of odorants. Consequently, such modulation constituted not an outcome of combinatorial coding but inhibition.

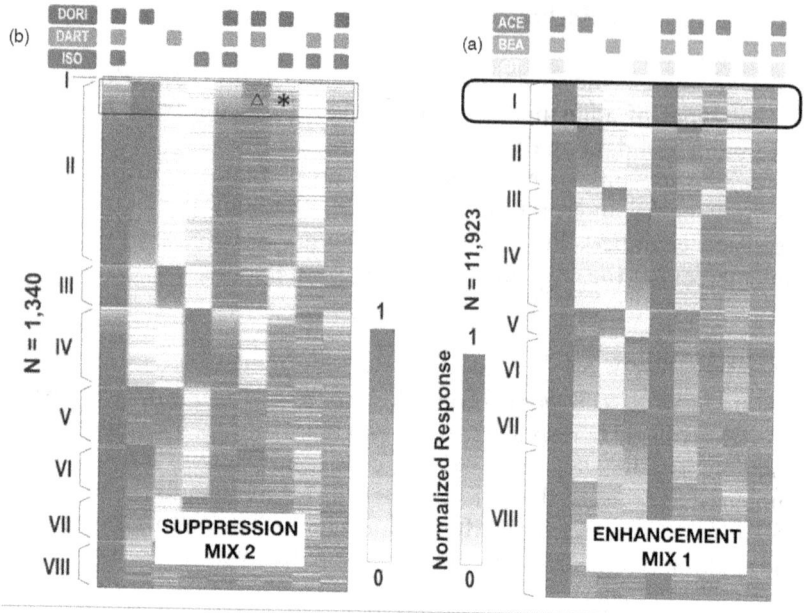

Figure 5 Averaged heat maps of olfactory sensory neurons responding to two sets of odor stimuli (in monomolecular solutions, binary and tripartite combinations). Cells show significant suppression (left) and enhancement (right) effects (Image modified from Xu et al. 2019).

These observations of inhibitory modulation at the periphery match with behavioral effects mentioned in several psychophysical studies (e.g., Cain 1974; Laing et al. 1984; Kay et al. 2005). Now there was clear evidence that these psychological effects were not necessarily produced by "higher-level" mechanisms in the central nervous system but already caused by interactions at the periphery. One key consequence of this insight is that the expression of perceptual quality and variation in response to an olfactory stimulus need not be an effect of cognitive bias (e.g., familiarity with a stimulus or cross-modal cues), but can also point to genetic divergence (e.g., in receptor expression).[9]

Even more remarkable was the realization that the functional role of an odorant, meaning whether it served as an agonist and an inverse agonist, depended on the mixture, instead of being a feature of the odorant in isolation. In other words, an odorant could play multiple interactive roles in varying ligand-binding contexts. Briefly, an odorant might act as (i) an agonist to one olfactory receptor (i.e., an odorant binds to a receptor to affect its basal activity), (ii) an inverse agonist to another receptor (i.e., odorant binds to a receptor to decrease its basal activity), and (iii) an antagonist (i.e., an odorant binds to a receptor to block other odorants from affecting its basal activity). Such functional promiscuity of odorants in mixture coding was quickly confirmed by other studies (Inagaki et al. 2020; Pfister et al. 2020).

4.2 Effect Two: Enhancement

The second effect Xu noted during the SCAPE experiment would pose a greater surprise. It would constitute a riddle for months to come. There also were enhancement effects (Figure 5, right). Some cells showed activity when exposed to the mixture but did not respond to any individual components! These cells only reacted to these compounds when combined and not in isolation! What did this effect mean? Firestein himself noted that these results seemed baffling: "I can't quite make sense of that part yet."

The breakthrough occurred a couple of days before Barwich had to submit her book manuscript on the science of olfaction to her publisher. The book featured a chapter on the SCAPE study (Barwich 2020a, Chapter 6). Firestein's first message in his email to Barwich was foreshadowing (August 16, 2019): "I think we now know that enhancement is real and that it makes sense. I will send you a copy of the manuscript we are about to submit – Lu is putting some finishing touches on it today." He continued in a follow-up email the day after (August 17, 2019):

So, attached is a confidential draft of the inhibitor/enhancement manuscript. We will submit by the middle of next week and then put it up on bioarxiv. You should pay attention to the introduction and the Discussion. Especially you might be interested in figure 7 (the last figure) [Figure 6 in this Chapter] which is a model of how this may work in olfactory perception. It's largely Lu's idea and I think it's very simple and very clever. It is explained pretty well in the discussion and in the figure legend but if you have any questions, I'll do my best to answer them.

Enhancement effects suggest a molecular mechanism at the receptor level that had never been observed at the sensory periphery, but that was known from pharmaceutical studies: allosteric modulation. The presence of an allosteric mechanism implies that a receptor has a potential binding site in addition to the activity-inducing binding pocket for ligands. A ligand binding to the allosteric site does not lead to receptor activation but results in a change of receptor conformation. In its new conformation, that receptor is now receptive to components with which it previously did not interact (Figure 7). By way of example, imagine a receptor {R1} does not interact with a specific odorant {O1} when O1 is administered individually; R1 remains silent. But when O1 is presented as part of a complex mixture with other odorants what happens is that another odorant {O2} changes the configuration of R1. Here, O2 attaches

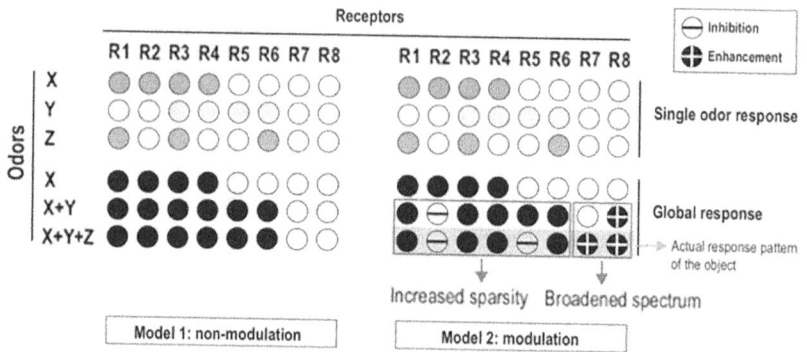

Figure 6 Receptor modulation model in olfaction. Xu's model of sparse coding in mixture detection at the sensory periphery in olfaction. Comparison between the received combinatorial model (left) and the new model of receptor modulation (right) (Image 7 in Xu et al. 2019).

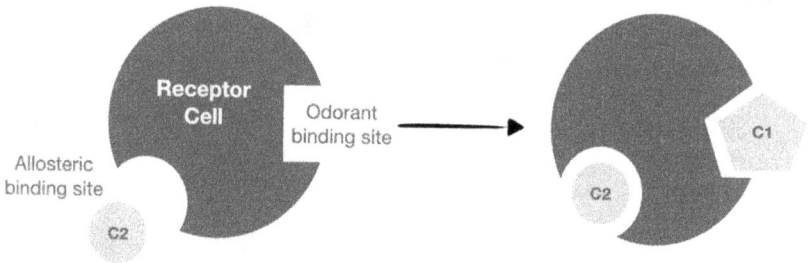

Figure 7 (Quite) simplified model illustrating the principle of allosteric interaction in receptor binding.

to the hypothesized allosteric site of R1 and modulates its activity, such that R1 receptor now interacts with O1.

What was the reasoning process behind the new receptor mechanism model? The challenge was to link cellular data with coding capacity:

> The idea of figure 7 [Figure 6 in this chapter] came up during a discussion between Stuart and me in his office. We were going through the manuscript. Everything seems to be there except for one piece missing – what's the significance of the modulation effect in the periphery? With so many flavors of mechanism (partial agonism, competitive antagonism, synergic enhancement, and probably also allosteric enhancement), it seems to make the odor-receptor interaction more complicated and less predictable. "It's ok if the modulation effect doesn't have any significance," said Stuart, "maybe it's

a flaw of the system." Inspired by this comment, I started thinking about what advantage this mechanism can possibly have. Reflecting on the way we calculated the modulation effect, I realized the existence of inhibition and enhancement is capable of flipping the valence of odor response – something that would never happen in a combinatorial coding scheme, where the only type of operation is addition.

When I got back home, I told Wenze about this idea and asked him what he thought about it. For half a minute, he didn't say anything. "This is so obvious," he finally replied, "but people would barely think of it in this way. Yet once you say it out loud everyone would think it's already in their mind." We then shared this idea with Elizabeth and all four of us gathered together to discuss it. During this process, this idea has been refined and finally evolved to the final model presented in our paper.

(It is a pity that we were not able to give strict mathematical proof of how much it can improve the coding capacity and the associated boundary conditions, such as the possibility and frequency of modulation effects.).[10]

In effect, these observations of various modulation effects explain how mixtures can adopt odor qualities different from their components' sensory qualities. Expertise in perfumery meets research in molecular biology. By having entirely new cells reacting to a complex mixture, they introduce distinct patterns of signals for the brain to compute into odor images. The whole is indeed more than the sum of its (chemical) parts.

4.3 There's no eSCAPE from Paradigm Shift

Meanwhile, these SCAPE findings offer more than an explanation of the emergence of some puzzling psychological effects in olfaction by way of presenting a molecular mechanism. They point toward a revolution in our understanding of the nature of odor coding and the conceptual thinking required for its scientific study.[11]

Xu et al.'s (2020) study highlights that the scientific puzzle of odor coding cannot be solved by an analytic chemical approach, comparing chemical features of odorants in isolation and separated from their binding interactions with the receptors at the sensory periphery. This analytic chemistry approach had defined large parts of olfaction research throughout the 20th century prior to the receptor discovery (Barwich 2015b). It still represents a popular, increasingly outdated understanding of stimulus-response modeling in olfaction today (Barwich 2020a). Xu's results now presented another damning piece of evidence to the analytic chemical approach. It suggested, in contrast, that olfaction must be approached as a biological system, not a chemical formula, with the complex forms of regulation that come with that shift in orientation.

Rather than chemistry, the data straightforwardly pointed to a biological explanation. Modulation effects did not originate from a chemical reaction since these organic chemicals are chemically inert under the above experimental conditions.

Indeed, these modulation effects revolutionize our understanding of odor coding. They reveal that combinatorial coding is not the only or even the principal mechanism by which mixture coding in olfaction operates. Think about it. The combinatorial coding of odor mixtures would result in an indistinguishable smear of activation across epithelium cells. Firestein remarked (in Barwich, 2020a):

> Making conservative estimates that any given odor molecule can activate 3–5 receptors at a medium level of concentration, then a blend of just 10 odors could occupy as many as 50 receptors, more than 10% of the family of human receptors. This will result in fewer differences between two blends of 10 similar compounds.

Meanwhile, many smells consist of hundreds of aromatic compounds (Maarse 1991). So how could the brain possibly know and distinguish what chemicals hit the nose?

> The SCAPE study presents a possible answer to the inherent neuro-computational challenge arising from combinatorial coding at the periphery: How does the brain discriminate different complex mixtures from widespread and overlapping receptor activity? Antagonistic modulation at the receptor level would facilitate sparse coding resulting in less ambiguous signal patterns. Aromatic blends, such as coffee or roses, are composed of hundreds of different components. The combinatorial code allows humans to detect various odorant features in such mixtures and respond to a complex and, in its constituents, unpredictable chemical environment. However, with combinatorial activation alone, receptor activation patterns quickly overlapped to form a broad and smudged signal, which would lose its distinctiveness. Modulation, antagonistic and allosteric, facilitates a unique receptor code for the discrimination of complex mixtures.
>
> (Kurian et al. 2021, 5)

This is why the significance of Xu et al. (2020) goes beyond mere technological finesse using a new tool to advance understanding of an old problem. The SCAPE study did not just provide some new details and more depth of observation. It facilitated the development of an entirely new theoretical approach to the study of odor coding, one that supplanted the analytical approach and assured a more biologically realistic conceptual orientation to the study of the olfactory system.

Xu's model, summarized in Figure B (and highlighted in Firestein's earlier email remarks) introduced a new model explaining how olfactory signals at the periphery are sufficiently differentiated for the brain to make sense of complex blends by showing either (i) a reduction of activity via inhibitory modulation that results in a sparser and thus differentiated signal, or (ii) an enhancement of cell activity that allows the brain to further distinguish complex mixture signals.

Crucially, the use of SCAPE in Xu et al. (2020) changed the chief target of explanation in theories of olfaction: explanations of odor coding are less about the chemistry of the stimulus and more about what signals actually reach the brain via the receptors.[12]

5 Discussion: Cognitive Scaffolding in Tool Use and Development

The value of SCAPE microscopy and its successful application in olfaction goes beyond mere technological affordances that probe unknown receptor behavior by allowing a scientist to "see more" or "look deeper" into layers and layers of cell tissue. It is the distinctly *cognitive* function that SCAPE played in the research process.

We want to suggest that to understand how tools facilitate new ideas in neuroscientific experiments, tools and technologies are best analyzed as a constitutive and active part of the reasoning process of scientists. This suggestion links to a range of modern theories in cognitive science associated with the label of "distributed cognition" (e.g., McClelland et al. 1986; Hutchins 1995). Theories of distributed cognition originated during the 1980s and have garnered increasing attention in the philosophical and scientific study of cognitive processes, especially over the past couple of decades (Clark and Chalmers 1998; Clark 2008). Thus, it is worthwhile implementing these theories further in philosophical accounts of scientific practice (as also proposed, for example, in the works Giere 2002; Giere and Moffatt 2003; Solomon 2007; Lui, Nersessian, and Stasko 2008).

Distributed cognition understands the cognitive capacities of scientists—and, naturally, other cognitive agents—as embedded and spread out in a broader system. It's a systems theoretical approach that is framing cognition primarily as a process, not in terms of its product. According to this view, technologies (like tools or instruments), scientific representations (such as formulas), social structures (such as institutes and funding organizations), as well as other scientists (such as collaborators and competitors) all are part of the cognitive process. Critical to distributed cognition is the thought that these various elements are more than causal factors *adding further information to the content* of an individual scientist's knowledge of a research situation. Instead, these elements are *causally integral to the cognitive process* in which the individual scientist partakes as an epistemic agent. In other words, these elements do not passively figure in an already well-defined and independent mental process (e.g., by enhancing, accelerating, or biasing the autonomous reasoning of the scientist). Instead, these elements often enable and actively structure the cognitive mechanisms in question in the first place.

A popular example to illustrate the workings of distributed cognition is mathematics (McClelland et al. 1986, 44–8). Unless you are a genius savant, complex calculations are often too complicated for most people to process in their heads alone. Say, what is the product of 456 × 789? Aiding the process of enacting such a calculation is an externalization of the various steps involved, traditionally on paper. This externalization structures the information so that, if one has learned the appropriate steps, the resulting symbol manipulations can be correctly and swiftly processed in the proper order. Other examples can be found in the history of science, for instance, with the manipulation of chemical formulas as externalized symbol structures to investigate the elemental dynamics in chemical reactions. The historian Klein (2003, 2–3) notably described Berzelian formulas as "paper tools," remarking:

> (...) that chemists began applying chemical formulas not primarily to represent and to illustrate preexisting knowledge, but rather as productive tools on paper or 'paper tools' for creating order in the jungle of organic chemistry. Berzelian chemical formulas... were tools for experimentally investigating organic chemical reactions and for constructing models of reactions and of the invisible constitution of organic substances.

In the case of SCAPE, we likewise encounter a cognitively significant structuring of steps in the reasoning process through the way in which this tool, in parallel with the presentation of new empirical data, serves as visualization and externalization of conceptual possibilities. What do we mean by that?

Xu's theorizing behind the novel sparse coding mechanism at the olfactory periphery was not merely a consequence of the instrument's theory-ladenness. The construction of SCAPE as a tool surely builds on previous technological advances and modeling assumptions, including genetically modified mice and fluorescent markers. These built-in modeling assumptions in tools, of course, shape the way in which data is produced and what can be seen (e.g., analysis of this issue with the example of protein synthesis in Rheinberger 1997). However, they cannot explain how the newly produced data is viewed and interpreted by the scientist. Recall Xu's description of trying to explain the modulation effects observed at the olfactory periphery. The model she came up with was far from obvious or a direct derivation from the tool's set-up. In other words, focus on the existing theoretical assumptions that are embodied and occasionally black-boxed by new technology remains insufficient to understand how new theoretical models are developed via the use of new gadgets and tools in scientific experimentation.

By way of example, some of the cognitively significant features structuring scientific reasoning we can observe in the application of SCAPE, without claims of exhaustiveness, are as follows:

1   Similar to the above example of mathematical calculation: the application of SCAPE allowed for an organization and division of otherwise incomprehensively complex data and data-points into several steps and combinations—e.g., cells responding to monomolecular, binary, and tertiary mixtures—that provided the basis for inference-making about the receptor activity patterns revealed.

2   Similar to the example of Berzelian formulas: the application of SCAPE facilitated the external visualization of proportions to compare elemental cell dynamics and interactive relationships. Moreover, these visualizations facilitated the possibility to abstract from the present data set (meaning, the specific stimuli used) to cell behavior toward mixtures in general.

3   Additionally, the application of SCAPE coordinated the use of various other techniques in tandem with this new microscopic technique (e.g., the development of algorithms, the selection of tissues and stimuli), as well as the coordination of collaborative activities between researchers in two laboratories. A similar point is found in Hutchins' (1995) analysis of coordination on a naval vessel as distributed cognition. Concretely, coordination adopts a cognitive task in how experimental information is translated into propositional structures to be communicated. This propositionalizing then scaffolds how the experimental data is integrated into the existing literature on the topic and how follow-up strategies concerning experimental adjustments and revision are designed.

4   Further, the iterative tinkering,[13] involving repeated adjustments and modifications in the application of SCAPE, facilitated new opportunities not only for data recording but also for theorizing about the data (and its scope). For example, initial challenges in sample mounting (Section 3.2) resulted in an experimental set-up that was a much closer match to the conditions involved in natural odor detection than previous tissue preparation.

Now, how did this re-organization, visual externalization, and coordination of data about the behavior of olfactory receptor populations promote fresh theorizing about odor coding?

Key to situating the theoretical impact of the SCAPE study in olfaction is the ontological shift that has taken place in this study:

> The SCAPE study is a demonstration [of] how new tools allow for a targeted reconsideration of causal elements as defined by the limits of previous technologies. Older technologies may have posited different elements as central and as partaking in different levels of causal mechanisms – e.g., the behavior of individual cells versus cell populations. The response of cells in the context of other cells as a population can now be modeled on one causal plane and integrated into a causal mechanistic explanation with fewer levels of hypothetical mechanisms.
>
> (Barwich 2020c, including a full analysis of the ontological shift from single cells to cell populations in odor coding. Also, see Figure 8)

Such ontological shift concerning the nature of causation at the olfactory periphery does not simply arrive with new data. It stems from new thinking. We can compare Xu's development of a sparse coding mechanism at the olfactory periphery to the case of chemists fiddling with chemical formulas or mathematicians playing with symbols combinations on paper.

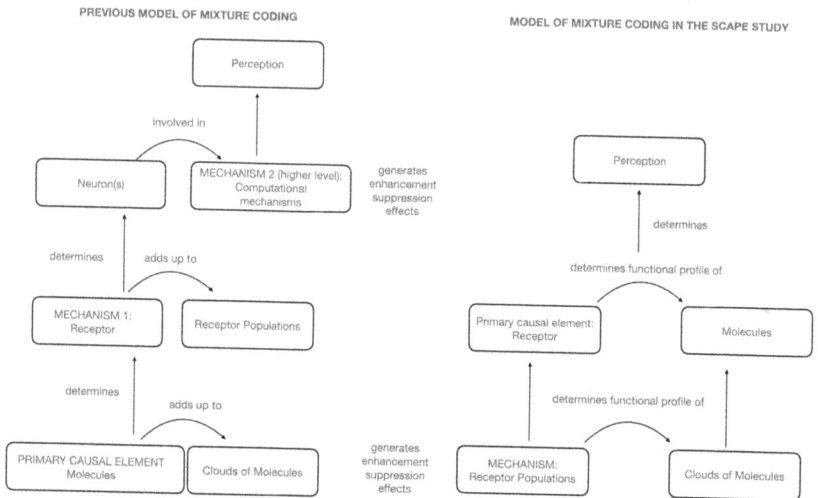

Figure 8 Comparison of the ontologies in between the different models of coding at the periphery. SCAPE changed the ontological structure of odor coding ad its fundamental components. Components (including their relevant features) are not defined in isolation but as causal units via their causal role within a mechanism. This means that the fundamental level in odor coding is not the {code = single odorant binding combinatorically to receptors} but {code = receptor populations responding to multiple odorants in combination}.

Tools in experimental practice in such contexts, therefore, present an extension of the thought process that allows for the creation of new patterns, new pattern conceptualizations and combinations, and, in further consequence, new inferences about the theoretical nature of this data.

The visual display of more comprehensive cell reactions to various combinations of chemical stimuli carried a powerfully suggestive power of *introducing new significances*, i.e., new causal relations and even new causal constituents (i.e., population behavior as representing the overall olfactory code, instead of single-cell calculations from individual stimuli). This display *restructured the intellectual framework* by introducing new concepts, relations, and avenues of further research (i.e., the shift from stimulus chemistry to receptor biology as a key determinant of odor coding). Moreover, SCAPE produced *new questions*: what kind of mechanism could cause enhancement effects, and to what potential purpose from a system's theoretical point of view?

The skeptic of distributed cognition may ask whether such a conceptual shift in thinking about odor coding *could* have also happened without SCAPE. Perhaps someone *could* have considered this mechanism, in principle. The point is, however, that it *did not* happen that way. To understand the realities of scientific reasoning, we need to look at what happens at the bench, instead of what is hypothetically conceivable in the armchair. Besides, a distributed account of cognition does not posit that those ideas are inconceivable without the appropriate technology. It asserts that technologies facilitate a broader and different perspective by being an integral part of the thinking process itself. In other words, technologies do more than produce data to align with hypotheses—their use co-creates mental structures in scientific reasoning. As the example of SCAPE illustrated, these mental structures include iterative procedures of conceptual refinement, the direction of attention to specific empirical observations (which may not always be transparent in their interpretation), and the combination of otherwise separately occurring phenomena on one observational place. (In a way, this can be compared with the use of language, where syntax and semantics afford meaningful but language-dependent creations, so much so that some works of poetry and especially humor are difficult to translate into another language without sufficiently similar syntactic structure.)

In conclusion, our brief discussion of the cognitive function of tools in neuroscientific experiments primarily serves as an invitation for philosophers and researchers to further consider the ways in which tools structure and actively contribute to scientific theorizing. For the analytically inclined philosopher, this discussion must remain wanting in conceptual detail and argumentative explication. Yet, given the constraints of this chapter—with its primary purpose (of providing a first-hand account of a new tool and in its theoretical impact)—the concluding remarks are best understood as a pointer toward the promise that targeted cognitive studies of tools in experimental practice yields for the study of scientific reasoning.

Acknowledgments

We are grateful to our colleagues in the Firestein and Hillman labs, especially Stuart Firestein and Wenze Li. Additional thanks belong to Carl Craver, John Bickle, and Marco Nathan for their constructive suggestions in the revision of this manuscript.

Notes

1 Review of the issues concerning the heterologous expression of olfactory receptors in Peterlin, Firestein, and Rogers (2014).
2 Notably, it took almost ten years to find the insect receptors after the mammalian receptors had been discovered because they are substantially different genetically (Clyne et al. 1999; Vosshall et al. 1999).
3 The "one neuron—one receptor gene" doctrine has been called into question recently (Mombaerts 2004).
4 This laborious type of work is currently under way, though, for example in the lab of Hiroaki Matsunami at Duke University.
5 See Passy (1895).
6 Personal communication.
7 The authors disagree on that verdict.
8 Peterlin was a postdoctoral researcher in Firestein's lab before she moved to work at Firmenich, Princeton.
9 Detailed analysis of the theoretical implications emerging from recent insights into receptor coding in olfaction in Barwich (2020a).
10 Analysis of the mechanisms of odor coding at the periphery, including the SCAPE study, and how it links to pattern recognition further downstream in the central nervous system in Barwich (2020a).
11 Revolution not necessarily in the Kuhnian sense.
12 Further elaboration and details about the implications of this study in the broader context of olfaction, and why smell needs to be modeled via the biological processes encoding chemical features (rather than stimulus chemistry), in Barwich (2020a, 2020b).
13 The notion of "tinkering" is adopted from Bickle's (this volume) analysis of historical examples that look at tool engineering as drivers of theorizing in neuroscience.

References

Avants, Brian B., Tustison, Nick and Song, Gang. 2009. "Advanced normalization tools (ANTS)." *Insight Journal* 2(365):1–35.
Axel, Richard. 2005. "Scents and sensibility: A molecular logic of olfactory perception (Nobel Lecture)." *Angewandte Chemie International Edition* 44:6110–27.
Barwich, Ann-Sophie. 2015a. "What is so special about smell? Olfaction as a model system in neurobiology." *Postgraduate Medical Journal* 92(1083):27–33.

Barwich, Ann-Sophie. 2015b. "Bending molecules or bending the rules? The application of theoretical models in fragrance chemistry." *Perspectives on Science* 23(4):443–65.

Barwich, Ann-Sophie. 2017. "Is Captain Kirk a natural blonde? Do X-ray crystallographers dream of electron clouds? Comparing model-based inferences in science with fiction." In: *Thinking about Science, Reflecting on Art*, ed. by Otávio Bueno, George Darby, Steven French, Dean Rickle. London: Routledge, pp. 62–79.

Barwich, Ann-Sophie. 2018. "How to be rational about empirical success in ongoing science: The case of the quantum nose and its critics." *Studies in History and Philosophy of Science* 69:40–51.

Barwich, Ann-Sophie. 2020a. *Smellosophy: What the Nose Tells the Brain*. Cambridge, MA: Harvard University Press.

Barwich, Ann-Sophie. 2020b. "What Makes a Discovery Successful? The Story of Linda Buck and the Olfactory Receptors." *Cell* 181(4):749–53.

Barwich, Ann-Sophie. 2020c. "Imaging the living brain: An argument for ruthless reductionism from olfactory neurobiology." *Journal of Theoretical Biology* 512:110560.

Barwich, Ann-Sophie and Bschir, Karum. 2017. "The manipulability of what? The history of G-protein coupled receptors." *Biology & Philosophy* 32(6):1317–39.

Bickle, John. 2016. "Revolutions in neuroscience: Tool development." *Frontiers in Systems* Neuroscience 10:24.

Bickle, John. 2019. "Linking mind to molecular pathways: The role of experiment tools." *Axiomathes* 29(6):577–97.

Bickle, John. 2020. "Laser lights and designer drugs: New techniques for descending levels of mechanisms 'in a single bound'?." *Topics in Cognitive Science* 12(4):1241–56.

Bickle, John. Forthcoming. " Research Tools in Relation to Theories." In: *The Tools of Neuroscience Experiment: Philosophical and Scientific Perspectives*, ed. by John Bickle, Carl Craver, Ann-Sophie Barwich. London: Routledge.

Bouchard, Matthew B., Voleti, Venkatakaushik, Mendes, César S., Lacefield, Clay, Grueber, Wesley B., Mann, Richard S., Bruno, Randy M. and Hillman, Elizabeth M. C. 2015. "Swept confocally-aligned planar excitation (SCAPE) microscopy for high-speed volumetric imaging of behaving organisms." *Nature Photonics* 9(2):113–9.

Buck, Linda B. 2005. "Unraveling the sense of smell (Nobel lecture)." *Angewandte Chemie International Edition* 44:6128–40.

Buck, Lind B. and Axel, Richard. 1991. "A novel multigene family may encode odorant receptors: A molecular basis for odor recognition." *Cell* 65(1):175–87.

Bushdid, Caroline, Magnasco, Marcelo O., Vosshall, Leslie B. and Keller, Andreas. 2014. "Humans can discriminate more than 1 trillion olfactory stimuli." *Science* 343(6177):1370–72.

Butterwick, Joel A., Del Mármol, Josefina, Kim, Kelly H., Kahlson, Martha A., Rogow, Jackson A., Walz, Thomas and Ruta, Vanessa. 2018. "Cryo-EM structure of the insect olfactory receptor Orco." *Nature* 560(7719):447–52.

Cain, William S. 1974. "Odor intensity—Mixtures and masking." *Bulletin of the Psychonomic Society* 4:244.

Churchland, Paul M. 1996. *The Engine of Reason, the Seat of the Soul: A Philosophical Journey into the Brain.* Cambridge: MIT Press.

Clark, Andy 2008. *Supersizing the Mind: Embodiment, Action, and Cognitive Extension.* New York: Oxford University Press.

Clark, Andy and Chalmers, David. 1998. "The extended mind." *Analysis* 58(1):7–19.

Clyne Peter J., Warr, Coral G., Freeman, Marc R., Lessing, Derek, Kim, Junhyong and Carlson, John R. 1999. "A novel family of divergent seven-transmembrane proteins: Candidate odorant receptors in Drosophila." *Neuron* 22(2):327–38.

Dey, Sandeepa, Zhan, Senmiao and Matsunami, Hiroaki. 2011, "Assaying surface expression of chemosensory receptors in heterologous cells." *Journal of Visualized Experiments* 48:e2405.

Firestein, Stuart. 2005. "A nobel nose: The 2004 Nobel Prize in physiology and medicine." *Neuron* 45:333–8.

Firestein, Stuart, Greer, Charles and Mombaerts, Peter. 2014. The molecular basis for odor recognition. *Cell Annotated Classic* (accessed 09/29/2021). https://els-jbs-prod-cdn.jbs.elsevierhealth.com/pb/assets/raw/journals/research/cell/libraries/annotated-classics/ACBuck.pdf

Gerkin, Richard C. and Castro, Jason B., 2015. "The number of olfactory stimuli that humans can discriminate is still unknown." *eLife* 4:e08127.

Giere, Ronald. 1988. *Explaining Science: A Cognitive Approach.* Chicago, IL: Chicago University Press.

Giere, Ronald. 2002. "Scientific cognition as distributed cognition." In: The Cognitive Basis of Science, ed. by Peter Carruthers, Stephen Stich, Michael Siegal. Cambridge: Cambridge University Press, p. 285.

Giere, Ronald N. and Moffatt, Barton. 2003. "Distributed cognition: Where the cognitive and the social merge." *Social Studies of Science* 33(2):301–10.

Hillman, Elizabeth M. C., Voleti, Venkatakaushik, Li, Wenze and Yu, Hang. 2019. "Light-sheet microscopy in neuroscience." *Annual Review of Neuroscience* 42:295–313.

Hutchins, Edwin. 1995. *Cognition in the Wild.* Cambridge: MIT Press.

Inagaki, Shigenori, Iwata, Ryo, Iwamoto, Masakazu and Imai, Takeshi 2020. "Widespread inhibition, antagonism, and synergy in mouse olfactory sensory neurons in vivo." *Cell Reports* 31(13):107814.

Kay, Leslie M., Crk, Tanja and Thorngate, Jennifer. 2005. "A redefinition of odor mixture quality. *Behavioral Neuroscience* 119:726–33.

Keller, Andreas and Vosshall, Leslie B. 2016. "Olfactory perception of chemically diverse molecules." *BMC Neuroscience* 17(1):55.

Klein, Ursula. 2003. *Experiments, Models, Paper Tools: Cultures of Organic Chemistry in the Nineteenth Century.* Stanford, CA: Stanford University Press.

Kurian, Smija M., Naressi, Rafaella G., Manoel, Diogo, Barwich, Ann-Sophie, Malnic, Bettina and Saraiva, Luis R. 2021. "Odor coding in the mammalian olfactory epithelium." *Cell and Tissue Research* 338: 445–456.

Laing, David G., Panhuber, H., Willcox, M.E. and Pittman, E.A., 1984. "Quality and intensity of binary odor mixtures." *Physiology & Behavior* 33(2):309–319.

Liu, Zhicheng, Nersessian, Nancy and Stasko, John. 2008. "Distributed cognition as a theoretical framework for information visualization." *IEEE Transactions on Visualization and Computer Graphics* 14(6):1173–80.

Maarse, H., 1991. Volatile compounds in foods and beverages (Vol. 44). New York: CRC Press.

Mainland, Joel D., Li, Yun R., Zhou, Ting, Liu, Wen LingL and Matsunami, Hiroaki. 2015. "Human olfactory receptor responses to odorants." *Scientific Data* 2:150002.

Malnic, Bettina, Hirono, Junzo, Sato, Takaaki and Buck, Linda B. 1999. "Combinatorial receptor codes for odors." *Cell* 96(5):713–23.

Matsunami, Hiroaki. 2016. "Mammalian odorant receptors: Heterologous expression and deorphanization" *Chemical Senses* 41(9):E123.

McClelland, James L., Rumelhart, David E. and PDP Research Group. 1986. *Parallel Distributed Processing*. Vol. 2. Cambridge: MIT Press.

Meister, Markus. 2015. "On the dimensionality of odor space." *eLife* 4:e07865.

Mombaerts, Peter. 2004. "Odorant Receptor Gene Choice in Olfactory Sensory Neurons: The One Receptor–One Neuron Hypothesis Revis- ited," *Current Opinion in Neurobiology* 14(1):31–36.

Mombaerts, Peter, Wang, Fan, Dulac, Catherine, Chao, Steve K., Nemes, Adriana, Mendelsohn, Monica, Edmondson, James and Axel, Richard. 1996. "Visualizing an olfactory sensory map." *Cell* 87(4):675–86.

Ohloff, Günther, Pickenhagen, Wilhelm and Kraft, Philip. 2012. *Scent and Chemistry: The Molecular World of Odors*. Zürich: Wiley-VCH.

Passy, Frédéric. 1895. *L'Année Psychologique*, second year, p. 380.

Peterlin, Zita, Li, Yadi, Sun, Guangxing, Shah, Rohan, Firestein, Stuart and Ryan, Kevin. 2008. "The importance of odorant conformation to the binding and activation of a representative olfactory receptor." *Chemistry & Biology* 15(12):1317–27.

Peterlin, Zita, Firestein, Stuart and Rogers, Matthew. 2014. "The state of the art of odorant receptor deorphanization: A report from the orphanage." *Journal of General Physiology* 143(5):527–42.

Pfister, Patrick, Smith, Benjamin C., Evans, Barry J., Brann, Jessica H., Trimmer, Casey, Sheikh, Mushhood, Arroyave, Randy, Reddy, Gautam, Jeong, Hyo-Young, Raps, Daniel A., Peterlin, Zita, Vergassola, Massimo and Rogers, Matthew E. 2020. "Odorant receptor inhibition is fundamental to odor encoding." *Current Biology* 30:2574–87.

Pnevmatikakis, Eftychios A., Soudry, Daniel, Gao, Yuanjun, Machado, Timothy A., Merel, Josh, Pfau, David, Reardon, Thomas, Mu, Yu, Lacefield, Clay, Yang, Weijian, Ahrens, Misha, Bruno, Randy, Jessel, Thomas M., Peterka, Darcy S., Yuste, Rafael and Paninski, Liam. 2016. "Simultaneous denoising, deconvolution, and demixing of calcium imaging data." *Neuron* 89(2):285–99.

Pnevmatikakis, Eftychios A. and Giovannucci, Andrea. 2017 "NoRMCorre: An online algorithm for piecewise rigid motion correction of calcium imaging data." *Journal of Neuroscience Methods* 291:83–94.

Poivet, Erwan, Peterlin, Zita, Tahirova, Narmin, Xu, Lu, Altomare, Clara, Paria, Anne, Zou, Dong-Jing and Firestein, Stuart. 2016. "Applying medicinal chemistry strategies to understand odorant discrimination." *Nature Communications* 7:11157.

Poivet, Erwan, Tahirova, Narmin, Peterlin, Zita, Xu, Lu, Zou, Dong-Jing, Acree, Terry and Firestein, Stuart. 2018. "Functional odor classification through a medicinal chemistry approach." *Science Advances* 4(2):eaao6086.

Rheinberger, Hans-Jôrg. 1997. *Toward a History of Epistemic Things: Synthesizing Proteins in the Test Tube.* Stanford, CA: Stanford University Press.

Rossiter, Karen J. 1996. "Structure-odor relationships." *Chemical Reviews* 96(8):3201–40.

Sell, Charles S. 2006. "On the unpredictability of odor." *Angewandte Chemie International Edition* 45(38): 6254–61.

Snogerup-Linse, Sara. 2012. "Studies of G-protein coupled receptors. The Nobel Prize in chemistry 2012. Award ceremony speech." *The Royal Swedish Academy of Sciences* (accessed 09/25/2014). http://www.nobelprize.org/nobel_prizes/chemistry/laureates/2012/advanced-chemistryprize2012.pdf

Solomon, Miriam. 2007. "Situated cognition." In: *Philosophy of Psychology and Cognitive Science* , ed. by Paul Thagard. Amsterdam: North-Holland, pp. 413–28.

Thagard, Paul. 2012. *The Cognitive Science of Science Explanation, Discovery, and Conceptual Change.* Cambridge: MIT Press.

Vaadia, Rebecca D., Li, Wenze, Voleti, Venkatakaushik, Singhania, Aditi, Hillman, Elizabeth M. C. and Grueber, Wesley B. 2019. "Characterization of proprioceptive system dynamics in behaving Drosophila larvae using high-speed volumetric microscopy." *Current Biology* 29(6):935–44.

van Fraassen, Bas. 1980. *The Scientific Image.* Oxford: Oxford University Press.

van Fraassen, Bas. 2008. *Scientific Representation: Paradoxes of Perspective.* Oxford: Oxford University Press.

Voleti, Venkatakaushik, Patel, Kripa B., Li, Wenze, Campos, Citlali Perez, Bharadwaj, Srinidhi, Yu, Hang, Ford, Caitlin, Casper, Malte J., Yan, Richard Wenwei, Liang, Wenxuan, Wen, Chentao, Kimura, Koutarou D., Targoff, Kimara L. and Hillman, Elizabeth M. C. 2019. "Real-time volumetric microscopy of in vivo dynamics and large-scale samples with SCAPE 2.0." *Nature Methods* 16(10):1054–62.

Vosshall, Leslie B., Amrein, Hubert, Morozov, Pavel S., Rzhetsky, Andrey and Axel, Richard. 1999. "A spatial map of olfactory receptor expression in the Drosophila antenna." *Cell* 96(5):725–36.

Xu, Lu, Li, Wenze, Voleti, Venkatakaushik, Hillman, Elizabeth M. C. and Firestein, Stuart. 2019. "Widespread receptor driven modulation in peripheral olfactory coding." *bioRxiv* 760330.

Xu, Lu, Li, Wenze, Voleti, Venkatakaushik, Zou, Dong-Jing, Hillman, Elizabeth M. C. and Firestein, Stuart. 2020. "Widespread receptor driven modulation in peripheral olfactory coding." *Science* 368(6487):eaaz5390.

Zhao, Haiqing, Ivic, Lidija, Otaki, Joji M., Hashimoto, Mitsuhiro, Mikoshiba, Katsuhiro and Stuart Firestein. 1998. "Functional expression of a mammalian odorant receptor." *Science* 279:237–42.

5 A Different Role for Tinkering

Brain Fog, COVID-19, and the Accidental Nature of Neurobiological Theory Development

Valerie Gray Hardcastle and C. Matthew Stewart

John Bickle and his colleagues are current drivers of the science-in-practice movement and its focus on the extra-theoretical aspects of science for philosophers (See, e.g., Ankeny et al. 2011). This movement grew out of an intellectual frustration with the near divorce of the philosophy of science from what scientists actually do in their day-to-day professional lives. Its adherents promote the detailed and systematic study of the activities of science, while still maintaining the traditional philosophy of science foci on rationality, justification, observation, evidence, and theory (and in contrast to prevailing tendencies in the social studies of science and technology, which focus almost exclusively on science as a human construct). Philosophers of science-in-practice explore the historical context and current practices that lead to a model or theory in an effort to better understand the scientific process.

Bickle holds that revolutions in neurobiology-in-practice are driven exclusively by new tool development, which he believes drives experimental design (2016) – as opposed to, say, Thomas Kuhn's (1962) model of scientific theory development as a paradigm shift. He argues that tool development is an analog of Ian Hacking's (1983) famous "microscopes" argument for the "relative independence" of "the life of experiment" from theory, further downgrading theory's purported centrality in science (Bickle 2018). And following Hacking, Bickle holds that engineering counts more than theory in the development of molecular and cellular neurobiology research tools. Indeed, according to Bickle,

> the genesis of every piece of theory [in neurobiology] … can be tied directly to the development of new research tools. Theoretical progress in this paradigmatic science of our times *is secondary to and entirely dependent upon* new tool development, both temporally and epistemically.
>
> (2021, p. 14, emphasis in the original)

DOI: 10.4324/9781003251392-7

The larger, and perhaps more controversial, point that Bickle wants to make is that tool development drives everything: not just theory development, but resource allocation, experimental design, and researchers' time and attention. Bickle notes that Hubel and Weisel's advancement in our understanding of the receptive field properties in striate and extra-striate cortex, which led to their theory of information processing in the visual cortex, and which garnered them the 1981 Nobel Prize in Physiology or Medicine, "rode on the back of Hubel's catch-as-catch-can, make-it-work, trial-and-error-tinkered invention of a new experiment tool, the metal microelectrode and hydraulic microdriver, and the new kinds of experiments it enabled" (2022, p. 18). If theories weren't diminished enough in their place in scientific practice, Bickle is further claiming that tool development in turn relies on what he calls "laboratory tinkering," and what Hacking calls "fooling around" (1983, p. 199). So, actually, "theory progress in neurobiology is thus doubly dependent, and hence tertiary in both epistemic and temporal priority" (Bickle 2022, p. 14). Tinkering in the lab leads to creating new tools for new experimental approaches, which, in turn leads to theoretical progress (see also Stix 2012).

Bickle goes on to surmise that perhaps this "double dependence" of theory on tinkering and new tool development might be true across all the bench scientific fields in the life sciences. These lessons taken from his examination of neuroscience-in-practice stand in direct contrast to the lament of many of the early authors in the philosophy of neuroscience: that there was no theoretical framework for understanding the brain (e.g., Crick 1979; Churchland 1986; Churchland and Sejnowski 1992). Still today, the lack of theory in neuroscience remains a concern among many (Gold and Roskies 2008; Churchland and Sejnowski 2016). And still today, there is no overarching theoretical framework in which to organize the brain sciences (Hardcastle and Hardcastle 2015; Hardcastle 2017).

Bickle suggests that the lack of theory in neuroscience should not be of great concern; instead, he follows Hubel's explanation that the activities of neuroscientists "seemed not to conform to the science that we are taught in high school, with its laws, hypotheses, experimental verification, generalizations, and so on" (1996, 312). The actual impact of theory on the day-to-day practice of neuroscience appears small. Instead, neuroscientists tinker around in their laboratories, intervening in the world as they can with the tools they have (or create) and then seeing what comes of it. As Hubel explains, they are akin to "15th century explorers, like Columbus sailing West to see what he might find" (1996, p. 312).

But is this how bench neuroscience works across the board? This chapter argues that the answer is yes and no. On the one hand, tool development and tinkering are fundamental aspects of the neuroscientific trade. But on the other hand, theories are just another tool that neuroscientists can utilize when poking about in the brain. Theories are not tertiary outcomes of neuroscientific practice; rather, they are a utensil, just like a microelectrode, with which we use to probe the brain. We illustrate this perspective by recounting two recent discoveries on the impact of COVID-19 in the brain, both of which were supported by the tinkering and practices of one scientist. In one case, theory clearly drove tool innovation; in the other, as with Columbus, he was just sailing West, hoping against hope to find something useful. But each case resulted in significant theoretical advancement. Sometimes novel tools drive theory, but other times, theory promotes novel tools. And both are ways that neuroscience advances.

1 COVID-19

On 31 December 2019, China notified the World Health Organization (WHO) about a cluster of cases of pneumonia in Wuhan City, home to 11 million. Less than two weeks later, there were 282 confirmed cases, with six deaths. Four of these cases were outside of China in neighboring countries. During this same timeframe, the virus responsible had been isolated and its genome sequenced. The cause of the novel pneumonia became known as COVID-19 (short for COronaVIrus Disease 2019), and it was a new coronavirus,[1] dubbed SARS-CoV-2 (Chaplin 2020; Lago 2020). Less than eight weeks after that, there were over 118,000 cases and almost 5,000 deaths across 114 counties, and the WHO calls it a pandemic. And now, at the time of this writing, a short 22 months later, the WHO reports over 230 million cases worldwide, with almost 5 million dead (https://covid19.who.int). Forty percent of those cases and half of the deaths have been in the Americas.

While it is not definitively known how or why the new coronavirus appeared in humans, genomic analysis suggests that it originated in bats and was transmitted to perhaps a pangolin, which was illegally sold at a wet market in Wuhan, where it was then transmitted to humans (Anderson et al 2020). SARS-CoV-2 is not the first coronavirus to have been passed from other animals to humans – six have been identified so far, four of which cause the common cold. A fifth is now known by SARS (Severe Acute Respiratory Syndrome), which also originated in China, likely also via bats (then perhaps through civets), in 2002. In the two years in which it was active, just over 8,000 cases were identified with roughly 10% of those infected dying. And the sixth, abbreviated as MERS (Middle Eastern Respiratory Syndrome), originated in Saudi Arabia in 2012, again likely via bats and then through camels. Unlike SARS, MERS continues to infect humans to this day, with roughly 2,500 known infections and 860 deaths. Both SARS and MERS cause a flu-like illness with symptoms ranging from asymptomatic infection to the sniffles to severe pneumonia to acute respiratory distress syndrome, septic shock, and multiorgan failure (Kahn and MacIntosh 2005; Chaplin 2020; Liu et al. 2020).

MERS now seems to appear most often as a result of animal to human transmission (perhaps as a function of tending to camels' birthing their young) and only secondarily through human spread. This coronavirus is not terribly contagious and requires very close contact between humans to be transmitted this way, such as occurs when one is caring for someone who is ill (Durst et al. 2018). MERS is transmitted via respiratory aerosol droplets and airborne particles, as is COVID-19. However, relative to MERS, COVID-19 appears more contagious. This is probably largely due to asymptomatic carriers and genetic mutations (Lago 2020). In the four weeks after 55 index cases had been identified of SARS in East Asia, an additional 3,000 cases had appeared (WHO 2003). But in the four weeks after the first 59 cases of COVID-19 were identified, 25,000 cases had been confirmed – an eight-fold increase in new cases (WHO 2020).

The COVID-19 pandemic is often compared to global flu outbreaks as a way of putting the disease in context. However, seasonal flus kill 250,000–650,000 annually, depending on the outbreak. And the H1N1 swine flu epidemic in 2009–2010 caused 280,000 deaths worldwide (Kelly et al. 2011). Obviously, these numbers do not compare with what we have seen with COVID-19. The closest is perhaps the H1N1 flu pandemic in 1918–1919, in which 50 million worldwide died, with 650,000 of those in the United States (Centers for Disease Control and Prevention 2019).

As with SARS and MERS, the clinical presentation of COVID-19 varies from asymptomatic infection to mild illness to severe disease and death. Sudden deterioration is common, most often in the second week of the disease, and attributed to cytokine "storms[2]" or hyperinflammation. Risk factors for severe disease include older age, immunosuppression, hypertension, diabetes, and cardiovascular disease, chronic respiratory disease, and kidney disease. Some of the risk factors could be explained by the virus's high affinity for binding to ACE2 (angiotensin-converting enzyme 2), which is expressed by the epithelial cells in lungs, intestines, kidneys, and blood vessels (Gouvea dos Santos, 2020).

2 COVID-19 in the Ear

Important to our discussion, the most common symptom of COVID-19 is a sudden loss of taste or smell, reported in 86% of those with mild cases and over a third with more severe cases (Lechien et al. 2021). Newly diagnosed COVID-19 patients are over 27 times more likely to complain of loss of smell as compared to non-COVID-19 patients (Wagner et al. 2020). Often it is used as the primary identifying symptom of the disease.

Evidence suggests that this loss of smell happens in the nasal epithelium in the upper nasal cavity, as neither the olfactory sensory neurons nor the olfactory bulb, which receives input from the olfactory sensory neurons, express the gene that encodes for the ACE2 receptor protein which SARS-CoV-2 uses to enter host cells (Brann et al. 2020). The olfactory epithelium is a specialized tissue in the upper nasal cavity that houses olfactory neurons and allows for odor detection. Both olfactory sustentacular cells, which provide structural and metabolic support to olfactory neurons, and olfactory basal cells, which act as stem cells that regenerate the olfactory epithelium after damage, in the olfactory epithelium express ACE2.

The hypothesis is that because olfactory mucosa is in such close proximity to olfactory bulb projections, infected olfactory mucosa will affect olfactory bulb processes (likely via an inflammatory response), even though the virus itself will not bind to cells in that region (Meinhardt et al. 2021). In any event, it quickly became obvious that otolaryngologists could not operate in the nose or mouth because of the potential for aerosol spray from infected nasal and throat passages. Indeed, some otolaryngologists in China, Italy, and Iran died from operating on patients early in the pandemic (Kulcsar et al. 2020).

COVID-19 has been billed as a respiratory illness (cf., WHO, 2021). This description is not entirely off the mark, as SARS-CoV-2 is primarily transmitted by breathing in the virus from the air, and it does indeed bind with the epithelial tissue found in the lungs. However, and the import of this point was originally missed in the first few months of the SARS-CoV-2 outbreak, epithelial respiratory tissue is found outside the lungs. Our respiratory tract does more than support breathing; it also removes waste brought into the body along with the atmospheric gases we need to function. Part of respiration includes a neurodigestive system, as it were.

For example, the epithelium in the upper nasal cavity comprises part of our respiratory tract; our sinuses are a component of this neurodigestive system. In addition to smelling the world around us, they move detritus into our gut to be digested. Sinuses make mucus, which traps dust, pollen, dirt, and other unwanted particles breathed up from the nose, and then sweeps this mucus to the back of the throat to swallow down as our own internal garbage disposal system. A similar process occurs in our lung epithelium. It consists of, among other cell types, goblet cells, which produce and secrete mucus to trap pathogens and debris within the airway, and ciliated cells, which help sweep the trapped debris across the airway tract to the back of the throat, where it too is swallowed down.

But the nasal passages and the lungs are not the only epithelial respiratory tissue in our bodies. Our middle ear and mastoid also have respiratory functions. The mastoid bone consists of a cell structure that contains air pockets and is lined by modified respiratory epithelium. The question of how the human tympanic cavity came to be lined by a continuous epithelial layer while the cavity is separated by ossicles, muscles, and nerves, has been debated for years. The respiratory-like epithelium was originally considered an extension of the upper respiratory tract, thought to have developed because the pharyngeal pouch was turned inside out in development, and the most recent evidence suggests that this hypothesis is still a good one (van Waegeningh et al. 2019). Regardless of how the epithelium came to be in the inner ear, the mastoid produces mucus and, in conjunction with the middle ear, sweeps ear detritus trapped in the mucus through the Eustachian tube to the back of the throat for swallowing, just as our other sinus cavities do.

We know that SARS-CoV-2 can infect the epithelial respiratory cells in the lungs, which causes shortness of breath. We know it can infect the epithelial respiratory cells in the sinuses, which causes the loss of smell.[3] And we know that SARS-CoV-2 can affect the olfactory system of the brain via the mucosa in the upper nasal cavity. It therefore stands to reason that SARS-CoV-2 could affect the epithelial respiratory cells in the ear too. In other words, the virus could migrate to the middle ear and infect the mastoid in COVID patients. And if it can infect the mastoid, then perhaps it could also impact the central nervous system in an analogous fashion to what happens between the nasal cavities and olfactory bulb projections. These are the hypothesis that Matt Stewart wanted to test.

There were some additional hints that these hypotheses might be true. For example, viral infections can cause hearing loss, vertigo, and occasionally tinnitus. Significant percentages of adults who have tested positive for COVID-19 do report sudden hearing loss (8% of all cases), vertigo (7%), or tinnitus (15%) among their symptoms, regardless of the level of severity of the disease (Almuffarrij and Munro 2021). We are starting to see longer-term effects on the auditory system for patients with "long-hauler" syndrome,[4] including earaches, vertigo, loss of hearing, and tinnitus, all persisting a month or more (Assaf et al. 2020). Problems with hearing or dizziness generally reflect a challenge in the inner ear, but tinnitus is not a peripheral phenomenon; it is a central one. Its sufferers perceive sounds when they are not present, and sound perception requires the involvement of auditory neurons.

Moreover, mouse data indicate that ACE2 is diffusely present in the Eustachian tube, middle ear spaces, and cochlea of the mouse ear. Intracellular entry of SARS-CoV-2 via ACE2 depends on spike protein cleavage mediated by Furin and spike protein priming by transmembrane protease serine 2 (TMPRSS2). Both Furin and TMPRSS2 are present in mouse ear tissue as well (Uranaka et al. 2020), suggesting that the mouse ear could harbor SARS-CoV-2, which in turn suggests that human ears could too.

In sum, there was evidence for both peripheral and central effects of COVID-19 on the auditory system, as well as evidence that SARS-CoV-2 would be able to bind with the epithelial tissues found in the inner ear. If these data were accurate, then the impact of SARS-CoV-2 could extend to the auditory system as well.

To test the hypothesis that SARS-CoV-2 can infiltrate the auditory system, one must examine the inner ears and brains of COVID-19 patients. But doing so presents immediate technological challenges, for there is no way to do this non-invasively in live patients. At the same time, there was no good way to do this in deceased patients either, for the normal protocol for accessing the brain in cadavers requires power tools, which, of course, could easily broadcast the virus throughout the autopsy theater. A new approach was needed – perhaps not new tools, but at least a different way to access brains that did not utilize contemporary Western methods for doing so. This was the challenge that confronted Stewart: If he wanted to test his hypotheses, then he would need to devise a way to access human brains that would not risk infecting himself or others with SARS-CoV-2. In this particular instance, theory and hypothesis-testing are driving tool development, instead of the other way around.

To cut to the end of the story, Stewart used essentially a hammer, a chisel, and a tiny scoop to access the middle ear and auditory neurons. These were not new tools, but rather old tools used in a novel way. These comprised the surgery equipment used by head and neck surgeons in developing countries, who do not have access to modern mastoid surgery drills or other power tools (Fagan and Jackler 2017). These tools in turn reflect surgery techniques from the 1930s in the United States (Portman et al. 1939) (See Figure 1 below).

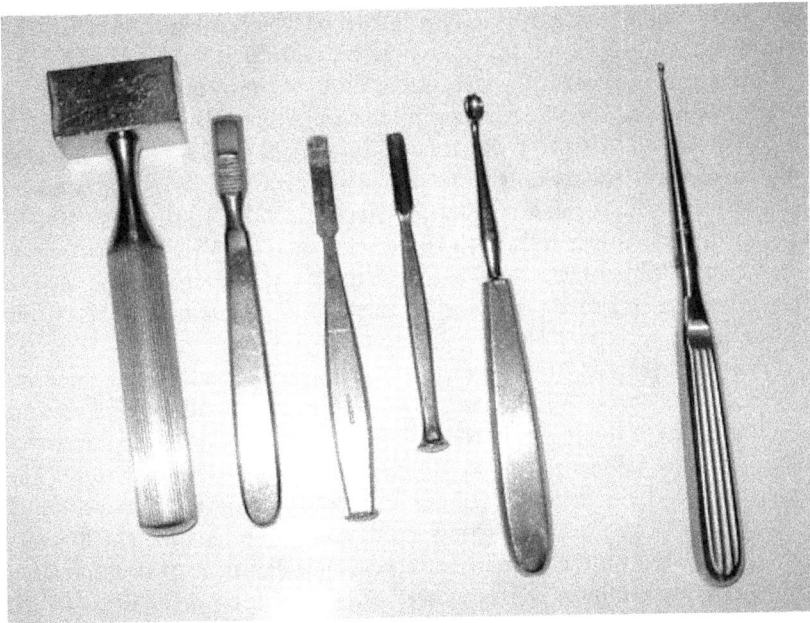

Figure 1 Mallet, rasp, chisels, curette, and gouge. From Fagan and Jackler (2017), p. 2.

Stewart partnered with the rapid autopsy program for inpatient COVID-19 deaths at Johns Hopkins School of Medicine, pioneering the use of hand tools as a safer method for autopsying the brains potentially infected with SARS-CoV-2. To investigate whether the virus could be found in the middle ear, he started with the usual method for detecting SARS-CoV-2: the PCR (polymerase chain reaction) swab test to search for genomic sequencing of SARS. He accessed the inner ear by trephining and curetting through the mastoid bone using a small hammer and a chisel and then swizzled in the middle ear with a tiny scoop or gouge.

He and his team discovered that decedents who had died from complications of COVID-19 exhibited a very strong positive result to the PCR test. Furthermore, this positive result continued to be evident for quite long postmortem intervals – up to 96 hours after death (Frazier et al. 2020). SARS-CoV-2 could be found in human ears. (As an aside, this discovery had immediate implications for medical care, because it was now clear that providers should not peer into ruptured ears as part of routine medical examinations because COVID-19 could potentially be transmitted that way.)

But there is more. Stewart and others had good reason to suspect that SARS-CoV-2 was infiltrating epithelial tissue in the inner ear. But to confirm this suspicion, they would need to determine whether ACE2 receptors are indeed present in the human tympanic cavity. The natural approach would be to use electron microscopy to examine which cells, if any, in the inner ear have ACE2 receptors, or other markers like Furin or TMPRSS2, which would promote binding with SARS-CoV-2.

This again is straightforward scientific hypothesis-testing. No ACE2 receptors, Furin, TMPRSS2, or similar would contraindicate the ability of SARS-CoV-2 to infect the inner ear, which would further suggest that the central effects that some patients with COVID-19 experienced would have to be secondary implications of COVID-19. If SARS-CoV-2 cannot directly infect cells in the inner ear, then COVID-19-related tinnitus could not be due to SARS-CoV-2 itself but perhaps instead due to inflammation or other responses by the immune system to fight off the infection.

But using electron microscopy to examine which cells from the tympanic cavity express ACE2 is not an easy protocol to adopt because our ear bones are among the hardest bones in our bodies. And, unfortunately, the decalcification process required to soften them enough to be able to slice them thin enough for microscopy examination normally takes ten months – much too long in our race to understand the impacts of SARS-CoV-2 on the human body. But once again, Stewart innovated by modifying techniques from other eras used for other purposes. In this instance, he reached back to his undergraduate studies and adapted the procedures he had learned in the chemistry lab to thinly section and decalcify rocks. Amazingly, using this novel method for decalcifying bones took only 13 days to soften the bones enough for microscopy examination.

At the time of this writing, Stewart is now harvesting the entire vestibular/cochlear part of the temporal bone for examination. While this work is still ongoing, enough is known to be able to conclude definitively that SARS-CoV-2 can infect the cochlear region. It is not just that there were viral proteins present in the inner ear of COVID-19 cadavers in the mucosa, but the bone tissue itself in the tympanic cavity can be infected. Just as SARS-CoV-2 is ubiquitous in the lungs, nasal passages, and vascular systems in patients with severe COVID-19, it is also present in the ears.

Once again, we see theory driving tool innovation and not the other way around. In this instance at least, instead of "the genesis ...of theory [in neurobiology] ...[being] tied directly to the development of new research tools" such that "theoretical progress ...*is secondary to and entirely dependent upon* new tool development, both temporally and epistemically" (Bickle 2022, p. 14), we are seeing that the confirmation of a neurobiological theory was tied directly to the development of new research techniques such that while theoretical progress was indeed temporally dependent upon new tool development, it was not epistemically.

However, we do not wish to push too hard on this conclusion or to try to generalize it very far. In our next case study, we see that the same researcher, still investigating the neurological implications of COVID-19, this time does not have a hypothesis to drive his innovation. In this next case, we see that theoretical progress was both temporally and epistemically dependent on tool innovation.

3 COVID-19 and the Brain

As a reminder: the primary symptom of COVID-19, the loss of smell, is neurological. Moreover, it is now very clear that many patients with COVID-19 – both those with severe cases and those with mild – develop additional neurological symptoms, often days or weeks after disease onset. These symptoms can include headache, chronic pain, confusion, memory loss, fatigue, insomnia, excessive drowsiness, alterations of consciousness, anxiety, depression, and even psychosis. Quite common is what is known as "brain fog," or more formally as dysexecutive syndrome (Couzin-Frankel 2020, Helms et al. 2020). Alarmingly, over a third of patients with COVID-19 receive a diagnosis for some psychiatric or neurological ailment within six months of getting infected with the virus (Zubair et al. 2020).

Other viruses have had this impact on our brains, most notably a variant of the measles virus and the strain of flu from the 2918 pandemic (Hoffman and Vilensky 2017; Garg et al. 2019). Very recent analysis suggests that the molecular neuropathologies found in decedents who had had COVID-19 roughly mimic those of Alzheimer's disease, multiple sclerosis, Huntington's disease, autism spectrum disorder, and other chronic CNS diseases. While the COVID-19 changes found in neurons were not exactly the same as these other disorders, the overlap between the two was striking (Yang et al. 2021).

These findings are worrisome, to put it mildly. A significant concern among neurologists and clinical neuropsychologists is the possibility that SARS-CoV-2 infection could lead to long-term cognitive dysfunction or decline (Pratt et al. 2021). While it is much too soon to be able to know definitely whether humanity will be struggling with the long-term effects of COVID-19 among a large proportion of our population for decades to come, at the moment, this does appear to be a real and very sobering possibility.

How might SARS-CoV-2 do this? One suggestion is that the virus could pass through the blood-brain barrier and infect the brain directly, as it apparently can in human's close biological cousin, the rhesus monkey (Jiao et al. 2021). Another possibility is that the inflammation associated with the release of cytokines by our immune system as it fights off SARS-CoV-2 could promote the accumulation of tau plaques in our brain, which perhaps could eventually lead to dementia or Parkinson's disease (see, e.g., Heneka et al. 2020). And, of course, both hypotheses could be true as well.

However, evidence for the viral RNA or proteins in the brain itself is extremely sparse, including in the olfactory bulb (Mukerji and Solomon 2021), which is the neural system closest to the primary infection site. Quantitative reverse transcriptase polymerase chain reaction tests (qRT-PCR) did find very low levels of viral RNA in some of the brains (Puelles et al. 2020, Solomon et al. 2020, Wichmann et al. 2020), but this was much, much less than what was detected in the nasal epithelium – and RNAscope and immunocytochemistry have not detected any viral RNA or proteins in any brains studies thus far (Thakur et al. 2021).

At the same time, neuropathological examination of a variety of brain areas from numerous patients who have died from SARS-CoV-2 shows evidence of ischemic strokes, both large and small, with areas of dead tissue, both globally and locally (Duarte-Neto et al. 2020, Reichard et al. 2020; Remmelink et al. 2020; see also Lee et al. 2021; Thakur et al., 2021). Given the minute levels of SARS-CoV-2 found in cadaver brains, there is no obvious way for the virus to cause the stroke damage found in the decedents. Clearly, something is happening in the brains of persons with COVID-19, but what and how?

Unlike in our previous case, there was no theory to guide this investigation. Somehow, SARS-CoV-2 was instigating deleterious changes in the brain. It was not doing this by direct infection; it likely was somehow causing multiple small stokes. But what that mechanism might be and how that mechanism was inducing ischemia was unknown. In this case,

Stewart had to just start looking around in the brains of patients who had died from COVID-19 to see if he could determine what might be causing the changes. He had no real theory to guide his investigation, just the tools he developed to autopsy COVID-19 cadavers and basic histopathology. This was tinkering in its purest form.

As before, the autopsies would have to proceed without the usual powered autopsy saw because of the potential for aerosol spray. Building upon the older surgical techniques Stewart used to dissect the inner ear, he attempted to access the temporal lobe without power tools. Needless to say, it was quite physically challenging to chisel through the skull in order to remove it and the dura while maintaining an adequate N95 facial seal!

The goal was to access the temporal lobe, which is not normally a target in autopsy, but the first attempts ended in a failed mess. With more practice, and a new PAPR (Powered Air Purifying Respirator), Stewart and his colleagues were able to successfully perform whole-brain extraction and dissect randomly targeted cortical areas. There they discovered an unexpected type of cell had clogged the capillaries in COVID-19 patient brains. Surprisingly, what they discovered were megakaryocytes, the extremely large cells that normally reside in bone marrow and make the platelets found in blood (see Figure 2) (Nauen et al. 2021).

It turns out that in times of inflammation, megakaryocytes can be stimulated to move from bone marrow plates and to start circulating in blood vessels. Because they are so large, they can directly block both small capillaries as well as end-organ vessels. Autopsies of decedents with COVID-19 had previously uncovered circulating megakaryocytes in the liver, kidney, heart, and lungs. (This can occur with other diseases as well.) These autopsies also showed that capillary blockage had occurred in these same organs – regardless of when in the course of the disease the patient died and sometimes despite full anticoagulation. The discovery of megakaryocytes along with platelet-infused thrombi in the liver, kidneys, heart, and lungs suggests that these cells are playing a role in the blockages. But megakaryocytes are not routinely found in the brain as part of any normal process (Duarte-Neto et al. 2020, Rapkiewicz et al. 2020). (A few rare genetic diseases are correlated with megakaryocytes in the brain, however.)

Nevertheless, a third of the brains that Stewart sampled contained these megakaryocytes (see also Jensen et al. 2020). Because brain autopsy sections sample only a small portion of the entire cortex, finding megakaryocytes at all indicates that the total number of them circulating in brains could be quite large. By tracing the impact of these occlusions through downstream tissue, Stewart and his colleagues determined that the megakaryocytes spilled platelets in the brain, which then initiated a thrombotic cascade. If large numbers of megakaryocytes block blood flow in this manner in capillaries across the brain, then they might be

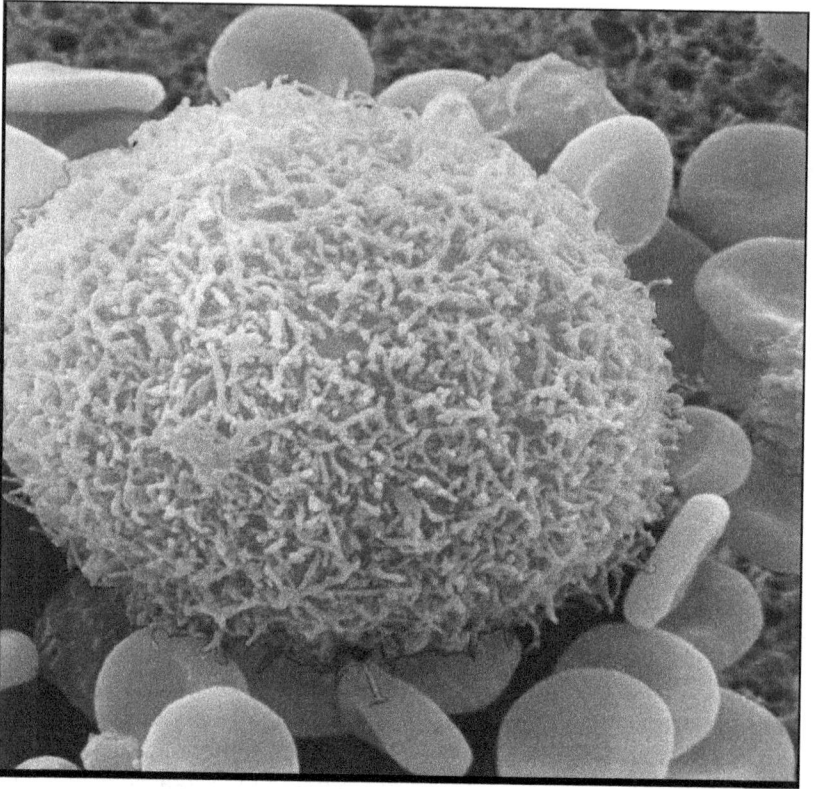

Figure 2 Scanning electron microscope image of a megakaryocyte in the marrow with red blood cells for comparison. BSIP SA.

creating a distinct pattern of ischemic destruction, which could potentially lead to a distinct type of COVID-19 neurologic impairment.

One of the big mysteries about the long-term CNS sequelae after recovery is the ongoing brain fog that occurs in a disturbingly large number of patients, given that finding viral RNA or active infection in the CNS is extremely rare and very limited. Recent comparison scans of almost 800 individuals pre- and post-SARS-CoV-2 infection indicate that there is a consistent and significant loss of grey matter across cortex, with the most profound effects being found a reduction of thickness and volume in the gustatory-, olfactory-, and memory-related regions of the brain (Douaud et al. 2021). Most disquieting is the limbic nature of the gustatory and olfactory systems, and their proximity to the hippocampus, which not only might account for the brain fog but also might indicate that one long-term consequence of COVID-19 could very well be dementia for some number of patients. And these changes could be wrought by multiple tiny strokes caused by megakaryocytes running rampant in our brains.

Of course, we do not yet definitely know whether megakaryocytes cause the neurological problems associated with long-hauler syndrome. Nevertheless, this case presents a clear case of technological innovation driving theory production: In this case, tinkering in the lab led to novel uses for older (now unused) tools that opened a new experimental approach, which, in turn led to at least the potential for theoretical progress.

4 Tool Innovation in Neurobiology-in-Practice

Increasingly, evidence suggests long-term brain involvement COVID-19. Acutely ill patients are often confused and exhibit what appear to be CNS disorders. Post-recovery, many patients complain of ongoing anxiety, depression, and difficulties with cognition. The challenge has been how to reconcile patient experience with hitherto inconclusive brain studies. Due to restrictions by the Centers for Disease Control and Prevention (and common sense), routine autopsies cannot be performed on the brains of COVID-19 patients because they involve instruments that generate aerosol spray. But, after tinkering with a variety of different approaches to get around this restriction, researchers at Johns Hopkins School of Medicine returned to the lessons from previous generations of practitioners and adapted old-fashioned manual surgery techniques. With these new protocols for autopsy, their dissections revealed both strong evidence for SARS-CoV-2 in the epithelial tissues of the inner ear and the presence of megakaryocytes in the brain tissue of COVID-19 decedents. Both of these discoveries have huge implications for our understanding of how SARS-CoV-2 affects the body, both over short-term and long-term periods.

Aside from being an ingenious solution, returning to hand-held tools for autopsying brains is a textbook case of How Science Works: researchers working to find the right tools that would allow them to peel the lid off of a black box and figure out what is going on. In these cases, the novel use of these tools is not informing theory per se; rather, the desperate need to uncover the causal-mechanistic chain behind the neurological sequelae of COVID-19 drove the innovative tool use. And then the innovative use helped to confirm a hypothesis in one instance and allowed for the development of a hypothesis in the other instance.

What do we learn from these case studies? In many respects, the lessons echo Barwich's example of how a tool was exploited to develop a new theoretical perspective in an otherwise rather hopeless circumstance. In the first case, contra Bickle's examples, this theoretical advance was both predicted and expected; but in the second case, as in Bickle's examples, the advance was essentially an accidental finding.

We agree that directed tinkering is indeed connected to significant conceptual theoretical advancement more often than not in neurobiology. But how it is connected can differ depending on the specifics of the case. Sometimes tinkering and novel tool use drive hypothesis-testing, and sometimes they drive hypothesis generation. As adumbrated by philosophers focused on science-in-practice, the processes by which researchers come to their theories are as important, if not more important, than the theories themselves. For, as many of the papers in this volume illustrate, technological advancement is the primary limiting factor in theory confirmation and advancement in neurobiology.

Notes

1 The name coronavirus is derived from the Latin word corona, which means crown or wreath. The name is due to the shape of virions on the surface of the virus as visualized by electron microscopy creates an image reminiscent of a crown (Chauhan 2020).
2 Cytokine literally means "cell mover," which is exactly what these storms do – they move cells from one part of the body to another.
3 We also know it can infect the epithelial cells in our blood vessels, but this fact is not part of our current story.
4 "Long haulers" refer to patients who previously tested positive for COVID-19 but continue to experience adverse symptoms weeks or months after the virus has been cleared from the body.

References

Almufarrij, I., and Munro, K.J. (2021). One year on: An updated systematic review of SARS-CoV-2, COVID-19, and audio-vestibular symptoms. *International Journal of Audiology*. doi: 10.1080/14992027.2021.1896793.
Anderson, K.G., Rambaut, A., Lipkin, W.I., Holmes, E.C., and Garry, R.F. (2020). The proximal origins of SARS-CoV-2. *Nature Medicine* 26: 450–452.
Ankeny, R., Chang, H., Boumans, M., and Boon, M. (2011). Introduction: Philosophy of science in practice. *European Journal of the Philosophy of Science* 1: 303–307.
Assaf, G., David, H., McCorkell, L., Wei, H., Brooke, O, Akrami, A., Low, R., Mercier, J., and other member of the COVID-19 Body Politic Slack Group. (2020). *Report: What does COVID-19 recovery actually look like? An analysis of the prolonged COVID-19 symptoms survey by patient-led research team*. Patient Led Research Collaborative. https://patientresearchcovid19.com/research/report-1/.
Bickle, J. (2016). Revolutions in neuroscience: Tool development. *Frontiers in Systems Neuroscience*, 10: 24 doi: 10.3389/fnsys.2016.00024.
Bickle, J. (2018). From microscopes to optogenetics: Ian Hacking vindicated. *Philosophy of Science* 85: 1065–1077.
Bickle, J. (2022). Tinkering in the lab. This volume, pp. 13–36.
Brann, D.H, Tsukahara, T., Weinreb, C. et al. (2020). Non-neuronal expression of SARS-CoV-2 entry genes in the olfactory system suggests mechanisms

underlying COVID-19-anosmia. *Science Advances* 6: eabc5801. doi: 10.1126/sciadv.abc580.

Centers for Disease Control and Prevention (2019). 1918 Pandemic (H1N1 virus). https://www.cdc.gov/flu/pandemic-resources/1918-pandemic-h1n1.html

Chaplin, S. (2020). COVID-19: A brief history and treatments in development. *Prescriber* May: 23–28.

Chauhan, S. (2020). Comprehensive review of coronavirus 2019 (COVID-19). *Science Direct Biomedical Journal* 43: 334–340.

Churchland, P.S. (1986). *Neurophilosophy*. Cambridge, MA: The MIT Press.

Churchland, P.S., and Sejnowski, T.J. (1992). *The Computational Brain*. Cambridge: MIT Press.

Churchland, P.S., and Sejnowski, T.J. (2016). Blending computational and experimental neuroscience. *Nature Reviews Neuroscience* 17: 567–568.

Couzin-Frankel, J. (2020). From "brain fog" to heart damage, COVID-19's lingering problems alarm scientists. *Science*. Published July 31, 2020. doi: 10.1126/science.abe1147.

Crick, F.H. (1979). Thinking about the brain. *Scientific American* 241: 219–232.

Douaud, G., Lee, S., Alfaro-Almagro, F., Arthofer, C., Wang, C. Lange, F., Andersson, J.L.R., Griffanti, L., Duff, E., Jbabdi, S., Taschler, B., Windkler, A., Nichols, T.E., Collins, R., Matthews, P.M., Allen, N., Miller, K.L., and Smith, S.M. (2021). Brain imaging before and after COVID-19 in UK biobank. Preprint posted at https://www.medrxiv.org/content/10.1101/2021.06 .11.21258690v1.

Duarte-Neto, A.N., Monteiro, R.A.A., da Silva, L.F.F., Malheiros, D.M.A.C., de Oliveira, E.P., Theordoro-Filho, T., Pinho, J.R.R., Gomes-Gouvea, M.S., Salles, A.P.M., de Oliveira, I.R.S., Mauad, T., Saldia, P.H.N., and Dolhnikoff, M. (2020). Pulmonary and systemic involvement in COVID-19 patients assessed with ultrasound-guided minimally invasive autopsy. *Histopathology* 77: 186–197. doi: 10.1111/his.14160.

Durst, G. Carvalho, L.M., Rambaut, A., and Bedford, T. (2018). MERS-CoV spillover at the camel-human interface. *eLife* 7: e31257. doi: 10.7554/eLife.31257.

Fagan, J., and Jackler, R. (2017). Hammer & gouge cortical mastoidectomy for acute mastoiditis. In J. Fagan (Ed.) *The Open Access Atlas of Otolaryngology, Head & Neck Operative Surgery*, pp. 1–14. https://vula.uct.ac.za/access/content/group/ba5fb1bd-be95-48e5-81be-586fbaeba29d/Hammer%20%20Gouge%20Mastoidectomy%20for%20acute%20mastoiditis-1.pdf.

Frazier, K.M., Hooper, J.E., Mostafa, H.H., and Stewart, C.M. (2020). SARS-CoV-2 isolated from the mastoid and middle ear: Implications for COVID-19 precautions during ear surgery. *JAMA Otolaryngology-Head & Neck Surgery* 146: 964–969.

Garg, R.K., Mahadevan, A., Malhotra, H.S., Rizvi, I. Kumar, N., and Uniyal, R. (2019). Subacute sclerosing panencephalitis. *Reviews of Medical Virology* 29: e2058. doi: 10.1002/rmv.2058.

Gold, I., and Roskies, A.L. (2008). Philosophy of Neuroscience. In M. Ruse (Ed.) *The Oxford Handbook of Philosophy of Biology*. New York: Oxford University Press, pp. 349–380.

Gouvea dos Santos, W. (2020). Natural history of COVID-19 and current knowledge on treatment and therapeutics. *Biomedicine and Pharmacotherapy* 129: 110493. doi: 10.1016/j.biopha.2020.110493.

Hacking, I. (1983). *Representing and Intervening.* Cambridge: Cambridge University Press.

Hardcastle, V.G. (2017). Thinking about the brain: What is the meaning of neuroscience knowledge and technologies for capital mitigation? In E.C. Monahan and J.J. Clark (Eds.) *Mitigation in Capital Cases: Understanding and Communicating the Life-Story.* Washington, DC: American Bar Association, Chapter 5.

Hardcastle, V.G., and Hardcastle, K. (2015). A new appreciation of Marr's levels: Understanding how brains break. *Topics in Cognitive Science* 7: 259–273.

Heneka, M.T., Golenback, D., Latz, E., Morgan, D., and Brown, R. (2020). Immediate and long-term consequences of COVID-19 infections for the development of neurological disease. *Alzheimer's Research & Therapy* 12: 69 doi: 10.1186/s13195-020-00640-3.

Helms, J., Kremer, S., Merdji, H., Clere-Jehl, R., Schenck, M., Kummerlen, C., Collange, O., Boulay, C., Fafi-Kremer, S., Ohana, M., Anheim, M., and Meziani, F. (2020). Neurologic features in severe SARS-CoV-2 infection. *New England Journal of Medicine* 382: 2268–2270. doi: 10.1056/NEJMc2008597.

Hoffman, L.A., and Vilensky, J.A. (2017). Encephalitis lethargica: 100 Years after the epidemic. *Brain* 140: 2246–2251.

Hubel, D.H. (1996). David H. Hubel. In L. Squire (Ed.) *The History of Neuroscience in Autobiography, Volume 1.* Washington, DC: Society for Neuroscience, pp. 294–317.

Jensen, M.P., Le Quesne, L., Officer-Jones, J., Teodiósio, A., Traventhiran, J. Ficken, C., Goddard, M., Smith, C., Menon, D., and Allinson, K.S.J. (2020). Neuropathological findings in two patients with fatal COVID-19. *Neuropathology and Applied Neurobiology* 47: 17–25 doi: 10.1111/nan.12662.

Jiao, L., Yang, Y., Yu, W., Zhou, Y., Long, H. Gao, J., Ding, K. Ma, C., Zhao, S., Wang, J., Li, H., Yang, M., Xu, J., Want, J., Yang, J., Kuang, ., Luo, F., Qian, X., Xu, L., Yin, B., Liu, W., Lu, S., and Peng, X. (2021). The olfactory route is a potential way for SARS-CoV-2 to invade the central nervous system of rhesus monkeys. *Signal Transduction and Targeted Therapy* 6: 169. doi: 10. 1038/s41392-021-00591-7.

Kahn, J.S., and MacIntosh, K. (2005). History and recent advances in coronavirus discovery. *The Pediatric Infectious Disease Journal* 24: S223–S227.

Kelly, H. Peck. H.A., Laurie, K.L., Wu, P., Nishiura, H., and Cowling, B.J. (2011). The age-specific cumulative incidence of infection with pandemic influenza H1N1 2009 was similar invarious countries prior to vaccination. *PLoS One* 6(8): e21828. doi: 10.1371/journal.pone.0021828.

Kuhn, T. (1962). *The Structure of Scientific Revolutions.* Chicago, IL: University of Chicago Press.

Kulcsar, M.A., Montenego, F.L., Arap, S.S., Tavares, M. R., and Kowalski, L.P. (2020). High risk of COVID-19 for head and neck surgeons. *International Archives of Otorhinolaryngology* 24: e129–e130.

Lago, M.N. (2020). How did we get here? Short history of COVID-19 and other coronavirus epidemics. *Head & Neck* 42:1535–1538.

Lechien, J.R., Chiesa-Estomba, C.M., Beckers, E., Mustin, V., M. Ducarme, M. Journe, J., Marchant, A., Jouffe, L., Barillari, M.R., Cammaroto, G., Circiu, M.P., Hans, S., and Saussez, S. (2021). Prevalence and 6-month recovery of olfactory dysfunction: A multicentre study of 1363 COVID-19 patients. *Journal of Internal Medicine.* doi: 10.1111/joim.13209.

Lee, M.H., Perl, D.P., Nair, G. Li, W., Maric, D., Murray, H., Dodd, S.J., Koretsky, A.P., Watts, J.A., Cheung, V., Masliah, E., Horkayne-Szakaly, I., Jones, R., Stram, M.N., Moncur, J., Hefti, M., Folkerth, R.D., and Nath, A. (2021). Microvascular injury in the brains of patients with Covid-19. *New England Journal of Medicine* 384: 481–483.

Liu, Y.-C., Kuo, R.-L., and Shih, S.-R. (2020). COVID-19: The first documented coronavirus in history. *Science Direct Biomedical Journal* 43: 328–333.

Meinhardt, J., Radke, J., Dittmayer, C. et al. (2021). Olfactory transmucosal SARS-CoV-2 invasion as a port of central nervous system entry in individuals with COVID-19. *Nature Neuroscience* 24: 168–175.

Mukerji, S.S., and Solomon, I.H. (2021). What can we learn from brain autopsies in COVID-19? *Neuroscience Letters* 742:135528.

Nauen, D.W., Hooper, J.E., Stewart, C.M., and Solomon, I.H. (2021). Assessing brain capillaries in coronavirus 2019. *JAMA Neurology* 78: 760–762. doi: 10.1001/jamaneurol.2021.0225.

Portmann, G., and Colleagues (1939). Translated by P. Voilé. *A Treatise on the Surgical Technique of Otorhinolaryngology*. Baltimore, MD: William Wood & Company, Medical Division, The Williams & Wilkens Co.

Pratt, J., Lester, E., and Parker, R. (2021). Could SARS-CoV-2 cause tauopathy? *The Lancet* 20: P506. doi: 10.1016/S1474-4422(21)00168-X.

Puelles, V.G., Lütgehetmann, M., Lindenmeyer, M.T. et al. (2020). Multiorgan and renal tropism of SARS-CoV-2. *New England Journal of Medicine* 38: 590–592.

Rapkiewicz, A.T., Mait, X., Carsons, S.E., Pittaluga, S., Kleiner, D. Berger, J., Thomas, S., Adler, N.M., Charytan, D.M., Gasmi, B., Hochman, J.S., and Reynolds, H.R. (2020). Megakaryocytes and platelet-fibrin thrombi characterize multi-organ thrombosis at autopsy in COVID-19: A case series. *EClinicalMedicine*. 24: 100434. doi: 10.1016/j.eclinm.2020.100434.

Reichard, R.R., Kashani, K.B., Boire, N.A., Constantopoulos, E., Guo, Y., and Lucchinetti, C.F. (2020). Neuropathology of COVID-19: A spectrum of vascular and acute disseminated encephalomyelitis (ADEM)-like pathology. *Acta Neuropathologica* 140: 1–6.

Remmelink, M., De Mendonca, R., D'Haene, N. De Clercq, S., Verocq, C., Lebrun, L., Lavis, P., Racu, M-L., Trepant, A-L, Maris, C., Rovive, S., Goffard, J-C., De Witte, O., Peluso, L., Vincent, J-L., Decaestecker, C., Taccone, F.S., and Salmon, I. (2020). Unspecific post-mortem findings despite multiorgan viral spread in COVID-19 patients. *Critical Care* 24: 495.

Solomon, I.H., Normandin, E., Bhattacharyya, S. Mukerji, S.S., Ali, A.S., Adams, G., Hormick, J.L. Padera, R.F., and Sabeti, P. (2020). Neuropathological features of Covid-19. *New England Journal of Medicine* 383: 989–992.

Stix, G. (2012). A Q&A with Ian Hacking on Thomas Kuhn's legacy as "the paradigm shift" turns 50. *Scientific American* (April). https://www.scientificamerican.com/article/kuhn/.

Thakur, K.T., Miller, E.H., Glendinning, M.D., Al-Dalahman, A., Banu, M.A., Boehm, A.K. et al. (2021). COVID-19 neuropathology at Columbia University Irving Medical Center/New York Presbyterian Hospital. *Brain*. doi: 10.1093/brain/awab148.

Uranaka, T., Kashio, A., Ueha, R., Sato, T., Bing, H.Ying, G., Kinoshita, M., Kondo, K., and Yamasoba, T. (2020). Expression of ACE2, TMPRSS2, and furin in mouse ear tissue and the implications for SARS-CoV-2 infection. *The Laryngoscope* 131: E2013–E217. doi: 10.1002/lary.29324.

Van Waegeningh, H.F., Ebbens, F.A., van Spronsen, E., and Oostra, R.-J. (2019). Single origin of the epithelium of the human middle ear. *Mechanisms of Development* 158: 103556. doi: 10.1016/j.mod.2019.103556.

Wagner, T., Schweta, F.N.U., Murugadoss, K. et al. (2020). Augmented curation of clinical notes from a massive EHR system reveals symptoms of impending COVID-19 diagnosis. *eLife* 9: e58227. doi: 10.7554/eLife.58227.

Wichmann, D, Sperhake, J.P., Lutgehetmann, M. et al. (2020). Autopsy findings and venous thromboembolism in patients with COVID-19: A prospective cohort study. *Annals of Internal Medicine* 173: 268–277.

World Health Organization (2003). Emergency preparedness, response. Update 83 – One hundred days into the [SARS] outbreak. https://www.who.int/csr/don/20030618/en.

World Health Organization (2020). Coronavirus disease 2019 (COVID-19). Situation report – 16. https://www.who.int/emergencies/diseases/novel-coronavirus-2019/situationreports.

World Health Organization (2021). Coronavirus. https://www.who.int/health-topics/coronavirus#tab=tab1.

Yang, A.C., Kern, F., Losada, P.M. et al. (2021). Dysregulation of brain and choroid plexus cell types in severe COVID-19. *Nature*. doi: 10.1038/s41586-021-03710-0.

Zubair, A.S., McAlpine, L.S., Gardin, T., Farhadian, S., Kuruvilla, D.E., and Spudich, S. (2020). Neuropathogenesis and neurologic manifestations of the coronaviruses in the age of coronavirus disease 2019: A review. *JAMA Neurology* 77: 1018–1027. doi: 10.1001/jamaneurol.2020.2065.

Section 2

Research Tools and Epistemology

6 Dissemination and Adaptiveness as Key Variables in Tools That Fuel Scientific Revolutions

Alcino J. Silva

1 Introduction

New tools have often been catalysts of scientific revolutions in neuroscience, from the role of the Golgi stain in the discovery of neurons to the recent transformation of systems neuroscience by both optogenetics and ground-breaking neuronal imaging methods. Sophisticated tools open doors to novel observations and ideas, but not all new tools are either feasibly adaptable to multiple related uses or equally accessible to neuroscientists. In this chapter, I will discuss the idea that the power of a new tool is not only dependent on its ability to reveal new potentially transformative phenomena but also on its adaptiveness, ease of use and transferability. The impact of prohibitively complex or inaccessible tools is often limited by the relatively small number of laboratories that eventually use them, while the power of accessible and nimble tools is amplified by their wide dissemination. The ability to carry out replication and convergent follow up experiments is at the very heart of scientific revolutions in biology, and therefore most of the tools that fuel innovative leaps in neuroscience, and in other biological disciplines, are almost without exception very flexible and easily accessible to the majority of practitioners in their respective fields. I will illustrate these ideas by using examples from the recent history of neuroscience, and I will finish the chapter by predicting that a new set of tools that has just become available to neuroscientists, and with the properties mentioned above, will have a significant impact on the field, including in bridging the current gap between molecular and systems studies in neuroscience.

2 The Molecular Genetics Revolution in Neuroscience: Some Personal Reflections

I still remember as a new graduate student in 1983 the sense of wonder of opening Maniatis, as we then called Tom Maniatis' highly influential Molecular Cloning Laboratory Manual (Maniatis, et al. 1982). That incredible blue book included simple protocols for most of the techniques I would use in the next five years of my Ph.D. studies in

DOI: 10.4324/9781003251392-9

the early days of the molecular biology and human genetics revolution (McConkey 1993). Naively, I assumed that the accessibility and adaptiveness inherent in most tools that fueled the molecular biology and genetics revolutions were common to all disciplines in biology. I quickly discovered that matters were very different in neuroscience, the field I decided to join. In the late eighties, there were deep divisions amongst neuroscience fields that could be easily traced back to the tools that individual labs had access to. Strange that it may seem to neuroscientists now, at that time neuroscience areas were mostly defined by the tools used. For example, memory was studied by behavioral neuroscientists, electrophysiologists and molecular biologists, but there was hardly any overlap between the approaches they used and consequently the results they published. For example, behavioral assays and brain lesion tools were used in behavioral neuroscience to define the brain structures involved in specific forms of memory (e.g., spatial memory), while electrophysiologists used electrodes to probe the synaptic mechanisms thought to underlie memory (e.g., long term potentiation or LTP), and molecular biologists were busy cloning the molecules (e.g., receptors, kinases) that they thought may mediate mechanisms of memory. The barriers between fields were so deep that there was even a deeply entrenched reluctance to cross them. I will never forget being reminded mockingly by a leading neuroscientist that my "amateurish efforts" to use molecular genetics, electrophysiology and behavioral neuroscience approaches in my new laboratory were naïve since I would be a "jack of all trades and master of none" (Nelson 2015)!

But all of this would eventually change with the wide use of transgenic tools in neuroscience research (Grant and Silva 1994; Silva and Giese 1994; Tonegawa, et al. 1995; Silva 1996; Silva, et al. 1997). These tools would break barriers between neuroscience fields and open the doors to the integrative studies that now dominate the field (Silva, et al. 1997). I still remember during my post-doctoral studies my first day in Jeanne Wehner's laboratory, and the excitement of starting behavioral studies of the alpha calmodulin kinase II knockout mice that I had generated in Susumu Tonegawa's laboratory. With her post-doctoral fellow Richard Paylor, we showed that these mutant mice had deficits in hippocampal learning (Silva, et al. 1992)! Then, I took the same knockout mice to Charles Stevens laboratory, where along with Yanyan Wang we discovered deficits in LTP induction(Silva, et al. 1992), thus tentatively connecting the loss of that synaptic kinase (Bennett, et al. 1983) with hippocampal LTP and hippocampal-dependent learning (Silva, et al. 1997). In my own laboratory in 1992, we managed to have behavioral neuroscientists, electrophysiologists and molecular biologists working side by side, and the same was starting to happen in other neuroscience laboratories (Silva, et al. 1997). Mutant mice served as bridges between previously separate fields in neuroscience, thus fueling a revolution that transformed the field (Mayford, et al. 1995; Silva, et al. 1997).

Transgenic mice, flies and worms are very flexible and easily disseminated tools, since mutants can be generated for almost every gene of interest, and then shared amongst laboratories. In the years that followed those early heady days, countless mutants were used as integrative tools by hundreds of laboratories to test or unravel molecular and cellular mechanisms of nearly every behavior that had ever been studied (Bickle 2016). Within a few years, viral vectors were introduced to mutate specific regions of the mammalian brain, so as to confer molecular, cellular and brain region specificity to studies of behavior (Chen, et al. 2019; Nectow and Nestler 2020). At the same time, mutant mice were also used in systems neuroscience studies (Rotenberg, et al. 1996; Cho, et al. 1998), and they were instrumental in establishing connections between this field and others in neuroscience, including molecular, cellular and behavioral neuroscience. It is now difficult to find neuroscience papers in high-profile journals that do not share the integrative character of these early mutant mouse studies. A flexible and easy to share tool (i.e., mutant mice) has essentially completely transformed neuroscience in a way that was difficult to predict at the time (Morris and Kennedy 1992). I will never forget the attacks that the field suffered in the early days of this integrative effort. Many of our colleagues thought implicitly or explicitly that nothing of consequence could be gained from studies that dared to bridge the gaps between fields as far afield as molecular biology and behavioral neuroscience (Nelson 2015). Their compelling arguments invoked the necessary superficiality of such studies, the "inevitable" lack of deep expertise involved, and the "unavoidable errors" that would come from such amateurism. Their arguments were not without merit, but everything had been changed by the irresistible prospect of making causal connections across neuroscience fields, from molecular mechanisms, to the cellular properties they regulated, to systems processes mediated by these cellular mechanisms, all the way to behavior. The ruthless reductionism (Bickle 2007) inherent in work with molecular genetic tools had opened new broad horizons in neuroscience and there was no going back. The power of these new tools was inextricably linked to their easy dissemination, adaptability and wide range of experimental applications (Bickle 2016).

3 The Optogenetics Revolution in Systems Neuroscience

The optogenetics revolution in systems neuroscience (Yizhar, et al. 2011; Goshen 2014) is another example of the power that easily disseminated and highly adaptive tools can have in a field (Bickle 2016). Before these tools completely transformed the field, systems neuroscience studies were heavily dependent on electrophysiological recordings and computational modeling (Yizhar, et al. 2011). For example, electro-physiological approaches record the profiles of action potentials of neurons under different conditions and computational modeling attempts to capture and account for these profiles in ways that are generative (i.e., lead to further experiments that test the validity of the models). These models are not necessarily explanatory causal statements (Buzsáki 2019), but instead mathematical formulations or computational simulations that attempt to capture the complexity of the brain systems studied. The discovery of proteins that can be used to either activate or inhibit neurons with light (i.e., opsins) changed all of this (Boyden 2011). With these methods, ideas and hypotheses could now be tested with a number of experiments that directly manipulated the activity state of specific neurons in targeted brain regions of behaving animals (Yizhar, et al. 2011)! The initial optogenetic tools were followed within an astoundingly short time by a large number of other opsins with special properties that allowed for previously unimaginable experiments (Rost, et al. 2017), such as the specific activation and inhibition of nerve terminals between two connected brain regions! The tsunami of papers that followed was only possible because these tools were easily disseminated and extremely flexible: opsin genes could be easily shared amongst laboratories, and widespread genetic methods resulted in the engineering of novel opsins with a wide range of different uses. The proliferation of experiments where specific neurons could be precisely activated or inhibited with a range of optogenetic tools changed fundamentally the epistemological nature of systems neuroscience since these powerful tools allowed the direct testing of causal explanations between neuronal phenomena and brain states and behavior (Bickle 2016). This epistemological approach had fueled the molecular biology revolution, and now it had made its way into systems neuroscience!

4 Tools for Defining and Connecting Phenomena in Neuroscience

With this historical context set, I will describe next in detail key aspects of this epistemology and how it could guide tool development. Tools can be used to define the properties of phenomena (e.g., the sequence of a gene, the shape of a synapse, the activation state of an ensemble of neurons, the behavioral state of an animal), and to test possible causal connections between these phenomena (e.g., whether a specific gene regulates changes in the shape of synapses, the activation of memory ensembles and memory formation itself) (Silva, et al. 2014; Bickle 2016). Understanding the rules of how phenomena are defined and connected can be useful in determining the tools that could have the biggest impact at any one time in a particular field. Convergent evidence is critical for both defining and establishing causal connections amongst phenomena, and therefore it is important to define rules for measuring the degree of convergence in any one set of experiments (see below). Consistency is also critical in defining and connecting phenomena, and it is a key consideration in evaluating any tool: the lower the variability between the outcomes of identical experiments, the higher the usefulness of a given tool (Silva, et al. 2014).

To better define the role of tools in testing convergence in experimental findings, I will start by introducing the different categories of experiments to test or establish causality (i.e., connection experiments) commonly carried out in neuroscience (Silva, et al. 2014; Matiasz, et al. 2017; Matiasz, et al. 2018). In Positive Intervention experiments ($\uparrow$), the quantity or probability of one phenomenon (i.e., an Agent) is actively increased, and the change or lack of change in another (i.e., the Target) is measured. In contrast, in a Negative Intervention experiment ($\downarrow$), either the quantity or probability of an Agent is actively decreased, and the impact on a Target is measured. In a Positive Non-Intervention experiment ($\varnothing\uparrow$), an increase in either the quantity or probability of the Agent is observed without intervention and the effects on a Target are measured, while in a Negative Non-Intervention experiment ($\varnothing\downarrow$), a decrease in either the quantity or probability of the Agent is observed without intervention and the effects on a Target are measured. Convergence (or lack of) between the results of experiments in the categories just outlined is commonly used to evaluate the strength of evidence for any potential causal connection in biology, including neuroscience. Neuroscientists and other biologists also commonly perform a fifth type of experiment, a Multi-Intervention (∇), in which more than one Agent is either positively or negatively manipulated simultaneously to determine whether one or more secondary Agents mediate the effect of some primary Agent on a given Target. This last type of experiment is critical in testing causal paths between multiple phenomena (Bickle and Kostko 2018). Research-Maps (Matiasz, et al. 2017, 2018), an online computational tool (researchmaps.org), uses these experimental categories to generate causal maps of biological phenomena.

The strength of evidence for causal connections depends on the availability of tools for Intervention and Non-Intervention experiments, and therefore it is easy to see how the categories outlined above are used explicitly or implicitly to guide tool development. For example, late in my graduate studies I became fascinated with the emerging literature of molecular changes associated with brain states and behavior (Kennedy 1983). These Non-Intervention studies were thought-provoking, and it became apparent that there was a great need for approaches (i.e., Intervention tools) that could manipulate these molecular processes to test whether they had meaningful effects on a number of other phenomena, including behavioral phenomena, such as learning and memory. Pharmacological manipulations were limited by the difficulty of developing drugs with the molecular specificity and toxicology profile required for neuroscience experiments. I had the good fortune of doing my Ph.D. studies next door to Mario Capecchi, one of the inventors of a set of tools that allow for the manipulation of any gene in mice (i.e., gene targeting) (Capecchi 1989), and I decided to use these gene Intervention tools in my post-doctoral studies in neuroscience. As described above, my Negative Intervention experiments with the newly developed gene targeting approach (Capecchi 1989) were critical in implicating the alpha calmodulin kinase II in synaptic plasticity and memory (Silva, et al. 1992; Silva, et al. 1992), and they complemented Non-Intervention experiments that suggested a role for this general class of molecules in plasticity and memory (Silva, et al. 1992). Mouse transgenic tools, such as gene targeting, continue to have a key role in neuroscience. Because of their wide application, these techniques can be used for Positive and Negative Intervention experiments to test the role of any gene in any other phenomena of interest.

Beyond connecting phenomena, tools are also critical for defining the identity or properties of phenomena (i.e., identity experiments) (Silva, et al. 2014; Bickle 2016). Just as with connection experiments, convergence and consistency are also critical for identity experiments: When the same method gives reproducible results, and multiple methods give convergent results concerning the properties of a given phenomenon, then we can be assured that the results of the identity experiments in question are reliable. For example, in defining spatial learning, neuroscientists use multiple methods including the Morris water maze (Morris 1981), where animals swim in a pool of water looking for a hidden platform, and the Barne's Maze (Barnes 1979), where rodents escape a brightly lit open field by learning to navigate to a hole with an escape box. These two behavioral tools are very different, but they have one thing in common: they measure spatial learning and memory performance. Therefore, finding that a given manipulation (genetic, pharmacological, systems, etc.) affects both tasks in the same way (e.g., performance is disrupted or enhanced) is compelling evidence that it affects spatial learning and memory. Similarly, hippocampal CA1 place cells can be defined with electrophysiological (O'Keefe and Nadel 1978) and imaging methods (Dombeck, et al. 2010): finding that manipulating phenomenon A in the hippocampal CA1region disrupts the ability of these cells to fire in a location-specific manner, measured with these two dramatically different methods, argues that phenomenon A has a role in place specific firing in that region. Thus, convergence and consistency are critical for tools used in both connection and identity experiments. Convergence and consistency are also critical in experiments designed for tool development and characterization (Silva, et al. 2014; Bickle 2016).

5 Tools for the Next Revolution in Neuroscience

Epistemological ideas, including those concerning the role of tools in discovery, can not only be used to account for previous revolutions in science, but more importantly, these ideas can hopefully be useful in predicting and guiding future scientific developments. Although this is by no means universally agreed to (see for example Chicharro and Ledberg 2012; Buzsáki 2019) many neuroscientists believe that the key goal of studies in Neuroscience is to account for brain states and behavior with causal explanations that include multiple levels of analyses (e.g., molecular, cellular, systems, brain regions, cognitive) (Silva, et al. 2014; Bickle 2016; Sudhof 2017). However, currently, there is a deep chiasm in neuroscience between molecular explanations of brain states and behavior (i.e., molecular neuroscience) and those explanations centered on brain systems (i.e., systems neuroscience). One of the reasons for this chiasm is the lack of tools to test molecular explanations of systems phenomena associated with brain states and behavior. Tools that address this problem could have a profound impact in neuroscience research (Callaway 2005; Sudhof 2017). Ideally, these tools would be able to track (i.e., for non-intervention experiments) and manipulate (i.e., for intervention experiments) molecular function with the appropriate temporal resolution, cellular and brain region specificity required for the study of circuits, and their impact on brain states and behavior. Remarkably, although these very tools (see below) have been developed for other purposes, such as cancer research, they have been rarely used in neuroscience. Below, I will review only a couple of examples from each category of novel tools that could be used to bridge the gap between molecular neuroscience and system neuroscience studies. This is not meant as a comprehensive review of this fast-growing field. Instead, the examples below were chosen to illustrate the types of tools that I believe could have a transformative impact in systems neuroscience. Again, the power of a new tool is critically dependent on its adaptiveness, ease of use and transferability. The classes of tools I will discuss next have these properties and this is one of the reasons I believe they will become central to neuroscience research.

5.1 Imaging Systems

Miniaturized head-mounted fluorescent microscopes, (miniscopes), capable of recording from hundreds of cells (including neurons) for days or weeks in freely moving and behaving mice and other animals (Ghosh, et al. 2011; Ziv, et al. 2013; Cai, et al. 2016; Liberti, et al. 2017; Jacob, et al. 2018; Aharoni, et al. 2019), are a powerful and easily disseminated tool. Single unit recording systems, commonly used in systems neuroscience studies, require significant expertise, considerable time investment, and can only stably record neuronal activity for hours. In contrast, miniscopes require no previous experience with *in vivo* recordings, laboratories can even manufacture these miniscopes themselves at very low costs and stable neuronal recordings can be routinely made for days or even weeks.

Although currently miniscopes have limited sensitivity and resolution, upcoming technological improvements promise to overcome these limitations. An important facet of miniscopes is the ongoing community-based improvement in their design, which continues to add new features, such as for example, the ability to activate optogenetic tools in the very fields of view (with closed-loop approaches [Potter, et al. 2014]) that are being imaged (Stamatakis, et al. 2018). This opened up the exciting possibility of simultaneously tracking and manipulating molecular function in specific cells and circuits of behaving animals, such as mice.

The inexpensive nature and considerable power of miniscope systems, and consequently their expected widespread use in neuroscience laboratories world-wide, promises to be a significant catalyst for innovation in systems neuroscience. Until recently, miniscopes have been almost solely used for imaging changes in calcium concentration in neurons *in vivo*. However, new molecular sensor developments (see below) promise to dramatically expand the range of biological applications for this class of imaging tools.

Recent advances in imaging go well beyond miniscopes, and include other major advances which employ much larger, more technologically complex and far more expensive microscopes used with head-fixed animals, such as the two-photon mesoscope (Sofroniew, et al. 2016) and holographic two-photon imaging (Yang, et al. 2018). However, these systems' cost and complexity preclude their easy dissemination, and therefore most likely will limit the impact that they could have on neuroscience research.

5.2 *Molecular Sensors and Reporters*

In parallel with novel imaging devices, there has also been considerable progress in molecular sensors and reporters that could be used to dramatically expand the scope of these imaging systems (Chen, et al. 2013; Wang, et al. 2018). Fluorescence, autofluorescence and bioluminescence have been used to engineer a plethora of different molecular reporters and sensors that could potentially be coupled with imaging technologies (see above) to track the activation of specific molecular mechanisms in a cell and circuit-specific manner in behaving mice, rats and other animals. For example, Synapto-pHluorin is a novel pH imaging sensor that includes the transmembrane synaptic vesicle protein VAMP2, and a specific pHluorin called ecliptic pHluorin (Granseth, et al. 2006;

Rose, et al. 2013). Within the low pH milieu inside of transmitter vesicles, synapto-pHluorin is non-fluorescent. When vesicles are released, however, and synapto-pHluorin is exposed to the neutral extracellular space, it is brightly fluorescent, thus allowing for visualization of synaptic release events in a circuit-specific manner. Since they are essentially molecular biology tools that can be delivered to specific cell populations in the brain with widely used viral vectors, these molecular sensors will be easily disseminated and easily adapted for the study of any behavior or brain state.

5.3 Light Activated Manipulation of Molecular Mechanisms

Optogenetic tools have also been recently developed to manipulate most intracellular signaling events, from ligand binding, receptor activation, associated intracellular signaling, all the way to activation/suppression of gene expression, and protein translation (Rost, et al. 2017; Kwon and Heo 2020). For example, optical modulation approaches combined with sophisticated genetic methods have been used to modulate receptor function in specific cells of targeted systems and in defined brain regions (e.g., Kim, et al. 2005; Airan, et al. 2009). Neurotransmitter receptors, such as those for noradrenaline, serotonin, glutamate, GABA, and dopamine, have had a key role in systems neuroscience, and these novel optical manipulation tools that have been used to control the function of receptors in real time, provide an unprecedented opportunity to modulate associated molecular signaling mechanisms in a cell, circuit and brain region-specific manner, thus allowing for experiments that could connect molecular properties associated with these receptors with cellular and circuit processes modulating brain states and behavior.

In addition to receptor function, there are also optogenetic approaches to control protein interaction, phosphorylation, cleavage, aggregation/disaggregation, allosteric changes, etc. (Kwon and Heo 2020). For example, to control protein-protein interactions optogenetically, several Light-Inducible Dimerization (LIDs) systems have been developed that employ light-sensitive domains, including Phy-PIF, DrBphP, LOV2, and CRY2-Cib (Zhang, et al. 2016; Klewer and Wu 2019; McCormick, et al. 2020). These domains change conformation after light activation, and this has been used to regulate specific protein-protein interactions and consequently their function (Kakumoto and Nakata 2013; Zhang, et al. 2014). In addition to controlling dimerization/aggregation, optogenetic approaches have also been used to control enzyme activity by taking advantage of light-triggered changes in protein conformation (Nguyen, et al. 2016).

Other than controlling intracellular signaling, opto-tools have also been engineered to modulate transcription. For example, site-specific recombinase systems, such as Cre/Loxp, Flp/FRT, have been widely used in viral vectors and in transgenic mice for modulating genes in a cell-type specific manner (Wang, et al. 2011). To improve the temporal regulation of these approaches, multiple variants were engineered that allow for tight regulation by light (Schindler, et al. 2015; Kawano, et al. 2016; Jung, et al. 2019; Yao, et al. 2020). Importantly, there are approaches that depend on infrared deep brain stimulation and ultrasensitive opsins that do not require cannulae implantation and associated damage of brain tissue (Chen, et al. 2018; Jung, et al. 2019; Gong, et al. 2020). Again, these genetic tools can be delivered to any cell population in the brain with widely used viral vectors, and they can be adapted to test their impact on any behavior or brain state.

6 Molecules, Systems and Behavior

The incredibly powerful imaging and manipulation tools mentioned above (and many others that we did not have space to review) will revolutionize systems neuroscience. It is important to acknowledge the seminal contributions that systems neuroscience has made despite the fact that until recently (see above) the majority of studies in the field were exclusively focused on a small subset of cellular properties (electrical properties such as action potentials) of a single brain cell type (neurons), and that they were carried out mostly with a single class (electrophysiology) of experimental approaches. This success is truly remarkable, since we now have overwhelming evidence that the complexity of brain states and behavior can be ascribed to nearly every cell type in the brain (e.g., glia [Stevens 2003]), and can be traced back to a wide range of biological mechanisms that go well beyond the electrical properties of neurons. Despite the continuing success of traditional neuroscience approaches, it is clear now that imaging and manipulating the very molecular properties that both shaped brain systems (not just neuronal circuits) during evolution, and that now account for and constrain much of their functionality, will open countless windows into the properties and mechanisms of the systems (neuronal, glial, etc.) that underlie the wonderful complexity of brain states and behavior.

7 Conclusion

In this chapter, I discussed how novel tools can be the catalysts of innovation, and reviewed key properties, including ease of dissemination and adaptability, that allow tools to open doors to ground-breaking observations and ideas. I argued that the potential usefulness of a new tool is not only dependent on its ability to reveal new potentially transformative phenomena, but also on its ease of use, adaptability and transferability.

The ability to readily carry out replication and convergent follow up experiments in many laboratories is at the very heart of scientific revolutions in biology, and therefore most of the tools that fuel innovative leaps in neuroscience, and in other biological disciplines, are frequently very flexible and easily accessible to practitioners in the field. I propose that molecular optogenetic tools, capable of optically tracking and manipulating a wide range of molecular phenomena in diverse cell types and systems in the brain of behaving animals, will be key catalysts for an upcoming wave of innovation in neuroscience. These nimble and easily disseminated tools will not only catalyze a much-needed synthesis between molecular and systems neuroscience, they will also move systems neuroscience away from its neurocentric roots to a more biological realistic inclusion of other cell types including for example astrocytes, glia and oligodendrocytes.

References

Aharoni, D., B. S. Khakh, A. J. Silva and P. Golshani (2019). "All the light that we can see: a new era in miniaturized microscopy." *Nat Methods* **16**(1): 11–13.

Airan, R. D., K. R. Thompson, L. E. Fenno, H. Bernstein and K. Deisseroth (2009). "Temporally precise *in vivo* control of intracellular signalling." *Nature* **458**(7241): 1025–1029.

Barnes, C. A. (1979). "Memory deficits associated with senescence: a neurophysiological and behavioral study in the rat." *J Comp Physiol Psychol* **93**(1): 74–104.

Bennett, M. K., N. E. Erondu and M. B. Kennedy (1983). "Purification and characterization of a calmodulin-dependent protein kinase that is highly concentrated in brain." *J Biol Chem* **258**(20): 12735–12744.

Bickle, J. (2007). "Ruthless reductionism and social cognition." *J Physiol Paris* **101**(4–6): 230–235.

Bickle, J. (2016). "Revolutions in neuroscience: tool development." *Front Syst Neurosci* **10**: 24.

Bickle, J. and A. Kostko (2018). "Connection experiments in neurobiology." *Synthese* **195**: 5271–5295.

Boyden, E. S. (2011). "A history of optogenetics: the development of tools for controlling brain circuits with light." *F1000 Biol Rep* **3**: 11.

Buzsáki, G. (2019). *The Brain from Inside Out*. New York, Oxford University Press.

Cai, D. J., D. Aharoni, T. Shuman, J. Shobe, J. Biane, W. Song, B. Wei, M. Veshkini, M. La-Vu, J. Lou, S. E. Flores, I. Kim, Y. Sano, M. Zhou, K. Baumgaertel, A. Lavi, M. Kamata, M. Tuszynski, M. Mayford, P. Golshani and A. J. Silva (2016). "A shared neural ensemble links distinct contextual memories encoded close in time." *Nature* **534**(7605): 115–118.

Callaway, E. M. (2005). "A molecular and genetic arsenal for systems neuroscience." *Trends Neurosci* **28**(4): 196–201.

Capecchi, M. R. (1989). "The new mouse genetics: altering the genome by gene targeting." *Trends Genet.* **5**(3): 70–76.

Chen, S., A. Z. Weitemier, X. Zeng, L. He, X. Wang, Y. Tao, A. J. Y. Huang, Y. Hashimotodani, M. Kano, H. Iwasaki, L. K. Parajuli, S. Okabe, D. B. L. Teh, A. H. All, I. Tsutsui-Kimura, K. F. Tanaka, X. Liu and T. J. McHugh (2018). "Near-infrared deep brain stimulation via upconversion nanoparticle-mediated optogenetics." *Science* 359(6376): 679–684.

Chen, S. H., J. Haam, M. Walker, E. Scappini, J. Naughton and N. P. Martin (2019). "Recombinant Viral Vectors as Neuroscience Tools." *Curr Protoc Neurosci* 87(1): e67.

Chen, T. W., T. J. Wardill, Y. Sun, S. R. Pulver, S. L. Renninger, A. Baohan, E. R. Schreiter, R. A. Kerr, M. B. Orger, V. Jayaraman, L. L. Looger, K. Svoboda and D. S. Kim (2013). "Ultrasensitive fluorescent proteins for imaging neuronal activity." *Nature* 499(7458): 295–300.

Chicharro, D. and A. Ledberg (2012). "When two become one: the limits of causality analysis of brain dynamics." *PLoS One* 7(3): e32466.

Cho, Y. H., K. P. Giese, H. Tanila, A. J. Silva and H. Eichenbaum (1998). "Abnormal hippocampal spatial representations in alphaCaMKIIT286A and CREBalphaDelta-mice." *Science* 279(5352): 867–869.

Dombeck, D. A., C. D. Harvey, L. Tian, L. L. Looger and D. W. Tank (2010). "Functional imaging of hippocampal place cells at cellular resolution during virtual navigation." *Nat Neurosci* 13(11): 1433–1440.

Ghosh, K. K., L. D. Burns, E. D. Cocker, A. Nimmerjahn, Y. Ziv, A. E. Gamal and M. J. Schnitzer (2011). "Miniaturized integration of a fluorescence microscope." *Nat Methods* 8(10): 871–878.

Gong, X., D. Mendoza-Halliday, J. T. Ting, T. Kaiser, X. Sun, A. M. Bastos, R. D. Wimmer, B. Guo, Q. Chen, Y. Zhou, M. Pruner, C. W. Wu, D. Park, K. Deisseroth, B. Barak, E. S. Boyden, E. K. Miller, M. M. Halassa, Z. Fu, G. Bi, R. Desimone and G. Feng (2020). "An ultra-sensitive step-function opsin for minimally invasive optogenetic stimulation in mice and macaques." *Neuron* 107: 38–51.

Goshen, I. (2014). "The optogenetic revolution in memory research." *Trends Neurosci* 37(9): 511–522.

Granseth, B., B. Odermatt, S. J. Royle and L. Lagnado (2006). "Clathrin-mediated endocytosis is the dominant mechanism of vesicle retrieval at hippocampal synapses." *Neuron* 51(6): 773–786.

Grant, S. G. and A. J. Silva (1994). "Targeting learning." *Trends in Neurosciences* 17(2): 71–75.

Jacob, A. D., A. I. Ramsaran, A. J. Mocle, L. M. Tran, C. Yan, P. W. Frankland and S. A. Josselyn (2018). "A compact head-mounted endoscope for *in vivo* calcium imaging in freely behaving mice." *Curr Protoc Neurosci* 84(1): e51.

Jung, H., S. W. Kim, M. Kim, J. Hong, D. Yu, J. H. Kim, Y. Lee, S. Kim, D. Woo, H. S. Shin, B. O. Park and W. D. Heo (2019). "Noninvasive optical activation of Flp recombinase for genetic manipulation in deep mouse brain regions." *Nat Commun* 10(1): 314.

Kakumoto, T. and T. Nakata (2013). "Optogenetic control of PIP3: PIP3 is sufficient to induce the actin-based active part of growth cones and is regulated via endocytosis." *PLoS One* 8(8): e70861.

Kawano, F., R. Okazaki, M. Yazawa and M. Sato (2016). "A photoactivatable Cre-loxP recombination system for optogenetic genome engineering." *Nat Chem Biol* 12(12): 1059–1064.

Kennedy, M. B. (1983). "Experimental approaches to understanding the role of protein phosphorylation in the regulation of neuronal function." *Annu Rev Neurosci* 6(493): 493–525.

Kim, J. M., J. Hwa, P. Garriga, P. J. Reeves, U. L. RajBhandary and H. G. Khorana (2005). "Light-driven activation of beta 2-adrenergic receptor signaling by a chimeric rhodopsin containing the beta 2-adrenergic receptor cytoplasmic loops." *Biochemistry* 44(7): 2284–2292.

Klewer, L. and Y. W. Wu (2019). "Light-induced dimerization approaches to control cellular processes." *Chemistry* 25(54): 12452–12463.

Kwon, E. and W. D. Heo (2020). "Optogenetic tools for dissecting complex intracellular signaling pathways." *Biochem Biophys Res Commun* 527(2): 331–336.

Liberti, W. A., L. N. Perkins, D. P. Leman and T. J. Gardner (2017). "An open source, wireless capable miniature microscope system." *J Neural Eng* 14(4): 045001.

Maniatis, T., E. F. Fritsch and J. Sambrook (1982). *Molecular Cloning: A Laboratory Manual.* Cold Spring Harbor, NY, Cold Spring Harbor Press.

Matiasz, N. J., J. Wood, P. Doshi, W. Speier, B. Beckemeyer, W. Wang, W. Hsu and A. J. Silva (2018). "ResearchMaps.org for integrating and planning research." *PLoS One* 13(5): e0195271.

Matiasz, N. J., J. Wood, W. Wang, A. J. Silva and W. Hsu (2017). "Computer-aided experiment planning toward causal discovery in neuroscience." *Front Neuroinform* 11: 12.

Mayford, M., T. Abel and E. R. Kandel (1995). "Transgenic approaches to cognition." *Curr Opin Neurobiol* 5(2): 141–148.

McConkey, E. H. (1993). *Human Genetics: The Molecular Revolution.* Boston, MA, Jones and Bartlett Publishers.

McCormick, J. W., D. Pincus, O. Resnekov and K. A. Reynolds (2020). "Strategies for engineering and rewiring kinase regulation." *Trends Biochem Sci* 45(3): 259–271.

Morris, R. G. M. (1981). "Spatial localization does not require the presence of local cues." *Learning Motivation* 12: 239–260.

Morris, R. G. M. and M. B. Kennedy (1992). "The Pierian spring." *Current Biology* 2(10): 511–514.

Nectow, A. R. and E. J. Nestler (2020). "Viral tools for neuroscience." *Nat Rev Neurosci* 21(12): 669–681.

Nelson, N. C. (2015). "A knockout experiment: disciplinary divides and experimental skill in animal behaviour genetics." *Med Hist* 59(3): 465–485.

Nguyen, M. K., C. Y. Kim, J. M. Kim, B. O. Park, S. Lee, H. Park and W. D. Heo (2016). "Optogenetic oligomerization of Rab GTPases regulates intracellular membrane trafficking." *Nat Chem Biol* 12(6): 431–436.

O'Keefe, J. and L. Nadel (1978). *The Hippocampus as a Cognitive Map.* London, Oxford University Press.

Potter, S. M., A. El Hady and E. E. Fetz (2014). "Closed-loop neuroscience and neuroengineering." *Front Neural Circuits* 8: 115.

Rose, T., P. Schoenenberger, K. Jezek and T. G. Oertner (2013). "Developmental refinement of vesicle cycling at Schaffer collateral synapses." *Neuron* 77(6): 1109–1121.

Rost, B. R., F. Schneider-Warme, D. Schmitz and P. Hegemann (2017). "Optogenetic tools for subcellular applications in neuroscience." *Neuron* 96(3): 572–603.

Rotenberg, A., M. Mayford, R. D. Hawkins, E. R. Kandel and R. U. Muller (1996). "Mice expressing activated CaMKII lack low frequency LTP and do not form stable place cells in the CA1 region of the hippocampus." *Cell* 87(7): 1351–1361.

Schindler, S. E., J. G. McCall, P. Yan, K. L. Hyrc, M. Li, C. L. Tucker, J. M. Lee, M. R. Bruchas and M. I. Diamond (2015). "Photo-activatable Cre recombinase regulates gene expression *in vivo*." *Sci Rep* 5: 13627.

Silva, A. J. (1996). Genetics and learning: misconceptions and criticisms. In *Gene Targeting and New Developments in Neurobiology*, ed. S. Nakanishi, A. J. Silva, S. Aizawa and M. Katsuki. Tokyo, Japan Scientific Societies Press, 3–15.

Silva, A. J. and K. P. Giese (1994). "Plastic genes are in!" *Curr Opin Neurobiol* 4(3): 413–420.

Silva, A. J., A. Landreth and J. Bickle (2014). *Engineering the Next Revolution in Neuroscience: The New Science of Experiment Planning*. New York, Oxford Press.

Silva, A. J., R. Paylor, J. M. Wehner and S. Tonegawa (1992). "Impaired spatial learning in alpha-calcium-calmodulin kinase II mutant mice." *Science* 257(5067): 206–211.

Silva, A. J., A. M. Smith and K. P. Giese (1997). Gene targeting and the biology of learning and memory. *Annu Rev Genet* 31: 527–546.

Silva, A. J., C. F. Stevens, S. Tonegawa and Y. Wang (1992). "Deficient hippocampal long-term potentiation in alpha-calcium-calmodulin kinase II mutant mice." *Science* 257(5067): 201–206.

Silva, A. J., Y. Wang, R. Paylor, J. M. Wehner, C. F. Stevens and S. Tonegawa (1992). "Alpha calcium/calmodulin kinase II mutant mice: deficient long-term potentiation and impaired spatial learning." *Cold Spring Harb Symp Quant Biol* 57: 527–539.

Sofroniew, N. J., D. Flickinger, J. King and K. Svoboda (2016). "A large field of view two-photon mesoscope with subcellular resolution for *in vivo* imaging." *Elife* 5: e14472.

Stamatakis, A. M., M. J. Schachter, S. Gulati, K. T. Zitelli, S. Malanowski, A. Tajik, C. Fritz, M. Trulson and S. L. Otte (2018). "Simultaneous optogenetics and cellular resolution calcium imaging during active behavior using a miniaturized microscope." *Front Neurosci* 12: 496.

Stevens, B. (2003). "Glia: much more than the neuron's side-kick." *Curr Biol* 13(12): R469–R472.

Sudhof, T. C. (2017). "Molecular neuroscience in the 21(st) century: a personal perspective." *Neuron* 96(3): 536–541.

Tonegawa, S., Y. Li, R. S. Erzurumlu, S. Jhaveri, C. Chen, Y. Goda, R. Paylor, A. J. Silva, J. J. Kim, J. M. Wehner and C. F. Stevens (1995). "The gene knockout technology for the analysis of learning and memory, and neural development." *Prog Brain Res* 105: 3–14.

Wang, H., M. Jing and Y. Li (2018). "Lighting up the brain: genetically encoded fluorescent sensors for imaging neurotransmitters and neuromodulators." *Curr Opin Neurobiol* 50: 171–178.

Wang, Y., Y. Y. Yau, D. Perkins-Balding and J. G. Thomson (2011). "Recombinase technology: applications and possibilities." *Plant Cell Rep* 30(3): 267–285.

Yang, W., L. Carrillo-Reid, Y. Bando, D. S. Peterka and R. Yuste (2018). "Simultaneous two-photon imaging and two-photon optogenetics of cortical circuits in three dimensions." *Elife* 7: e32671.

Yao, S., P. Yuan, B. Ouellette, T. Zhou, M. Mortrud, P. Balaram, S. Chatterjee, Y. Wang, T. L. Daigle, B. Tasic, X. Kuang, H. Gong, Q. Luo, S. Zeng, A. Curtright, A. Dhaka, A. Kahan, V. Gradinaru, R. Chrapkiewicz, M. Schnitzer, H. Zeng and A. Cetin (2020). "RecV recombinase system for *in vivo* targeted optogenomic modifications of single cells or cell populations." *Nat Methods* 17(4): 422–429.

Yizhar, O., L. E. Fenno, T. J. Davidson, M. Mogri and K. Deisseroth (2011). "Optogenetics in neural systems." *Neuron* 71(1): 9–34.

Zhang, K., L. Duan, Q. Ong, Z. Lin, P. M. Varman, K. Sung and B. Cui (2014). "Light-mediated kinetic control reveals the temporal effect of the Raf/MEK/ERK pathway in PC12 cell neurite outgrowth." *PLoS One* 9(3): e92917.

Zhang, Y., S. A. Sloan, L. E. Clarke, C. Caneda, C. A. Plaza, P. D. Blumenthal, H. Vogel, G. K. Steinberg, M. S. Edwards, G. Li, J. A. Duncan, 3rd, S. H. Cheshier, L. M. Shuer, E. F. Chang, G. A. Grant, M. G. Gephart and B. A. Barres (2016). "Purification and characterization of progenitor and mature human astrocytes reveals transcriptional and functional differences with mouse." *Neuron* 89(1): 37–53.

Ziv, Y., L. D. Burns, E. D. Cocker, E. O. Hamel, K. K. Ghosh, L. J. Kitch, A. El Gamal and M. J. Schnitzer (2013). "Long-term dynamics of CA1 hippocampal place codes." *Nat Neurosci* 16(3): 264–266.

7 Toward an Epistemology of Intervention

Optogenetics and Maker's Knowledge[1,2]

Carl F. Craver

1 Introduction

The biological sciences, like other mechanistic sciences, comprise both a modeler's and a maker's tradition. The aim of the modeler, in my narrow sense, is to describe correctly the causal structures—the mechanisms—that produce, underlie, maintain, or modulate a given phenomenon or effect.[3] These models are expected to save the phenomena tolerably well (that is, to make accurate predictions about them) and, in many cases at least, to represent the components and causal relationships composing their mechanisms. The aim of the maker, in contrast, is to build machines that produce, underlie, maintain, or modulate the effects we desire.[4]

The works of both maker and modeler depend fundamentally on the ability to intervene into a system and make it work differently than it would work on its own. My goal is to identify some dimensions of progress (or difference) in the ability to intervene in biological systems.

This project complements Alan Franklin's (1986, 1990, 2012) pioneering work on *the epistemology of experiment*. Franklin focuses on detection instruments and, specifically, on distinguishing "between a valid observation or measurement and an artifact created by the experimental apparatus" (see 1986, 165, 192; 1990, 104). He argues that scientists defend new detection techniques by showing that they detect known magnitudes reliably, that their results conform to the expectations of a well-confirmed theory, and that their findings agree tolerably well with those of other, more or less causally independent detection techniques.[5] Scientists sometimes defend their instruments directly by appeal to their well-supported design principles and by showing their results cannot be explained by known sources of error.[6] Yet by focusing on detection specifically, Franklin neglects a crucial aspect of causal experiments: interventions. My goal is to take some preliminary steps toward an epistemology of intervention by characterizing the norms by which improvements in intervention methods are measured.[7]

In pursuit of this goal, I examine aspects of the early history of optogenetics. This technique matured and made its way into the neurosciences

DOI: 10.4324/9781003251392-10

around the turn of the Twenty-first century and subsequently has been adopted widely and rapidly as an improved intervention method. Numerous biologists have won awards for inventing and describing the key components of this triumph of biological maker's knowledge (including Ernst Bamberg, Ed Boyden, Karl Diesseroth, Peter Hegemann, Georg Nagel, and Gero Miesenböck, according to the latest Wiki update), and the technique is currently featured in over 800 research articles per year (see Kolar et al. 2018). By exploring why this technique was adopted so readily and widely, we get a glimpse of the epistemic norms that make one intervention technique better than another and into the arguments by which such claims are defended.[8]

Optogenetics allows researchers to control the electrophysiological properties of neurons with light.[9] Researchers insert bacterial genes for light-sensitive ion channels into target cells in a given brain region. The virus that inserts this construct into cells commandeers the cell's protein synthesis and delivery mechanisms to assemble the light-sensitive channels and install them in the membrane. The light delivered through a fiber-optic cable then activates or inactivates the channels, changing the ionic current across the membrane and thereby modulating, producing, or blocking neural signals.[10]

In what follows, I first present a schema for thinking about causal experiments and complicate it to accommodate the complexity of optogenetics. I then discuss eleven dimensions of progress or difference in the ability to intervene into brain function. These give us a sense of the epistemic norms guiding the assessment of progress in intervention. I close reflecting on how and why makers and modelers differ in their assessment of the norms of intervention.

2 Causal Experiments

Figure 1 represents a simplified, standard causal experiment. A given causal hypothesis or mechanism schema is instantiated in a *target system*. The target system is the subject, organism, or system in which one performs the experiment.[11] One *intervenes* in the system to change one or more *target variables* (T) and *detects* the resulting value of putative *effect variables* (E).

The *intervention technique* is a means of changing one or more target variables in the mechanism. In the simple case, one sets T to a value. Sometimes, as in Kettlewell's famed experiments on moth populations, the researcher identifies natural circumstances that set the variable to a value, but here I focus on interventions under researchers' control.

Intervention checks detect the value of the target variable to see if the intervention succeeded in setting T to the desired value. In lesion experiments, for example, one confirms the location of the lesion using CT scans

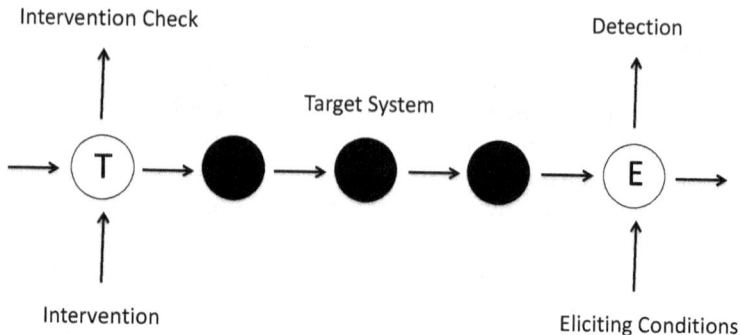

Figure 1 A standard form of causal experiment.

or post-mortem inspections. In pharmacological experiments, one might measure the plasma concentration of the drug. Intervention checks can also be used to compensate for unreliable intervention techniques; one grounds inferences on the measured, rather than the intended, value of *T*.

On the other side of this schema, the *detection technique* is a device or process that takes some feature or magnitude (here, *E*) in the experimental system as an input and returns a reading or measure as an output. Detection techniques indicate a variable's value: Litmus paper indicates pH; an osmometer detects ionic concentrations; and functional MRI (arguably) detects dendritic field potentials. Franklin focuses primarily on the reliability of detection techniques (1990, 2009).

Eliciting conditions are interventions required to prepare the putative effect variable for detection. In microscopic studies, experimenters stain tissues. In classic PET studies, they inject radiolabeled substances. Eliciting conditions are causal interactions with the target system, but they interact with the putative effect rather than the putative cause.[12]

3 Dimensions of Progress in Intervention

According to Woodward's (2003) account of causal relevance, the claim that *T* causes *E* amounts roughly to the claim that there exists an *ideal intervention* on *T* that changes the value of *E*. Importantly, an intervention need not be ideal in this sense to probe causal relationships. Nonetheless, the ideal case is a good starting point for thinking about progress in intervention.

Figure 2 summarizes Woodward's criteria for ideal interventions. Unidirectional arrows represent causal relations, the bidirectional dotted arrow represents correlation, and bars across arrows indicate that the relation must be absent. The depicted intervention is designed to test whether *T* makes a difference to the effect variable, *E*. An ideal

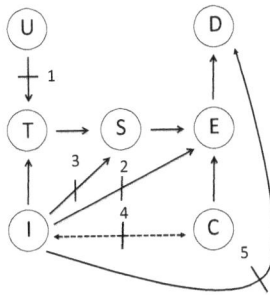

Figure 2 Constraints on an ideal intervention (cf. Woodward 2003).

intervention, *I*, fixes the value of *T*, rendering it independent of all other causal influences, *U* (1). This intervention changes *E* but only via the change in *T*. That is, the effect is neither mediated directly (2) nor induced by changing a variable, *S*, intermediate between *T* and *E* (3). Nor does *E* change simply because *I* is correlated with some other variable, *C*, that is causally relevant to *E* (4). Nor does I influence the detection apparatus (*D*) used to measure *E* (5).[13] Such conditions ensure, in short, that any observed change in *E* can be attributed to the change *I* induces in *T* and not to some other change wrought by or correlated with *I*. The use of placebos in drug trials and sham surgeries in lesion studies exemplify these ideals. Ideally, one contrives control conditions that mimic the intervention in all respects except for the change to *T*. Such controls allow one to assess whether the changes observed in *E* are due to the changes in *T* or to some other unanticipated effect of *I* upon (or some correlation of I with) some other variable causally relevant to *E*.[14]

Consider now how the schemas in Figures 1 and 2 might have to be complicated to describe more adequately the complexity of experiments as they occur in the "wild." First, *I* is typically an extended causal sequence (as in Figure 3a). For example, I might involve an experimenter's choice (*A*), an action or procedure based on that choice (*B*), a device or machine (*C*), which can also be decomposed into separate components, that makes an alteration to the system (*D*) in which the target variable (*T*) is located. Even Figure 3a is misleadingly simplified in representing only a single intervention sequence. As optogenetics illustrates, the intervention might involve a confluence of many tributary interventions (see Figure 3b). Different sequences are involved, for example, in building the genetic construct for the channels (determining *what* is delivered), in targeting the intervention to specific cell populations (determining *where* it is delivered), and in turning the channels on with light (determining *when* it is activated). Some of these tributary interventions are what Fred Dretske (1988) calls *structuring causes*; they build the mechanisms that

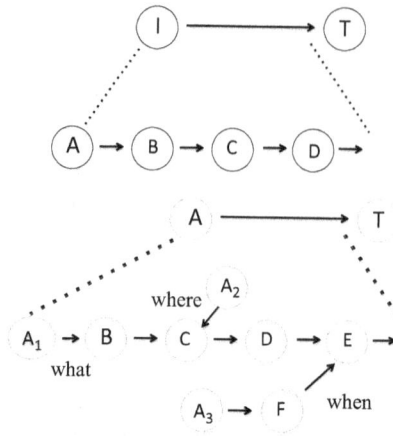

Figure 3 (a) Interventions are themselves complex mechanisms. (b) Tributary interventions affecting what, where, and when optognetic influence is delivered.

allow the experimenter to control neurons with light. Others, such as the light, are *triggering causes*.

Many experiments involve more than one complex structural cause. The target system, for example, may be surgically prepared or pre-treated to make the experiment possible or convenient. The animal might have been trained on a task or acclimated to an experimental setting. The target system might be set into a baseline state against which the experimental effect is evaluated. In an experiment discussed below, researchers first intervene to stimulate the basolateral amygdala (BlA) with direct current; they do so in order to test the effects of a second intervention, optogenetic inhibition of BlA terminals in the central amygdala (CeA), on indicators of anxiety.

This brief example illustrates that to represent experimental interventions as a single arrow into a single target *T* is often an extreme idealization. Different ways of organizing multiple interventions give different experiments their power to answer different kinds of questions about the causal structure of the target system. Precisely because such causal organization of experimental systems is key to their epistemic power, an adequate philosophy of experiment must move beyond this idealized simplification (See Craver and Darden 2013).

An adequate philosophy of experiment also must avoid assuming that idealized constraints represented in Figure 2 must be satisfied for an experiment to be epistemically valuable. Progress in intervention sometimes involves discovering previously unrecognized violations of such principles and correcting them, but not always. In some experimental setups, it is impossible or undesirable to change *T* in a way that makes its value independent of T's other causes (as required in 1). One might wish, for example, to increase the amount of dopamine in a system while allowing endogenous dopamine to vary under the influence of its typical, physiological causes. Interventions are also frequently ham-fisted, changing many potentially relevant variables at once, if only because technology does not permit a more surgical intervention. I discuss below some situations in which ham-fisted interventions might be preferred. And for the purposes of maker's knowledge, a useful intervention might be non-ideal and nonetheless uniquely useful.

These preliminaries in place, let us consider some dimensions[15] along which one evaluates the quality of an intervention method. Table 1 lists 11 epistemically relevant dimensions along which intervention techniques might vary from one another. I discuss each in turn, using early work on optogenetics as illustrative examples.

3.1 Number of Variables

Perhaps the most obvious dimension of progress in intervention concerns the number and diversity of variables a researcher can control. Many researchers believe the theta rhythm in the hippocampus is causally relevant to hippocampal function. Yet this claim will remain somewhat speculative in the absence of a means of intervening to change the theta rhythm in a controlled experiment. The same can be said for distributed cortical representations generally. For many areas of the cortex, researchers presently have no idea how to intervene on the cortex to produce physiologically relevant patterns of activation across widely distributed brain networks (perhaps involving millions of neurons). The development of such a technique would be real progress and would help to

Table 7.1 Eleven dimensions of virtue in intervention

- Which variables?
  - Number of (relevant) variables controlled
  - Selectivity
  - Physiological relevance
- Within variables
  - Range
  - Grain
- Nature of change
  - Valence
  - Reversibility
  - Physiological relevance
- Level of control
  - Efficacy
  - Dominance
  - Determinism

put talk of "codes" and "representations" on firmer epistemic footing.[16] So, beginning with the obvious: we make progress in intervention as we expand our ability to manipulate more and more of the variables that potentially make a difference to how things we care about work.

3.2 Selectivity among Variables

A second dimension, *selectivity among variables*, is more relevant to the explosion of optogenetics in neuroscience. Deisseroth explains:

> What excites neuroscientists about optogenetics is control over defined events within defined cell types at defined times—a level of precision that is most likely crucial to biological understanding beyond neuroscience.

> (Deisseroth 2010)

Optogenetics achieves this selectivity using genetic mechanisms that determine which cells express the channels. Boolean combinations of promoters and inhibitors in gene regulatory constructs allow researchers to target the channels at specific cells, with specific chemical signatures, specific morphologies, or specific topological connectivity. Only infected cells with the desired signatures initiate expression and become light-responsive.

This is a clear advantage over both electrophysiological and many pharmacological techniques for intervening in electrophysiological behaviors of cells. Using a traditional electrode, the injected current spreads through brain tissue, exciting all the cells in a region (e.g., excitatory and inhibitory, neurons and glia) with no regard for different cell (or neuronal) types. Given that different cell types plausibly act differently in neural mechanisms, an intervention technique that fails to distinguish them is impotent to evaluate a broad range of causal hypotheses.

Optogenetics is also more selective than population-level pharmacological interventions. Pharmacological interventions can be quite a bit more selective than electrophysiological stimulation because agonists and antagonists can be used to interfere with or stimulate specific ion channels and intracellular molecular cascades. However, pharmacological techniques are often non-specific in the sense that a given drug might work on many systems at once (e.g., on all cells with dopamine receptors).

The more selective an intervention technique is among potentially causally relevant variables, the more the technique allows one to test independently whether those variables make a difference. For example, the nucleus accumbens, a brain structure associated with cocaine reward, contains two types of dopaminergic projection neurons: one populated with D1 receptors, and the other populated with D2 receptors.

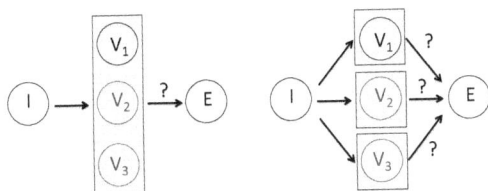

Figure 4 Selectivity among variables.

Optogenetic stimulation of the D1 subtype enhances the reward value of cocaine; stimulating the D2 subtype diminishes its reward value (Lobo et al. 2010). Pharmacological intervention with dopamine alone cannot reveal this mechanistically relevant difference.

More abstractly (as represented in Figure 4) suppose a modeler is testing the hypothesis that variable T makes a causal difference to E. The experimental goal is to intervene on T and to detect the consequences of this intervention (if any) on the value of E. Now imagine a set of alternative hypotheses, each of which asserts a different putative cause variable for E, V_1, V_2, and V_3, as in Figure 4. Clearly, an intervention that changes V_1, V_2, and V_3 at the same time cannot alone discriminate their causal contribution to E. Progress along this dimension would allow one to *change the putative cause without changing other putative causes at the same time.* In short, the more selective one's intervention, the more one can eliminate a certain class of artifacts and confounds (Craver and Dan-Cohen 2021). Greater selectivity among variables is also valuable for makers because more selective interventions can eliminate undesired side effects of ham-fisted interventions.[17]

3.3 Grain and Range among Values of a Variable

Given selective control over a single variable, an intervention method that affords more precise control over the value of that variable might be preferred to one that affords less precise control. And a technique that affords such precise control over a larger range of potentially relevant values of that variable will likewise be preferred to a technique with a restricted range.

First-generation optogenetic techniques gave researchers control over the firing rates of action potentials with mean interspike intervals around 100–200 ms. By 2012, scientists had modified the channel protein to produce action potentials reliably with a mean interspike interval around 5 ms (see Gunaydin et al. 2010). As Boyden, et al., describe it: "This technology thus brings optical control to the *temporal regime* occupied by the fundamental building blocks of neural computation" (Boyden et al., 2005; italics in original). The technique was intentionally modified so it could be used to explore the rates and patterns of electrophysiological activity across the entire range of activity neurons exhibit in their natural environments.

More abstractly, suppose two techniques target the same variable. A technique is an improvement over its predecessor if it allows one to explore more fully the variable's space of plausible *switch-points* (or *transition zones*). A switch-point in the value of a variable is a difference in the value of the variable that makes a difference to the effect variable (Craver 2007). Zero degrees Celsius is a switch-point (or, more accurately, a transition zone, i.e., an imprecise switchpoint) in temperature that makes a difference to whether water is liquid or solid. Switchpoints might be analog, where each increment in the cause variable (no matter how small) makes some difference to the effect variable (e.g., mass and gravitational attraction), or they might be digital, with a *minimally effective difference* in the cause variable.

For this reason, it is valuable to be able to set the putative cause variables to the widest *range* of relevant values. In testing theories of heat, for example, scientists sought ways to produce (and reliably detect) extremely high and low temperatures (see Chang 2004). Likewise, if one is interested in exploring the effects of mean firing rate on the behavior of a population of neurons, one would want control over at least the observed spectrum of that firing rate, or perhaps even simply a plausible range of known firing rates. The greater the range of the intervention technique, the more modelers can use it to explore the space of possible switch-points and transition zones. For similar reasons, the maker can use such interventions to find the buttons and levers that might be exploited in the pursuit of maker's knowledge.

An additional dimension of progress concerns the *grain* or *precision* of the intervention: the smallest change the technique can reliably induce in the putative cause variable. The ideal grain of an intervention varies with the system in question and with the pragmatic uses to which the intervention is to be put. Pharmacological interventions, for example, give one the ability to influence the chemical environments of neurons in ways that can directly affect neuronal activity. However, their effect is imprecise compared to that induced by optogenetics. Pharmacological antagonists increase or decrease the probability of neuronal activity, but they do not precisely regulate mean firing rates, let alone precise temporal patterns. Systems-level pharmacology thus affords comparatively coarse control over electrophysiological activities. If one thinks precise rates or temporal codes are relevant to neural mechanisms, as seems likely, one would then have reason to prefer exploring those possibilities with optogenetic interventions over pharmacological interventions.

These ideas are represented abstractly in Figure 5. At the top left is an intervention into T that covers its entire range of values at a very fine grain (i.e., very high precision). In the limit, I can be used to set T to any

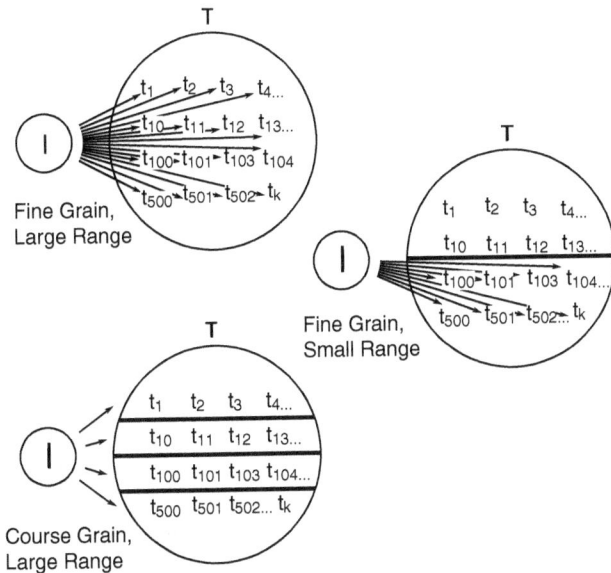

Figure 5 Interventions with different grains and ranges.

value it can take. To the right is an intervention technique that allows the researcher to set the putative cause variable to only part of the range of possible values. The grain is the same, but its range is diminished relative to the case just mentioned. On the bottom is a technique that covers the same range as the first but at a coarser grain. The technique can set the variable only to a value somewhere within a block of values.

3.4 *Physiological/Ecological Relevance*

Modelers and makers differ with respect to whether interventions must be physiologically and ecologically relevant or, perhaps more accurately, how physiologically and ecologically relevant they must be. The modeler's goal is to understand how a biological system works in its standard operating conditions. She necessarily enforces a distinction between how a system in fact works and how it might be made to work under extreme or otherwise unusual conditions. Modelers therefore tend to prize intervention techniques that can be used to manipulate physiologically relevant variables in ways and within ranges that are similar to the ways and ranges at which those variables operate in normal circumstances. Modelers also often prize interventions that are ecologically relevant, i.e., appropriate to the normal environment in which the organism lives or in which the system functions. Of course, modelers sometimes are interested in system behavior outside ecological and physiological ranges, but their interest extends to these conditions precisely because such behaviors reveal clues about underlying mechanisms in the normal or typical case.

To put this point abstractly, from the modeler's perspective, one kind of progress in intervention involves improving the ability to mimic the types of change one normally sees in the target system. Some aspects of this assessment include: (i) whether the intervention targets the *variables* operative in the system as it typically works, (ii) whether the values to which the target variable can be set are within the *range* those variables take in the system's normal or typical behavior, (iii) whether the stimulus values change at *rates* or in *manners* comparable to the ways they change during the system's normal or typical functioning, (iv) whether the changes in the stimulus values are induced via a *mechanism* similar to the mechanism by which the changes are produced in the system's normal or typical behavior.

Many early papers on optogenetics emphasize the method's physiological relevance. They note that the technique is targeted at electrophysiological properties known to be relevant to the function of the nervous system (i). As discussed in Section 3.3, the technique targets the temporal range of observed electrophysiological function (ii and iii). Given that optogenetically induced spike trains can be timed specifically, and given that these spike trains have a high degree of replicability trial to trial (see below), researchers can produce electrical signals in neurons that resemble closely the very signals neurons produce when they work. Although optogenetics does not produce action potentials by precisely the same mechanisms by which cells typically produce action potentials, the mechanism is more like the physiological case, involving the flux of ions through a membrane-spanning channel (iv), than is direct electrophysiological stimulation.[18]

The terms "normal," "physiological," and "ecological" imply a teleological orientation, a focus on how things work when they are working properly or as they typically do in the healthy life of the organism in the environment it is supposed to inhabit.[19] Makers care less than modelers about how something typically or normally behaves; they focus instead on how something might be made to serve our aims. Makers might care about promoting health, life, and the good of the species, but they recognize other ends as well, even those that run counter to these teleological goals. They might actively change the environment. They recognize a set of buttons and levers inside and outside organisms available to be pushed and pulled for purposes that might be irrelevant in (or even contrary to) evolutionary or physiological contexts (see Craver 2010, 2014).[20] Though the maker must take practical constraints into consideration, she is not generally constrained to intervene within the limits of normal or typical functioning in this teleological sense. For the maker, teleological biology offers only a blinkered view of the space of possible causal structures that can be used for engineering.

3.5 Reversibility

A further dimension for evaluating intervention techniques is the capacity to reverse the intervention. A clear example involves lesion techniques in experimental neuropsychology, where one uses a scalpel, a vacuum, or an electrical current to remove brain tissue. Because brain tissue cannot be restored, the experimenter has to compare lesioned animals to non-lesioned animals, or, alternatively, pre-lesioned animals to post-lesioned animals. In response to this epistemic limit, researchers have invented methods, such as cooling and transcranial magnetic stimulation, to produce reversible, functional lesions. These techniques allow one to change the value of the target variable from "on" to "off" and back again, allowing one to run experimental and control conditions in the same animals and in whatever order or sequence one desires.

Pharmacological interventions are typically reversible, but only on long timescales. In standard optogenetics applications, light opens or closes the channel. In more advanced applications involving *step function opsins*, however, one wavelength of light activates the channel, allowing ions to diffuse across the membrane, and another wavelength turns it off. The reversal is, for practical purposes, instantaneous.

The value of reversibility is illustrated dramatically in a set of experiments on the role of the BlA and the CeA in anxiety (Tye et al. 2011). Reversible intervention allows one to test the effects of activating and inactivating the BlA on anxiety (operationalized as the tendency to avoid open spaces) in the same mice over time. One can make a mouse even more anxious (i.e., less likely to enter open spaces) by stimulating its BlA. The BlA sends axonal projections to the CeA (among other structures). By inhibiting those projections to the CeA, one can nullify the effect of the stimulation. Tye et al. report the effect of electrophysiological stimulation in the BlA with or without optogenetic inhibition of terminals in the CeA. The latter optogenetic stimulation can be turned on and off at will, convincingly demonstrating a gating effect of the CeA on the BlA's contribution to anxious behavior.

Reversible intervention in such physiological systems allows one to avoid confounds that result from comparing two groups of organisms that might differ in innumerable and unmeasured ways. It also allows one to test whether the observed effects of the intervention result from order effects.

3.6 Bivalence

A related, but distinct, dimension of progress in intervention is to move from interventions that can manipulate the value of a variable only in one direction to interventions that can manipulate the value of the variable in both directions. Lesion studies, for example, remove but cannot

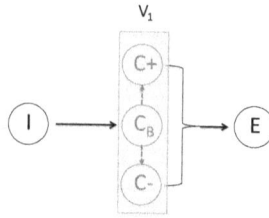

Figure 6 Bivalent interventions can increase and decrease the value of a variable in the same target system.

stimulate brain tissue. Optogenetic methods, for reasons just described, allow one to both stimulate and inhibit neuronal activity, raising it or lowering it from baseline. Bivalence is represented in Figure 6.

Bivalence is a virtue because it facilitates the search for switch-points and transition zones. A bivalent intervention can raise or lower the value of the putative cause variable. Bivalent interventions can be used to explore whether the cause variable and the effect variable vary concomitantly across the spectrum of their values and perhaps to describe that concomitant variation mathematically. Bivalent interventions also allow one to explore higher-order differences produced by different kinds of change: to assess the effect of increases and decreases, different rates of increase or decrease, and different patterns of increasing and decreasing. Bivalent intervention techniques thus allow one to explore a wider range of values, and a wider range of changes to the value of the relevant target variables, than do univalent intervention techniques. If one combines two univalent techniques, one for stimulation and one for inhibition, one inevitably introduces experimental differences between conditions that are avoided if bivalence is packaged in a single technique.

3.7 Efficacy

As noted in Section 2, interventions are typically complex causal sequences, starting with an action and ending with the change in the target variable. Just as an experimenter's efforts to *detect* a given variable can be complicated by, for example, failures anywhere in the detection apparatus or in the process by which the results are stored and manipulated, the effort to *intervene* into a target system might be complicated by failures anywhere in the complex causal chain in the intervention method.

An experimenter might fail to take the appropriate action. Or she could take the appropriate action, but her device might glitch and so fail to initiate the causal sequence. Or the target system might somehow foil the would-be intervention. In a drug trial, for example, the subject might forget to take the pill, or the patient might have a stomach enzyme that degrades the drug before it enters the blood. Bracketing experimenter error, the efficacy of an intervention technique is the reliability with which the intervention technique produces the desired change to the target variable.

Efficacy is in part a matter of objective frequency: given that an experimenter decides to set T to a target value (or target range), and given that she has activated her instruments to initiate the chosen intervention, what is the probability that T actually takes the target value (or falls within the target range)? Or for non-binary values, what is the variance in the value of T given the intervention to set T to a particular value?

In the case of optogenetics, two measures of efficacy have been particularly important. One is the extent to which the technique succeeds in causing the expression of rhodopsin channels in the membranes of all and only the target cells. Tsai et al (2009) describe one such result as follows:

> Greater than 90% of the TH immunopositive cells were positive for ChR2-EYFP near virus injection sites and more than 50% were positive overall, demonstrating a highly *efficacious* transduction of the TH cells.
>
> (2009)

TH, tyrosine hydroxylase, is a marker for dopaminergic cells. ChR2-EYFP is a marker for the expression of the Channel-Rhodopsin 2 gene. Tsai et al. thus use intervention checks to establish the efficacy of their intervention. This aspect of efficacy for optogenetics varies considerably across different brain regions and in different experimental organisms.

Another measure of efficacy for optogenetics, focused on a distinct tributary intervention, is the frequency with which pulses of light produce action potentials in the target cells. The first paper to describe optogenetic interventions (Boyden et al. 2005) is largely dedicated to this measure. They show that light induces stable ionic currents with very rapid activation kinetics. They explore different stimulus durations to fine-tune the technique to deliver trains of action potentials reliably. They characterize how many cells in a population produce action potentials. They show that the same (or almost the same) patterns of action potentials can be repeated time and again in the same neuron and across different neurons by delivering the same light stimulus.

These distinct arguments about the efficacy of optogenetics address different parts of the complex intervention mechanism. The first (expression rates) concerns the efficacy of the relationship between delivery of the virus and channel expression in the target cell population. The second concerns the efficacy of the relationship between light and electrophysiological activity in the neurons. More generally, efficacy can be understood in terms of the variance of the target variable given that one initiates an intervention to fix its value. Given that one has decided to set a magnitude T to a particular value t, efficacy is the probability that T takes a value within a range around t. One could determine the efficacy of a technique by summing the squared distances between the intended and the actual value on a number of trials and dividing by the number of trials. Efficacy is improved by shrinking variance: bringing more of the actual values closer to the intended value.

Efficacy is clearly desirable if one hopes efficiently to replicate one's experimental interventions. However, an intervention need not be perfectly efficacious to be useful, either for the modeler testing a causal hypothesis or for the maker hoping to effect some practical outcome. Whether an intervention is efficacious enough for a given epistemic or practical objective depends on the variable in question and on the relevant switch-points for the effect variable. For the modeler, even a very inefficacious intervention can be useful so long as appropriate intervention checks determine whether or not the intervention has produced the desired outcome in T. For the maker, however, failures are failures, even if one can tell that the failure can be blamed on the equipment. This is another significant difference between modeling and making.

3.8 Dominance

The dominance of an intervention is the extent to which it satisfies condition (4) in Woodward's account of ideal interventions (see U in Figure 2). In an ideal intervention, the intervention technique sets T to a value independent of T's other causes. Such an intervention screens the value of T off from all T's other causes.

Woodward includes this requirement because T's other causes might change T's value in unintended ways, foiling the causal inference. Suppose, for example, one intervenes to reduce the value of T and fails to notice a change in E. Perhaps this is because other causes of T compensate for the intervention or coincidentally raise the value of T, erasing the effect of the intervention. In that case, one should not conclude that the induced change is causally irrelevant to the effect.[21]

But interventions need not screen T off from its other causes to be useful, as Eberhardt (2009) demonstrates in his consideration of hard and soft interventions. Hard interventions remove all causal arrows into T besides the intervention. T's value is influenced, if at all, only by the intervention. Soft interventions do not fix T's value; rather, they change the conditional probability distribution over T's values. In other words, hard interventions are arrow-breaking, eliminating the influence of T's other causes; soft interventions are arrow-preserving, leaving at least some of the parental influence on T intact.

Optogenetic interventions have been used in both hard and soft interventions. A single neuron in a dish, for example, can be removed from its cellular context leaving the light stimulus as the only exogenous determinant of cellular activity.[22] That would be a hard intervention. In contrast, researchers using step function opsins simply raise the membrane potential to make it more probable that an incoming signal will in fact lead to the generation of an action potential in the post-synaptic cell. This is a soft intervention.

Eberhardt and Scheines (2007) discuss some of the advantages of hard interventions for learning about a system's causal structure. First, if one uses a hard intervention, one can easily infer that the observed correlation between T and the putative effect variable is not due to the action of a common cause. By definition, a hard intervention severs the effect of any such common cause on T. Second, hard interventions allow one to assess the direction of causal influence between two correlated variables, i.e., to distinguish cases in which A causes B from cases in which B causes A. Finally, because hard interventions allow the experimenter to set the value of the cause variable, it gives the researcher information that might be used, for example, to characterize the strength of the causal relationship.

In other cases, hard interventions are either impossible or undesirable. They are practically impossible when we don't know how to break all the causal arrows into T. They are undesirable in cases in which one wants to leave the causal structure of the system intact, for experimental or practical reasons. The value of non-dominating interventions is perhaps most apparent in the domain of maker's knowledge. Many standard medical interventions are non-dominating. Insulin injections for diabetes, for example, augment rather than replace endogenous insulin production. L-Dopa treatments for Parkinson's disease augment rather than replace endogenous dopamine levels. In such cases, one intervenes to boost residual capacities of the system and/or to encourage it to compensate for its weaknesses, not to replace it with an artificial control system (as a heart and lung machine replaces hearts and lungs while they are off-line).

Modelers can also usefully deploy soft interventions. Eberhardt and Scheines (2007) demonstrate, for example, that there are conditions in which multiple simultaneous soft interventions on a system suffice to determine the system's causal structure in a single experiment (unlike hard interventions). They show further that if only a single intervention is allowed per experiment, then the choice between hard and soft interventions makes no difference to the rate at which the data from the series of experiments will converge on the correct causal structure (Eberhardt and Scheines 2007). These results, however, are bracketed by the assumption that one knows all the variables sufficient to determine the value of the effect variable. If there are possibly unmeasured common-cause confounds, as is likely the case in most biological experiments, then hard, dominating interventions have the clear advantage in trying to learn the system's causal structure.

The move from soft interventions to hard interventions (or vice versa) is not necessarily a form of progress in the ability to intervene in a system. Hard and soft interventions should rather be seen as distinct intervention strategies that can be used to solve different kinds of experimental and practical problems. But in many discovery contexts, there is a clear reason to prefer dominating interventions.

3.9 Determinism

The last dimension I consider is determinism. Some interventions are deterministic. Others are probabilistic. In a deterministic intervention, the intervention technique is used to set the value of the target variable to one and only one value. In indeterministic interventions, one allows a range of possible interventions around a mean, for example. In different contexts, deterministic or indeterministic interventions might be warranted.

In several of the early optogenetic experiments, researchers intervened by stimulating cells with pulses of light spaced around a mean interspike interval (e.g., 100 ms). They allowed the precise timing of the spikes to vary in a normal distribution around that mean.

Which sort of intervention is most appropriate depends on the hypothesis under test. In these experiments, researchers wanted merely to demonstrate that the method could generate action potentials at rates in the approximately physiological range and, crucially, that they could do so without presuming any particular pattern of stimulation. One might, however, hypothesize that mean interspike interval is the difference-making variable for the effect of interest (i.e., the system functions with a rate code). In that case, the experimenter might choose an indeterministic intervention to rule out the confounding possibility that observed effects are due to a particular spike sequence (e.g., regularly spaced spikes at 20 Hz).

Interventions, it should be acknowledged, are typically *de facto* indeterministic because complex intervention mechanisms might always fail. Most real-world interventions are probabilistic to some extent, if only due to differences in efficacy and dominance. People make mistakes. No intervention instrument is perfect. Experimental subjects might have individual differences in how they respond to the intervention. Any formal treatment of the epistemology of interventions must accommodate the fact that interventions are often chancy affairs, and that chance can enter into a complex intervention mechanism at many different stages.

3.11 Summary

Table 1 lists the epistemically relevant ways one intervention might differ from another discussed above. In some cases, movement from one end of that dimension to another is meaningfully interpreted as progress. In other cases, any preference along that dimension depends fundamentally on the empirical or practical problem the researcher faces. Such context-relativity, however, is underwritten by a deeper sense that there are distinct kinds of causal question and that distinct forms of intervention can be used most appropriately or efficiently to address them.

4 Conclusion: Makers and Modelers Revisited

Progress in the ability to intervene just is progress in the ability to control and produce phenomena with whatever reliability and precision we desire. In medical contexts, for example, the dream is to deploy maker's knowledge to cure and prevent diseases, to build prosthetic devices (such as artificial hearts and brain-machine interfaces), and to encourage recovery and reorganization in such systems after damage or disease. This growth in human know-how is one of the primary fruits that Bacon envisioned for science (1620; see Sargent 2001, 2012).

Maker's knowledge is a potent stimulus to the search for modeler's knowledge (see Carrier 2004). In the laboratory, especially in sciences such as neuroscience, the growth of knowledge about causal systems depends fundamentally on inventing new ways to intervene in those systems and control their behavior. Detection techniques, such as functional imaging and single-unit recording, are indispensable in the search for causes. Yet observation and detection alone are demonstrably incapable of disambiguating even relatively simple causal structures (Eberhardt 2009). Advances in intervention, such as optogenetics, make irreplaceable contributions to our ability to search efficiently through the space of possible mechanisms for a given phenomenon.

More than that, progress in intervention often brings with it new conceptual tools, allowing researchers to envision previously occluded parts of the space of possible mechanisms. Just as the telescope allowed Galileo and Kepler to see new things, developments in intervention techniques have the capacity to open new worlds and envision previously undreamt of causal variables. Optogenetics will likely transform in subtle and not-so-subtle ways how researchers think about the transmission of information through neural circuits.

Although makers and modelers often overlap, as evidenced by the invention of optogenetics itself, the fact that they have different goals places different demands on their methods. The modeler, in my restricted sense, starts with the task of understanding how a given biological mechanism normally or typically works. They chose a phenomenon of teleological interest and try to understand how the different parts of a mechanism are organized together so the phenomenon occurs. The model of the mechanism includes only the variables that make a difference to that phenomenon in the normal or typical conditions. The modeler is paradigmatically the reverse engineer.

Makers, in contrast, are engineers simpliciter. They begin with an engineering problem: something they would like to do or make. That problem might involve getting a biological system to do something utterly unnatural or unusual as viewed from an evolutionary or physiological perspective (such as driving a robotic arm or playing PONG with EEG waves). Makers are free to use any available components whatsoever, not merely those evolution has managed to cobble together. The optogenetics mechanism is a nice example: it involves infecting cells with artificially contrived viruses bearing DNA that would not, under any typical ecological and evolutionary conditions, ever make its way into the brains of mice and rats. The contrivance is, in this sense, altogether unnatural and atypical.

Makers and modelers also have different epistemologies. The solution to an engineering problem wears success on its sleeve: There is nothing more to "getting it right," for a maker, than producing the right input-output relationship within design constraints. The engineered solution need not be pretty (though elegance is an engineering value); the solution need not mirror a natural system; it simply needs to work. Modelers cannot rest comfortably with simply *producing* a phenomenon. Their goal is to understand how some naturally occurring phenomenon is produced. They therefore have the additional epistemic burden of describing a real phenomenon, building a model that "saves" that phenomenon, and making sure the model describes the mechanism that typically or normally produces that phenomenon in physiologically and ecologically relevant conditions. Modelers, in other words, have commitments to mirroring tolerably well the causal structure of the system. Makers must respect the causal structure of the world, of course, but they are not constrained to emulate it.

The science of genetics has always included both maker's and modeler's traditions (see Waters 2008, 2014; Allen forthcoming). Today, the science of genetics is arguably more about making than it is about modeling. In contrast, much of the work in cognitive neuroscience over the last 30 years has been driven primarily by the modeler's aspirations. The development of optogenetics, however, marks a significant step in the coming ascendancy of maker's knowledge of the brain. Optogenetics is a potent reminder that that brains will soon be under our control far more than we could have dreamed even a few years ago. Optogenetics makes salient the extent that science progresses not only by properly describing the world but, perhaps even more importantly, by developing new ways to change it.

Notes

1 Thanks to the Minnesota Causality and Biology workshop for comments on early drafts, especially John Beatty, David Danks, Christopher Hitchcock, Sarah Roe, Roberta Millstein, Ken Waters, and Marcel Weber. Thanks also to Andreas Hütteman's Research Group on Causality and Explanation at

the Universität zu Köln for helpful discussion in Spring 2011. Paul Stein and Mark Alford offered comments on a draft. Pamela Speh assisted with figure production. Marshall M. Weinberg and the Molecular, Cellular, & Developmental Biology Department at the University of Michigan provided funds and a workshop that called my attention to this interesting topic in the first place.

2 This paper was initially produced in August 2012, in the early days of optogenetics. The technique has since become a standard tool in neuroscience. I do not review all subsequent developments; but perhaps a focus on the early days is justified as especially important for illustrating the epistemic norms that determine whether a technique is accepted.

3 Not all models are mechanistic models (see Bogen 2005; Craver 2007; Kaplan and Craver 2011). Here I focus on mechanistic modelers, reverse engineers. Makers, in contrast, are engineers.

4 Martin Carrier (2004) discusses the relationship between applied and basic science, which is related to the narrower distinction between modelers and makers I have in mind. I take no stand on whether one kind of knowledge is more fundamental than the other and am content to note only that they are distinct when it comes to an epistemology of intervention. Sometimes, the modeler and the maker combine, as in the use of hybrid models, to deliver theoretically motivated interventions based on modeler's knowledge (e.g., Prinz et al. 2004).

5 Chang (2004) discusses aspects of detection validity in history of the thermometer.

6 Franklin (1990) grounds his account of these strategies in Bayesian statistics. Mayo (1996) provides an alternative analysis grounded in error statistics and severity of testing. Weber (2012) reviews some of the advantages and disadvantages of these and other approaches to the epistemology of detection.

7 Franklin (2009) describes on two biological experiments: Kettlewell's experiments on moths and the Meselsohn-Stahl experiment demonstrating the semi-conservative nature of DNA replication. In Kettlewell's experiments, the intervention (industrial pollution) is out of the experimenter's hands. The primary interventions in the Meselsohn-Stahl experiment are (a) the radiolabeling of Nitrogen, and (b) the replication of bacteria. The first of these interventions is entirely in the service of detecting the difference between parental DNA and offspring DNA (it is an eliciting condition). The second is left to the bacteria themselves; the experimenter decides only when to stop the process. His exemplars thus do not afford much opportunity to consider interventions.

8 My focus on epistemic norms contrasts with other pragmatic and other concerns such as cost, ease of use, learning curves, moral norms, technological demands, public acceptance, which obviously also influence which techniques thrive and which founder.

9 Some use the term optogenetics to describe both intervention and detection techniques (e.g., Wiens and Campbell 2018). Optogenetic detection techniques, for example, use gene constructs to make cells fluoresce when they express a protein, for example. Others are used to activate intracellular signaling molecules or to uncage biologically active molecules. Here I focus on interventions involving channel-rhodopsins inserted into neural membranes.

10 For accessible reviews, see Deisseroth (2010, 2011), and Fenno et al. (2011). An early paper presenting the technique is Zhang et al. (2006). For a discussion of application in nonhuman primates, see Diester et al. (2011).

11 Rheinberger uses the term "experimental system" to refer to include for example, the experimental subject, the intervention and detection techniques,

lab protocols, preparatory procedures, storage devices, data analysis techniques, and the like (see Weber 2005; Rheinberger 1997). Rheinberger describes experimental systems as the least unit of experimental analysis. I focus exclusively on intervention techniques, leaving the rest of Rheinberger's experimental system as background.

12 They are not interventions on T with respect to E (see Woodward 2003). Hacking (1983) uses staining as an example of the role of intervention in the growth of scientific knowledge. But eliciting conditions do not play the same epistemic role as interventions into putative causes. Kästner (2017) captures this useful point by distinguishing interventions, in Woodward's technical sense, from mere interactions.

13 Woodward's account of an ideal intervention does not include requirement (5), as it is not irrelevant to the semantics of causal claims. It is, however, relevant to how causal claims are tested and how artifacts are avoided (see Craver and Dan-Cohen 2021). Likewise, in experiments crucially involving an intervention check, one would want to know if the intervention influences the intervention check independently of the change induced in the target variable T.

14 Not all useful interventions are ideal in Woodward's proprietary sense: Woodward's goal is to provide a semantics of causal claims (that is, an answer to the question, "What do we mean when we assert that X causes Y?"). He does not provide, nor does he intend to provide, an account of the constraints that an experiment must satisfy to reveal useful information about the causal structure of a system. Nor does he intend his account to serve a model of all causal experiments.

15 The term dimension is intended informally. Still, it conveys the key idea that the usefulness of an intervention might depend on a number of independently varying features of the intervention.

16 This idea underlies Hacking's (1983) use of interventions as arguments for realism.

17 One problem with current-generation optogenetics is that different cells express the opsin molecules to a different extent, yielding a differential response to the same light stimulus and perhaps altering system-level behavior. See Heitmann et al. (2017). This difference might explain the early failures of optogenetic stimulation of primate motor cortex to initiate the required movements (see Lu et al. 2015).

18 Optogenetic stimulation does differ from physiological mechanisms in ways that might prove important. The temporal properties of the action potentials produced by bacterial rhodopsins are not precisely the same as in standard action potentials. As noted above, optogenetic stimulation drives the population of neurons all at once, more or less synchronously. Because populations of neurons interact in virtue of patterns of activation and inactivation across populations, the inability to produce such distributed patterns is a potential physiological limitation of the present-day method.

19 Judgments of typicality presuppose a choice of a reference class (think, for example, of the normal cancer cell or the typical mammalian cell expressing bacterial rhodopsin). Judgments of normality are inherently tinged by a preference for health, life, the good of the species, or some such valued end (see Craver 2014).

20 Jacques Loeb revealed himself as a paradigmatic "maker" when he wrote to Mach:

> The idea is now hovering before me that man himself can act as a creator even in living nature, forming it eventually according to his will. Man

can at least succeed in a technology of living substance. Biologists label that the production of monstrosities; railroads, telegraphs, and the rest of the achievements of the technology of inanimate nature are accordingly monstrosities. In any case, they are not produced by nature; man has never encountered them.

(in Pauly 1987, p. 51)

21 One can use intervention checks to confirm the intended value of the target variable. Tye et al. (2011) use this approach. They record from the CeA during two major interventions. The first stimulates the BlA. The second inhibits the cells of the CeA onto which the cells of the BlA project. The detection technique located in the CeA is designed to check that the interventions (electrophysiological stimulation in the BlA and light inhibition of the CeA) changed the activity of CeA cells as desired.

22 Even under such circumstances, one might still expect occasional "noise" in the system. Ion channels are chancy machines; one might inhibit electrical activity in a cell significantly and still see occasional spikes. In other experiments, however, the light pulses are added in addition to the inputs at dendrites that might generate spikes on their own.

References

Allen, G. (forthcoming). *A History of Genetics, 1880–1980: Its Economic, Social and Intellectual Context.*

Bacon, F. (1620). The New Organon. In G. Rees (ed.). *The Oxford Francis Bacon* (Vol. 11). Oxford: Clarendon Press. Revised 2004.

Bacon, F. (1626). *The New Atlantis. From Ideal Commonwealths.* New York: P.F. Collier & Son. (c)1901 The Colonial Press, expired. Prepared by Kirk Crady from scanner output provided by Internet Wiretap. This book is in the public domain, released August 1993. http://oregonstate.edu/instruct/phl302/texts/bacon/atlantis.html.

Bogen, J. (2005). Regularities and Causality; Generalizations and Causal Explanations. In C. F. Craver and L. Darden (eds.), Mechanisms in Biology, *Studies in History and Philosophy of Biological and Biomedical Sciences,* 36: 397–420.

Boyden, E.S., Zhang, F., Bamberg, E., Nagel, G., Deisseroth, K. (2005). Millisecond-timescale, genetically targeted optical control of neural activity. *Nature Neuroscience,* 8: 1263–1268.

Carrier, M. (2004). Knowledge and Control: On the Bearing of Epistemic Values in Applied Science. In P. Machamer and G. Wolters (eds.), *Science, Values and Objectivity.* Pittsburgh, PA: University of Pittsburgh Press; Konstanz: Universitätsverlag, 275–293.

Chang, H. (2004). *Inventing Temperature: Measurement and Scientific Progress.* New York: Oxford University Press.

Craver, C.F. (2007). *Explaining the Brain: Mechanisms and the Mosaic Unity of Neuroscience.* Oxford: Clarendon Press.

Craver, C.F. (2010). Prosthetic Models. *Philosophy of Science,* 77: 840–851.

Craver, C.F. (2014). Functions and Mechanisms: A Perspectivalist Account. In P. Hunneman (ed.), *Functions: Selection and Mechanisms.* Springer, Synthese Press, 133–158.

Craver, C.F. and Dan-Cohen, T. (2021). Experimental Artifacts. *British Journal for the Philosophy of Science.* doi: 10.1086/715202.

Craver, C.F. and Darden, L. (2013). *The Search for Mechanisms: Discoveries across the Life Sciences.* Chicago, IL: University of Chicago Press.

Deisseroth K. (2010). Controlling the Brain with Light. *Scientific American,* 303: 48–55.

Deisseroth, K. (2011). Optogenetics. *Nature Methods,* 8: 26–29.

Diester, I., Kaufman, M.T., Mogri, M., Pashaie, R., Goo, W., Yizhar, O., Ramakrishnan, C., Deisseroth, K., Shenoy, K.V. (2011). An Optogenetic Toolbox Designed for Primates. *Nature Neuroscience,* 14: 387–397. Epub Jan 30.

Dretske, F. (1988). *Explaining Behavior: Reasons in a World of Causes.* Cambridge: MIT Press. A Bradford Book.

Eberhardt, F. (2009). Introduction to the Epistemology of Causation. *The Philosophy Compass,* 4(6): 913–925.

Eberhardt, F., Scheines, R. (2007). Interventions and Causal Inference. *Philosophy of Science,* 74: 981–995.

Fenno, L.E., Yizhar, O., Deisseroth, K. (2011). The development and application of optogenetics. *Annual Review of Neuroscience,* 34: 389–412.

Franklin, A. (1986). *The Neglect of Experiment.* Cambridge: Cambridge University Press.

Franklin, A. (1990). *Experiment, Right or Wrong.* Cambridge: Cambridge University Press.

Franklin, A. (2012). Experimentation in Physics. *Stanford Encyclopedia of Philosophy.* Available online at http://plato.stanford.edu/entries/physics-experiment/.

Gunaydin, L.A., Yizhar, O., Berndt, A., Sohal, V.S., Deisseroth, K., Hegemann, P. (2010). Ultrafast Optogenetic Control. *Nature Neuroscience,* 13: 387–392.

Hacking, I. (1983). *Representing and Intervening.* Cambridge: Cambridge University Press.

Heitmann, S., Rule, M., Truccolo, W., Ermentrout, B. (January 2017). "Optogenetic Stimulation Shifts the Excitability of Cerebral Cortex from Type I to Type II: Oscillation Onset and Wave Propagation". *PLOS Computational Biology,* 13(1): e1005349.

Kaplan, D.M., Craver, C.F. (2011). The Explanatory Force of Dynamical Models. *Philosophy of Science* 78: 601–627.

Lobo, M.K., Covington, H.E., Chaudhury, D., Friedman, A.K., Sun, H., Damez-Werno, D., Dietz, D.M., Zaman, S., Koo, J.W., Kennedy, P.J., Mouzon, E. (2010). Cell Type–Specific Loss of BDNF Signaling Mimics Optogenetic Control of Cocaine Reward. *Science* 330(6002): 385–390.

Lu, Y., Truccolo, W., Wagner, F.B., Vargas-Irwin, C.E., Ozden, I., Zimmermann, J.B., May, T., Agha, N.S., Wang, J., Nurmikko, A.V. (June 2015). Optogenetically Induced Spatiotemporal Gamma Oscillations and Neuronal Spiking Activity in Primate Motor Cortex. *Journal of Neurophysiology,* 113(10): 3574–3587.

Kästner, L. (2017). *Philosophy of Cognitive Neuroscience: Causal Explanations, Mechanisms & Empirical Manipulations.* Berlin: Ontos/DeGruyter.

Kolar, K., Knobloch, C., Stork, H., Žnidarič, M., Weber, W. (2018). OptoBase: A Web Platform for Molecular Optogenetics. *ACS Synthetic Biology,* 7: 1825–1828. doi: 10.1021/acssynbio.8b00120.

Mayo, D.G. (1996). *Error and the Growth of Experimental Knowledge*. Chicago, IL: University of Chicago Press.

Pauly, P.J. (1987). *Controlling Life: Jacques Loeb and the Engineering Ideal in Biology*. New York: Oxford University Press.

Prinz, A., Abbott, L.F., Marder, E. (2004). The Dynamic Clamp Comes of Age. *Trends in Neurosciences* 27: 218–24. doi: 10.1016/j.tins.2004.02.004.

Rheinberger, H.-J. (1997). *Toward a History of Epistemic Things*. Stanford, CA: Stanford University Press.

Sargent, R.-M. (2001). Baconian Experimentalism: Comments on McMullin's History of the Philosophy of Science. *Philosophy of Science* 68: 311–317.

Sargent, R.-M. (2012). Bacon to Banks: The Vision and the Realities of Pursuing Science for the Common Good. *Studies in History and Philosophy of Science* 43: 82–90.

Tsai, H.C., Zhang, F., Adamantidis, A., Stuber, G.D., Bonci, A., de Lecea, L., Deisseroth, K. (2009). Phasic Firing in Dopaminergic Neurons Is Sufficient for Behavioral Conditioning. *Science*, 324: 1080–1084.

Tye, K.M., Prakash, R., Kim, S.Y., Fenno, L.E., Grosenick, L., Zarabi, H., Thompson, K.R., Gradinaru, V., Ramakrishnan, C., Deisseroth, K. (2011). Amygdala Circuitry Mediating Reversible and Bidirectional Control of Anxiety. *Nature*, 471: 358–362.

Waters, K. (2008). How Practical Know-How About Experimentation Contextualizes Theoretical Knowledge. *Philosophy of Science*, 75: 707–719.

Waters, K. (2014). Shifting Attention from Theory to Practice in Philosophy of Biology. In M.C. Galavotti, D. Dieks, W.J. Gonzalez, S. Hartmann, T. Uebel, M. Weber (eds.) *New Directions in the Philosophy of Science*. Berlin: Springer International Publishing, 121–139.

Weber, M. (2005). *Philosophy of Experimental Biology*. Cambridge: Cambridge University Press.

Weber, M. (2012). *Experimentation in Biology*. Stanford Encyclopedia of Philosophy. Available online at http://plato.stanford.edu/entries/biology-experiment/.

Wiens, M.D., R. Campbell. (2018). Surveying the Landscape of Optogenetic Methods for Detection of Protein–Protein Interactions. *Wiley Interdisciplinary Reviews. Systems Biology and Medicine*. doi: 10.1002/wsbm.1415.

Woodward, J. (2003). *Making Things Happen*. New York: Oxford University Press.

Zhang, F., Wang, L.P., Boyden, E.S., Deisseroth, K. (2006). Channelrhodopsin-2 and Optical Control of Excitable Cells. *Nature Methods*, 3: 785–792.

8 Triangulating Tools in the Messiness of Cognitive Neuroscience

Antonella Tramacere

1 Why Triangulating Tools?

Imagine you are Gina, a four-year-old child playing in the kitchen and finding a piece of brown stuff on the ground. At first glance, the stuff does look attractive. It could be a piece of chocolate, which survived from your last Easter egg. But it could also be a piece of soil coming from an apartment plant, or a piece of dried excrement from Leon, the house cat. Continuing to observe it is not going to give you any conclusive information; therefore, you decide to touch the undefined object and to inspect its texture. You are still unsure of its identity. You bring it to the nose to smell it, but the dryness has wiped any significant odor out. Finally, you decide to compare the touch and the smell of the object with those of the soil of other plants present in the apartment, and of Leon's feces in the litter. Now, the suspicion becomes somewhat real; the object is probably a piece of excrement from Leon.

This is not a classical textbook example, but it is still a case of triangulation, namely the use of multiple information sources to identify an object, supplying for the limitations of each source. Confronted with the task of identifying an undefined object, Gina *triangulates* on it by employing more than one sensory modality. The combination of vision, touch, and smell has helped her to investigate the object from different angles, and to supply for the limitation of each sensory modality. Gina eventually refined the initial hypothesis, by minimizing the bias of each modality, and through focused observations. Finally, she avoided eating a potentially harmful thing. The child has unwittingly employed an epistemic strategy, which has been used by scientists and discussed by philosophers for decades, perhaps centuries.

In the philosophy of science, triangulation is defined as the use of two or more lines of determination to validate the existence or the properties of objects (Wimsatt, 2012). Consider objects in a wide sense to be phenomena, entities, regularities, research results and so on. According to this definition, objects that have been validated through multiple lines of determination are more likely to be *robust*, that is they are more likely to be real, to be reliable and trustworthy, and to generalize across different

DOI: 10.4324/9781003251392-11

experimental situations (Culp, 1994; Wimsatt, 2012). Triangulation has received considerable attention in the literature (Soler et al., 2012). Various case studies have shown that scientists (at least sometimes) appeal to triangulation to determine the degree of robustness about objects, and thereby validate their hypotheses.

I will discuss triangulation in cognitive neuroscience. Identifying the role of brain processes and mechanisms underlying cognition is the goal of cognitive neuroscience. To make a parallel with Gina's case, neuroscientists aim to identify some yet undefined object. But in the case of cognitive neuroscience, the undefined stuff is constituted by brain processes, operations, and functions in cognition. Additionally, like in Gina's case, pursuing this goal is made difficult by the limitations of each one of the methods that can be used to investigate the object of interest.

In fact, in cognitive neuroscience, the role of brain mechanisms underlying cognition can only be indirectly investigated, because of the intrinsic limitations of experimental interventions, and of techniques used to measure the variable (Weichwald & Peters, 2021). Neuroscientists study brain activity and connectivity by using various tools (widely understood as methods, techniques, or procedures), providing data that are correlative in nature, and dependent on confounding factors that may produce partial or contradictory results. Not only may the different tools yield different outputs at the level of raw data, but they may not even focus on the same aspects of the phenomenon, thus making it unclear whether they provide evidence for the same hypothesis.

Using different methods or tools for investigating the role of the brain in psychological phenomena inevitably produces a considerable amount of diverse data that await to be integrated and validated. Integration and validation are needed because we want to know how data and findings produced by different tools relate to each other and to what extent they provide support for inferences bridging neural data to psychological phenomena. Given the *limitations of tools* leading to diverse (types of) data and potentially discordant results, could triangulation help with integrating findings and validating hypotheses about the role of the brain in cognition?

This is not a trivial question. To date, much philosophical ink has been spilled on the question of whether and to what extent triangulation warrants belief in the triangulated-upon object, but less attention has been paid to the ways that discordance is itself epistemically valuable.

This is the goal of this chapter. I will first present a case study, where triangulating different tools (call this *methodological triangulation*) has successfully increased the confidence in our understanding of a causal relation. Specifically, I will analyze research on the causal role of high values of systolic blood pressure in coronary heart disease. I will then present a comparatively messy case from cognitive neuroscience to analyze the epistemic force of triangulation when data and findings are inconsistent and divergent. Specifically, I will focus on research about the role of the mirror neuron system in autism spectrum disorder. By comparing this case study to the previous one, I will show that triangulating tools has comparable value in both cases.

Triangulation is useful when tools have limitations independently of whether results are concordant or not because incoherence and divergence are not insurmountable problems for validation of robustness. As in Gina's story, the utility of triangulation is not necessarily conditioned on reaching the same conclusion with all information sources, but rather on acquiring multidimensional information on objects and a modest unification of phenomena.

2 Triangulation to Robustness

Triangulation refers to the use of multiple independent lines of determination to ascertain whether an object is robust, namely, to exclude that it is an artifact of a particular method. The more a phenomenon is confirmed under *multiple independent lines of determination*, the more it is likely to be robust (Wimsatt, 2012). Triangulation as multiple determination connects to an epistemic conception of robustness, as it is used to deliver reliable connections between a claim and some fact about the world. This conception of robustness is particularly relevant to methodological triangulation because multiple tools for inquiring into a phenomenon may or may not produce the same results or consistent information. Consequently, it is important to ascertain whether and how various lines of evidence point to the same conclusion despite different modalities or experimental procedures.

Robustness is not an all-or-nothing construct, because it comes in degrees and depends on the *context of validation*. This means that objects or conclusions are evaluated against a set of contextual factors, depending on the question asked by scientists, the formulated hypothesis, and the specific methods used in the experimental setting. I will say more about the context-dependent features of robustness throughout the article.

Many philosophers apply the term "robustness" strictly in the context of debates about models and model outcomes (see Odenbaugh & Alexandrova, 2011; Orzack & Sober, 1993; Weisberg, 2006). According to these philosophers, the term 'robustness' indicates that model outcomes do not change with a fixed body of data when assumptions are varied. I do not use robustness in this sense. I am instead concerned with robustness understood as a form of validation of phenomena through triangulation of different tools (see Cartwright, 1991; Woodward, 2006) for analyses of varieties of robustness).

Because *independence* is a condition of possibility for robustness (but see Stegenga & Menon 2017 for a critical discussion), scholars have largely discussed what makes one tool independent from another. According to a widely used notion, tools are independent when they have unrelated sources of potential biases or confounding factors (Kuorikoski & Marchionni, 2016; Munafò & Smith, 2018; Woodward, 2006). When the possibility to incur an error using one tool is unrelated to the possibility of errors with another tool, these tools can be defined as independent. This implies that, to counterbalance the flaws or the weakness of one tool with the strengths of another, various tools relying on independent assumptions are needed.

Remember Gina's case. She used different sensory modalities to triangulate on the undefined object, because one single modality, such as vision, could not provide conclusive evidence. On the contrary, the combination of different modalities helped to counterbalance the weakness of each one. In one sense, the sensory modalities are independent because they are subjected to different sensory biases. Nevertheless, the sensory modalities pertain to the same subject, that is Gina, and are therefore dependent on potential cognitive biases that she may have. This suggests that the independence of different tools is always contextual and depends on the type of tool. Triangulation for different questions, with different tools or with different subjects would require different criteria of independence.

Triangulation also requires that evidence is commensurable, namely tractable within a consistent set of background assumptions. Since different methods often use "different languages" to generate data, it is possible that scientists are not able to amalgamate them to validate empirical claims about objects. Correctly individuating independence, while avoiding incommensurability, has been considered a *hard problem* for triangulation (Stegenga, 2009). Using different methods to inquire into an object could increase the chance of errors, and since different methods often rely on different sets of assumptions, any attempt to combine them may lead to confusion.

Consequently, it seems that triangulation relies on *integrating* commensurable and reliable data. We need to scrutinize data that depend on limitations of tools or study design, and we need to know whether and how different data pertains to the question under investigation. It has been noted however that, if practitioners knew that the methods used produce reliable and commensurable data about an investigated phenomenon, they would not need triangulation (Hudson, 2013; Stegenga, 2009). They could simply use one single method for investigating the phenomena, chosen for its precision and reliability.

These observations have produced skepticism about the value of triangulation. If triangulation requires that evidence is reliable and commensurable, the use of multiple independent methods would be restricted to specific situations. More specifically, triangulation would be valuable only when we know that the different methods produce reliable evidence that can be amalgamated. But if scientists knew it in advance, they would not need to triangulate methods. This is a serious criticism, but I think that the skepticism for triangulation can be mitigated if we consider it as neither a necessary nor a sufficient strategy for robustness.[1] Triangulation is only one possible strategy to minimize confounders and bias when we observe, measure, and thereby interpret and understand objects, reaching a modest and local level of scientific unification.

In what follows, I will try to mitigate the criticisms addressed to triangulation, by describing it as a way for minimizing the limitations of tools and for contributing to the integration of data and findings. When we don't trust methods, evidence concordance works as a regulative ideal to conduct research. Irrespective of the concordance of the evidence, triangulation can be valuable to merging disparate sources of data obtained through available methods and be instrumental to the validation of empirical claims by assessing the robustness of data-to-phenomena inferences.

I will discuss a case from etiological epidemiology to analyze how triangulation can be used to increase the confidence in the *causal role* of specific variables in the emergence of a disease. I will show how the robustness of a causal relation can be assessed in ideal cases of evidence concordance, and how multiple lines of determination can help in determining the reliability of the methods, through analysis of the assumptions and possible limitations of tools used in the experimental interventions and manipulation of variables. Later, I will use this example to analyze the case of evidence discordance in cognitive neuroscience.

I will leave aside the issue of what makes a causal claim causal, and when causality can be inferred with reasonable certainty from data, as this has been already the object of numerous investigations. Note that I rely on interventionism (Cartwright, 2006; Hausman & Woodward, 1999), as an account of causation which illustrates (and problematize) the ways scientists uncover the causal structure of the world through focused interventions (Eberhardt & Scheines, 2007; Spirtes & Scheines, 2004). Questions asked by scientists are often causal and aimed at event prediction, even when single experiments can only highlight correlations among variables (Nathan, this volume). Because experiments and interventions are important to validate causal inference about phenomena, analyzing the value of methodological triangulation is important to correctly identify the causal story behind the data.

3 A Case of Convergence from Epidemiology

In the *International Journal of Epidemiology*, Lawlor and colleagues (2016) discuss whether triangulation of different statistical methods can clarify the effect of lowering high blood pressure (BP) on the occurrence of coronary heart disease (CHD).

One method is the good old prospective cohort study. This is an observational study which follows over time a group of similar individuals differing with respect to certain factors (e.g., level of BP), to determine how these factors affect certain outcomes (e.g., coronary accidents). By conducting and meta-analyzing various observational studies, epidemiologists have calculated the number of fatal and non-fatal CHD in individuals with different values of blood pressure across time (Lawlor et al., 2016). The results showed that individuals with 10mmHg lower in BP were less affected by CHDs.

Can we be confident that lowering high blood pressure decreases the incidence of CHD? Not really. Observational studies have limitations. It is possible that lowering high BP has no direct effects on CHD, because individuals with higher values of BP have typically more metabolic comorbidities, and adiposity could for instance confound the observed effect. This means that higher levels of BP *per se* might not directly increase the risk of cardiovascular injuries; other factors such as obesity could produce elevated values of BP, thus leading to a cycle of accumulating vascular injury through time.

Epidemiologists also used another tool to investigate the relation between BP and CHD. The use of another technique to inquire into the same causal question contradicts some criticisms that have been raised against triangulation. Hudson (2013), for example, claimed that when scientists compare one tool with the measurement of another tool, they base this on the assumption that one tool is reliable, and the comparison serves to check the reliability of the second tool. On the contrary, epidemiologists added another line of determination for checking the reliability of the phenomenon, and not the tool.

Specifically, epidemiologists utilized randomized control trials (RCTs) to inquire into the effect of a higher level of BP. Participants are randomly assigned to the experimental group (treated with a drug) or to the control group (treated with placebo). The experimental group has been treated with an antihypertensive drug, to reduce BP by 10mmHg, while the control group has only taken a saline solution. A decrease in cardiovascular accidents in the group treated with the drug would support the hypothesis that lowering high values of BP causes a reduction in the risk of CHD.

Interestingly, many RCT studies have been conducted on this question. Later, the various results were integrated and meta-analyzed (Law et al., 2009), supporting the hypothesis that lowering high BP of 10 mmHg effectively reduces risks of cardiovascular accidents. Is this result robust enough to support the investigated causal hypothesis, and eventually guide preventive intervention in the population? Not yet.

Despite being considered the goal standard of epidemiologists, RCT studies also present limitations. This is because the hypertensive drug might not *exclusively* affect BP. The same drug could have several additional effects, making it unclear whether the reduced incidence of CHD in the experimental group is due to the target intervention or to other independent factors. For instance, commonly used antihypertensive drugs interfere with given regulative hormonal loops, which could have cardioprotective effects independently from its known effect on BP.

Epidemiologists have inquired about the relation between BP and CHD through a third line of determination (Ference et al., 2014). Specifically, they have looked at genetic variability through a technique called Mendelian randomization (MR). They were able to inquire into the endogenous genetic variation associated with lower values of BP in large samples of individuals while controlling for Body Mass Index and other confounders. The results of MR largely converged with the other lines of determinations, providing additional independent support that 10mmHg lower BP significantly reduces the risk of cardiovascular accidents.

This seems to be successful, but there is still some problem. We now know that lowering high values of BP decreases CHD in the population. But how much should BP be lowered to save the highest number of individuals? Looking closer, the three lines of studies differed in respect to the magnitude of the benefits of reducing high values of BP. Specifically, it seems that the benefit of lowering BP of 10mmHg is greatest for genetic studies, intermediate for observational studies and least for the RCTs. Which method should we trust more?

Contrary to the criticism developed by Stegenga (2009, 2012), for which multiple determination is not valuable with discordance of evidence, additional analyses propose a solution for the apparently discordant results. Scientists analyzed conditions of the study design, and samples of individuals involved in each of the approaches. Specifically, they have compared the duration of exposure to the risk factor (i.e., higher level of systolic blood pressure) in the target population, noting that they differ among the various studies. When these differences are taken into account, the three sets of results are broadly consistent with each other and can provide more precise information for quantifying the benefits of reducing BP of 10mmHg in the population.

Various aspects of this case study are relevant for answering the criticisms addressed to the value of triangulation. Before analyzing these aspects, however, I will present a case from cognitive neuroscience, which does not have such a happy ending, because the results of various tools eventually are incongruent and do not converge. By comparing the two cases, I will show that triangulation is beneficial also in situations of evidence discordance.

4 A Case of Discordance from Cognitive Neuroscience

Considerable efforts have been devoted to the identification of the neural bases causing the cognitive deficits observed in autism spectrum disorder

(ASD). Although a conclusive answer to this question has not been provided, progress has been made.

ASD is a multidimensional psychiatric disorder presenting a spectrum of behavioral and cognitive impairments, such as difficulties with verbal and non-verbal communication, repetitive or restrictive behaviors, abnormal social interaction, and restrictive specialized interests (Myers et al., 2007). ASD has risen in the last decades, with more diagnoses across countries and categories of subjects, perhaps due to an increased awareness and knowledge of the disease. Consequently, ASD has become one of the most studied neuropsychiatric disorders.

During about the last 20 years, the discovery of mirror neurons has boosted new lines of investigations on the specific neural mechanisms underlying ASD (Williams et al., 2001). Mirror neurons are motor neurons that activate during both the execution and perception of the same or similar actions (Gallese et al., 1996), and that are organized in functional spots in frontal-parietal areas. These neurons are embedded in the so-called mirror neuron system (MNS), a network of interconnected neural areas crucially implicated in social functions, such as mimicry, empathy, imitation, non-verbal communication, and language (Ferrari & Rizzolatti, 2015).

Interestingly, these functions overlap with the social cognitive symptoms in patients with ASD, motivating the formulation of the *broken mirror hypothesis* (Ramachandran & Oberman, 2006), which states that dysfunction of key nodes of the MNS is at the basis of the social deficits observed in ASD. The broken mirror hypothesis has been tested through multiple indirect tools because MNS dysfunction in patients with autism cannot be investigated directly by putting electrodes in their brains. Scientists have used a specific electroencephalogram (EEG) measurement, called the *mu wave*, which is blocked anytime a person makes a voluntary muscle movement and also when a person watches someone else performing the same action.

Mu wave is insufficient to identify the role of mirror neurons in ASD because EEG provides a good temporal resolution at the expense of the spatial localization of neural activation. Functional magnetic resonance (fMRI) has also been used. While offering a rough temporal characterization of neural activation through blood oxygenation level-dependent measure in specific brain areas, fMRI allows better spatial localization of the neural activation during specific tasks. But neither EEG nor fMRI can provide a measurement of the motor potential to identify disturbance of mirror neurons' activity. Using Transcranial Magnetic Stimulation (TMS) during observation of others' actions could do this, at the expense of the localization of brain activation.

The use of the three techniques has produced inconsistent and discordant results. Some EEG studies did support (Oberman et al., 2005; Palau-Baduell et al., 2011), while others did not support the relation between MNS and ASD (Fan et al., 2010; Raymaekers et al., 2009). The same has occurred with fMRI, insofar as some studies have observed reduced activity in the MNS in ASD patients (Dapretto et al., 2006; Fishman et al., 2014; Martineau et al., 2010), while other studies have not (Dinstein et al., 2010). In a similar way, some studies conducted with TMS did (Enticott et al., 2012), while others did not support the existence of the relation between mirroring mechanisms and ASD symptoms (Enticott et al., 2013).

As a consequence, scientists asked whether the various techniques are really investigating the same phenomenon; some questioned whether considering the mu wave in EEG experiments is suitable for identifying the activity of the MNS (Hobson & Bishop, 2016) because mu suppression could also be an index of differences in attentional engagements. Others questions whether the experimental method (i.e., repetition suppression) used with the fMRI can detect motor activation (Fuelscher et al., 2019). Repetition suppression occurs when neural activity is suppressed within a population of neurons following repeated activation by the successive presentation of stimuli to which these neurons are sensitive. Since the populations of mirror neurons activated during both observation and execution of movements, repetition suppression effects are expected in both conditions during repeated presentations of stimuli. The mixed results offered by fMRI investigations have led scientists to delve deeper into the neurophysiological mechanisms of repetition suppression and to refine the statistical methods used to analyze areas of activations.

Scientists also have analyzed the degree of independence of the approaches, the particular aspects of the experimental intervention, such as the types of stimuli, and of the subject samples, such age and severity of the symptoms, trying to determine whether and how all these factors could play a role in the inconsistency and divergence of the observed findings (Khalil et al., 2018; Yates & Hobson, 2020). For instance, it has been noted that experimental conditions using stimuli with low or null social relevance are incapable of detecting the activity of the MNS. Further, disturbance of mirroring mechanisms is more consistent in younger autistic subjects compared to adults.

Note that scientists utilized multiple tools *within the same experimental setting* to investigate the role of MNS in some of the cognitive deficits shown in ASD. This practice is progressively spreading in contemporary neuroscience (see Cichy & Oliva, 2020), and I will have more to say about it later. For example, both TMS and EEG have been used to inquire into the activation of the MNS in ASD, providing moderate support for the existence of the relation between the neural network and the symptoms of the disease (Cole et al., 2018). The combination of multiple tools within the same experimental setting has also been utilized to inquire into the role of MNS activations in facial mimicry (Likowski et al., 2012), a phenomenon in which the causal role of the MNS is now considered relatively more robust.

Together, the analyses of limitations, confounders and contextual conditions have led to the refinement of the initial hypothesis. The novel hypothesis integrates diverse results obtained through previous experiments, by stating that the observed inconsistencies could depend on the MNS affecting social cognition by means of the interactions with other brain regions, such as the prefrontal cortex and temporoparietal junctions (Yates & Hobson, 2020). Consequently, scientists are reasoning, only interventions using certain types of inputs (i.e., stimuli with social significance) may detect MNS dysfunction. Also, this prediction seems to hold only for children with ASD, because adults with autism do not consistently display both behavioral impairments and atypical MS activity during tasks typically associated with MNS functioning.

The research on this question is ongoing, and likely more experiments will be conducted in the future. Regardless of the answer, it is important to ask what we can learn about the value of triangulation by comparing this messy case with the previous one, where triangulation has successfully helped to establish the existence of a causal relation. What is the value of triangulation in cases of evidence discordance? Can the scientific practices I have described help to mitigate the criticisms addressed to triangulation?

5 Concordance as a Regulative Ideal

The rationale of triangulation is intuitive, at least in the case of evidence concordance. Multiple determined evidence typically provides greater support to a hypothesis (even though this is not always the case, see Hudson, 2013; Rasmussen, 2001 for discussions). By triangulating various methods, epidemiologists have provided support for the claim that higher values of BP cause a higher occurrence of CHD because the evidence is concordant. But multiple tools have produced inconsistent and divergent results in the neuroscientific case study, leaving us with the uncertainty of whether disturbance of the MNS causes deficits in ASD. What would triangulation prescribe in this case? How could it help us with answering the research question?

Some philosophers have claimed that triangulation is far less significant or frequent than commonly assumed (see Hudson, 2013), that scientists typically resist examining alternative procedures, and use only one method to inquire into phenomena, chosen because of its reliability. Others (such as Stegenga, 2009, 2012) claimed that, even when triangulation is used, findings are often inconsistent and/or divergent. In these situations, triangulation has no epistemic value, and can provide no guidance for deciding which evidence is reliable, and which should therefore be amalgamated to validate empirical claims. The only recommendation that triangulation would provide, critics would continue, is to conduct more experiments till convergence is reached, but this recommendation is simply too general. No scientist would need such a vague maxim.

I think these criticisms do not take into consideration that triangulation is used when tools are not trusted and that in this case, triangulation allows to achieve a series of epistemic goals with both concordance and discordance of evidence. In what follows, I will show that, irrespective of the concordance of the evidence, multiple determination is used and useful for error minimization, it requires (and thus promotes) integration of data and findings, it leads to refining hypotheses and eventually explanations, and therefore contributes to achieve a better understanding of objects and phenomena.

Let me explain this bold claim, by starting with the role of triangulation for *error minimization*. Triangulation of tools requires controlling for the reliability of the processes through which evidence is generated. For example, inquiring about the relation between BP and CHD did not stop with *prima facie* confirmation with one tool. Validating the strength of the relation, and the magnitude of the estimated effect also required controlling for bias, potential limitations, and residual confounders of each of the methods. In a similar way, the investigation of the relation between MNS and ASD did not stop with inconsistency and discordance of results. The lack of convergence did not produce a stalemate or led to abandoning the hypothesis, and rather motivated the analysis of why concordance is not reached.

These practices suggest that multiple determination involves analyzing background conditions, confounding variables and auxiliary hypotheses of the methods and tools used to address the research question (Bogen & Woodward, 1988). This is in line with Kuorikoski and Marchionni (2016) analysis of triangulation, for which the latter involves reasoning about the particular context of validation, about the processes that generate the data, and it is thereby useful for error minimization in both cases of evidence concordance and discordance. This is also in line with previous statements that robustness is always contextual because evidence is evaluated against a set of contextual factors, depending on the question asked by scientists, the formulated hypothesis, and the specific methods used in the experimental setting.

Also note that, to conduct these analyses, epidemiologists and neuroscientists have scrutinized (i.e., eliminating statistical artifacts), selected and processed raw data. They have analyzed the refined data and contrasted their value with results from different methods in the light of the investigated question. *Integration* has occurred while pre-processing and selecting raw data, while analyzing them, while interpreting the results of these elaborations, and while comparing these results with those from different measures. Processing, merging, and processing data, understanding whether and how they produce results that may finally be used to explain a phenomenon is a value in science because the more the data (and then results) are integrated, the more the science is unified.[2]

You may wonder how *unification* is even possible in case of inconsistent and divergent evidence, for unification requires coherence. But if you take unification to modestly mean interconnection between items within and across sub-field (Grantham, 2015) all you need is to reciprocally connect findings produced by different experimental procedures. Evidence is unified in the light of an updated hypothesis stating that ASD in young subjects is due to dysfunctional activation in neural areas beyond the MNS. The novel hypothesis connects and thus integrates a sub-set of previous findings in a coherent way and leads to novel rounds of experimentation that are thought to better address the original research question. Comparing multiple evidence often relies on meta-analyses and integrative reviews from multiple tools, on which scientist's base for conducting new experiments.

Critics of triangulation (such as Stegenga 2009) are right in saying that we lack principled criteria to quantify in advance the weight of each line of determination eventually converging on a conclusion; they are also right in claiming that we lack ways to assess the degree of robustness of a hypothesis when multiple determination is made and show inconsistencies. It is also impossible to consider and compare all the background conditions, potential biases, and auxiliary assumptions of tools, which may eventually undermine the independence of the determination, and consequently the robustness of claims. Robustness attributions to phenomena are always open to revision.

But this is not a sufficient reason to dismiss the epistemic value of triangulation, which is always contextual and dependent on the research question. Accordingly, triangulation on tools has value, because it requires mutual comparison and adjustment of results obtained by different experimental groups using various experimental procedures. Consequently, triangulation can contribute to (local and modest) integration and unification of findings because multiple evidence comparison involves checking whether the data themselves 'make sense', how it relates to data from other tools, how they depend on common or independent sources of error, and how well the data produced by a particular technique pertain and support the initial hypothesis.

That triangulation can be understood as a valuable, context-dependent practice for minimizing errors and biases is additionally confirmed by the simultaneous use of multiple tools within the same experiment described in the previous section. Call this *simultaneous methodological triangulation*. This practice contradicts criticisms that, not only triangulation is not common in science, but it is also not used to validate phenomena in daily scientific practice (Hudson, 2013).

In contrast, I have shown that neuroscientists explicitly and simultaneously direct a range of methods at a particular cognitive system or research problem about cognition, to gain a multidimensional understanding of how the system works. As such, simultaneous triangulation is a confirmation that evidence concordance *guides* the comparison, the mutual adjustments of independent evidence and eventually their integration. In other words, scientists conduct experiments with different tools and expect (or better, they hope!) that the results of the experiments will converge and be unified.

Simultaneous triangulation also provides support for the view that error minimization depends on the nature of the research question. Consider again the case of the causal role of SBP in CHD. In this case, using different statistical methods with the same samples of participants was considered a violation of independence, because it could increase the chances of biases in recruiting and allocating participants. On the contrary, using multiple tools with the same subject's sample and in the same experimental setting in cognitive neuroscience is (at least in some cases) desirable; it can clarify how different tools highlight (same or compatible) aspects of the relation between neural components and cognition, and for minimizing confounders due to interindividual brain variability.

In conclusion, while discordance of results may be a serious problem for a notion of triangulation that aims to provide quantifiable criteria for assessing robustness, it does not undermine the value of triangulation as a regulative ideal for conducting research. I thus agree with those (Coko, 2020; Trizio, 2012) who suggest that multiple determinations can guide scientists in evaluating the conditions for allocating confidence in empirical claims, where these evaluations are contextual, depending on the methods which have been used to address the research question, and not dependent on a priori criteria. Concordance thus plays the role of a "methodological attractor"—i.e., "an idealized logical scheme guiding the efforts of experimenters and technicians, and at the same time, playing a crucial role in the acceptance of a result by the scientific community" (Trizio 2012, p. 120).

6 Discussion and Conclusion

Let us wrap up the journey we have done so far, before concluding with general thoughts about the value of tool triangulation and the undefined brown stuff that Gina found on the ground.

By taking into consideration a case of success and a case of (at least temporary) failure, I tried to address criticisms stating that philosophers have too often focused on scientific success, disregarding that "the lovely paths of truth in the valleys of scientific struggle are often discordant" (Stegenga, 2009, p. 656). The discussion of only two examples of triangulation with different conclusions and different epistemic forces, cannot make up entirely for this tendency. Nonetheless, I hope that I have added reasons to claim that triangulation is effectively employed in different sub-fields of science, and in different epistemic situations.

As Lawlor and colleagues have noted (2016), the term triangulation (or any other synonym used in the philosophical literature) is not necessarily mentioned, but the conducted analyses are often in line with principles and requirements: multiply determine the existence or property of a phenomenon to validate it, thereby assessing its degree of robustness. In both cases of methodological triangulation discussed here, the rationale is similar: where methods and tools have limitations and are not sufficiently reliable, multiple determination is a valuable strategy, because it allows the researcher to control the process of evidence production.

Scientists in different sub-fields pursue multiple lines of determination and combine techniques to disambiguate unclear findings, conscious of the fact that tools do produce results which are affected by confounders. We are, especially with a novel and difficult discipline like cognitive neuroscience, in a sort of "drunkard's search." We cannot directly reach the entities that we need to measure, we often do not know whether and how obtained measures are critical for our questions, we measure only things that we can measure, trying to find some meaningful and reliable patterns in there.

Bechtel stated this almost 20 years ago (2002)

> In the cognitive neurosciences, where a major goal is to relate neural structures to cognitive operations, no one technique can reveal what cognitive operation is performed by a given brain area, but integrating the results from multiple techniques can provide a much better understanding.

Neuroscientists will often find themselves in the situation of not knowing what to trust. In a situation like this one, it is not even possible to be a purist of the method. Using multiple methods to address a causal question in neuroscience is a rational strategy to analyze how results of observations relate to each other through a process of selection, mutual adjustment and integration of data and findings. This process is always contextual and relative to the research question, tool, and context of validation. But, despite its contextual and local aspect, it serves to highlight reciprocal constraints between (psychological) phenomena and underlying brain processes, therefore aiding our understanding of how the mind works.

In the valley of neuroscientific struggle to understand how the mind works, we are like Gina, a four-year-old child unsure of whether what we are observing is chocolate, excrement, or something not properly exciting, like dry soil, which after all can be molded to do something else.

We can proceed step-by-step; we can assume (or hope!) a consilience of induction (Whewell & Butts, 1968), namely that what we discover in one situation through the tools that we possess, will hold for novel situations with same or different tools. Probably, we will not reach any unified and orderly word where few principles hold for explaining things within and beyond our mind, but we can still see how far we can go.

Acknowledgment

I would like to thank Francesco Bianchini, Marco Nathan, Adrian Spohr and Alfredo Vernazzani for critical comments and discussions on an early version of the chapter.

Notes

1 Triangulation is neither necessary nor sufficient for robustness. Triangulation is only one among the many possible epistemic strategies for assessing robustness about objects, based on the assumption that it is at best unlikely that multiple seemingly independent methods provide the same conclusion. This is known as the no miracle argument (Hacking, 1983). Triangulation is also not necessarily connected to integration of data and findings, because integration can be reached through different strategies, and does not even depend on the presence of a hypothesis to validate (O'Malley & Soyer, 2012).

2 This use of unification does not refer to classical ideals of intertheoretic and hierarchical disciplinary reductions. Classic philosophical works on unification have focused on interfield or disciplinary integration, aiming at a reduction between neuroscience and psychology (Bickle, 1996; Churchland, 1986; Schaffner, 1993). I here acquire conceptions of modest unifications (Grantham, 2015), understood as local interconnection between experimental results (other than concepts and theories) within and across sub-fields of science.

References

Bechtel, W. (2002). Aligning multiple research techniques in cognitive neuroscience: Why is it important? *Philosophy of Science, 69*(S3), S48–58. https://doi.org/10.1086/341767

Bickle, J. (1996). New wave psychophysical reductionism and the methodological caveats. *Philosophy and Phenomenological Research, 56*(1), 57–78. https://doi.org/ppr199656116

Bogen, J., & Woodward, J. (1988). Saving the phenomena. *The Philosophical Review, 97*(3), 303–52. https://doi.org/10.2307/2185445

Cartwright, N. (1991). Replicability, reproducibility, and robustness: Comments on Harry Collins. *History of Political Economy, 23*(1), 143–55. https://doi.org/10.1215/00182702-23-1-143

Cartwright, N. (2006). From metaphysics to method: Comments on manipulability and the causal Markov condition. *The British Journal for the Philosophy of Science, 57*(1), 197–218.

Churchland, P. S. (1986). *Neurophilosophy: Toward A Unified Science of the Mind-Brain.* Cambridge: MIT Press.

Cichy, R. M., & Oliva, A. (2020). A M/EEG-fMRI fusion primer: Resolving human brain responses in space and time. *Neuron, 107*(5), 772–81. https://doi.org/10.1016/j.neuron.2020.07.001

Coko, K. (2020). The multiple dimensions of multiple determination. *Perspectives on Science, 28*(4), 505–541. https://doi.org/10.1162/posc_a_00349

Cole, E. J., Barraclough, N. E., & Enticott, P. G. (2018). Investigating mirror system (MS) activity in adults with ASD when inferring others' intentions using both TMS and EEG. *Journal of Autism and Developmental Disorders, 48*(7), 2350–67. https://doi.org/10.1007/s10803-018-3492-2

Culp, S. (1994). Defending robustness: The bacterial mesosome as a test case. *PSA: Proceedings of the Biennial Meeting of the Philosophy of Science Association, 1994*(1), 46–57. https://doi.org/10.1086/psaprocbienmeetp.1994.1.193010

Dapretto, M., Davies, M. S., Pfeifer, J. H., Scott, A. A., Sigman, M., Bookheimer, S. Y., & Iacoboni, M. (2006). Understanding emotions in others: Mirror neuron dysfunction in children with autism spectrum disorders. *Nature Neuroscience, 9*(1), 28–30. https://doi.org/10.1038/nn1611

Dinstein, I., Thomas, C., Humphreys, K., Minshew, N., Behrmann, M., & Heeger, D. J. (2010). Normal movement selectivity in autism. *Neuron, 66*(3), 461–9. https://doi.org/10.1016/j.neuron.2010.03.034

Eberhardt, F., & Scheines, R. (2007). Interventions and causal inference. *Philosophy of Science, 74*(5), 981–995. https://doi.org/10.1086/525638

Enticott, P. G., Kennedy, H. A., Rinehart, N. J., Bradshaw, J. L., Tonge, B. J., Daskalakis, Z. J., & Fitzgerald, P. B. (2013). Interpersonal motor resonance in autism spectrum disorder: Evidence against a global "mirror system" deficit. *Frontiers in Human Neuroscience, 7*, 218. https://doi.org/10.3389/fnhum.2013.00218

Enticott, P. G., Kennedy, H. A., Rinehart, N. J., Tonge, B. J., Bradshaw, J. L., Taffe, J. R., Daskalakis, Z. J., & Fitzgerald, P. B. (2012). Mirror neuron activity associated with social impairments but not age in autism spectrum disorder. *Biological Psychiatry, 71*(5), 427–33. https://doi.org/10.1016/j.biopsych.2011.09.001

Fan, Y.-T., Decety, J., Yang, C.-Y., Liu, J.-L., & Cheng, Y. (2010). Unbroken mirror neurons in autism spectrum disorders. *Journal of Child Psychology and Psychiatry, 51*(9), 981–8. https://doi.org/10.1111/j.1469-7610.2010.02269.x

Ference, B. A., Julius, S., Mahajan, N., Levy, P. D., Williams, K. A., & Flack, J. M. (2014). Clinical effect of naturally random allocation to lower systolic blood pressure beginning before the development of hypertension. *Hypertension, 63*(6), 1182–8. https://doi.org/10.1161/HYPERTENSIONAHA.113.02734

Ferrari, & Rizzolatti, G. (2015). *New Frontiers in Mirror Neurons Research.* New York: Oxford University Press.

Fishman, I., Keown, C. L., Lincoln, A. J., Pineda, J. A., & Müller, R.-A. (2014). Atypical cross talk between mentalizing and mirror neuron networks in autism spectrum disorder. *JAMA Psychiatry, 71*(7), 751–60. https://doi.org/10.1001/jamapsychiatry.2014.83

Fuelscher, I., Caeyenberghs, K., Enticott, P. G., Kirkovski, M., Farquharson, S., Lum, J., & Hyde, C. (2019). Does fMRI repetition suppression reveal mirror neuron activity in the human brain? Insights from univariate and multivariate analysis. *The European Journal of Neuroscience, 50*(5), 2877–92. https://doi.org/10.1111/ejn.14370

Gallese, V., Fadiga, L., Fogassi, L., & Rizzolatti, G. (1996). Action recognition in the premotor cortex. *Brain: A Journal of Neurology, 119*(Pt 2), 593–609.

Grantham, T. (2015). Conceptualizing the (dis)unity of science. *Philosophy of Science 71*(2): 133–55. https://doi.org/10.1086/383008.

Hacking, I. (1983). *Representing and Intervening: Introductory Topics in the Philosophy of Natural Science.* Cambridge: Cambridge University Press.

Hausman, D. M., & Woodward, J. (1999). Independence, invariance and the causal Markov condition. *British Journal for the Philosophy of Science, 50*(4), 521–83. https://doi.org/10.1093/bjps/50.4.521

Hobson, H. M., & Bishop, D. V. M. (2016). Mu suppression—A good measure of the human mirror neuron system? *Cortex: A Journal Devoted to the Study of the Nervous System and Behavior, 82*, 290–310. https://doi.org/10.1016/j.cortex.2016.03.019

Hudson, R. (2013). *Seeing Things: The Philosophy of Reliable Observation.* New York: Oxford University Press.

Khalil, R., Tindle, R., Boraud, T., Moustafa, A. A., & Karim, A. A. (2018). Social decision making in autism: On the impact of mirror neurons, motor control, and imitative behaviors. *CNS Neuroscience & Therapeutics, 24*(8), 669–76. https://doi.org/10.1111/cns.13001

Kuorikoski, J., & Marchionni, C. (2016). Evidential diversity and the triangulation of phenomena. *Philosophy of Science, 83*(2), 227–247. https://doi.org/10.1086/684960

Law, M. R., Morris, J. K., & Wald, N. J. (2009). Use of blood pressure lowering drugs in the prevention of cardiovascular disease: Meta-analysis of 147 randomised trials in the context of expectations from prospective epidemiological studies. *BMJ, 338*, b1665. https://doi.org/10.1136/bmj.b1665

Lawlor, D. A., Tilling, K., & Davey Smith, G. (2016). Triangulation in aetiological epidemiology. *International Journal of Epidemiology, 45*(6), 1866–86. https://doi.org/10.1093/ije/dyw314

Likowski, K. U., Mühlberger, A., Gerdes, A. B. M., Wieser, M. J., Pauli, P., & Weyers, P. (2012). Facial mimicry and the mirror neuron system: Simultaneous acquisition of facial electromyography and functional magnetic resonance imaging. *Frontiers in Human Neuroscience, 6*, 214. https://doi.org/10.3389/fnhum.2012.00214

Martineau, J., Andersson, F., Barthélémy, C., Cottier, J.-P., & Destrieux, C. (2010). Atypical activation of the mirror neuron system during perception of hand motion in autism. *Brain Research, 1320*, 168–75. https://doi.org/10.1016/j.brainres.2010.01.035

Munafò, M. R., & Smith, G. D. (2018). Robust research needs many lines of evidence. *Nature, 553*(7689), 399–401. https://doi.org/10.1038/d41586-018-01023-3

Myers, S. M., Johnson, C. P., & American Academy of Pediatrics Council on Children with Disabilities. (2007). Management of children with autism spectrum disorders. *Pediatrics, 120*(5), 1162–82. https://doi.org/10.1542/peds.2007-2362

O'malley, M. A., & Soyer, O. S. (2012). The roles of integration in molecular systems biology. *Studies in History and Philosophy of Science Part C: Studies in History and Philosophy of Biological and Biomedical Sciences*, 43(1), 58–68. https://doi.org/10.1016/j.shpsc.2011.10.006

Oberman, L. M., Hubbard, E. M., McCleery, J. P., Altschuler, E. L., Ramachandran, V. S., & Pineda, J. A. (2005). EEG evidence for mirror neuron dysfunction in autism spectrum disorders. *Cognitive Brain Research*, 24(2), 190–8. https://doi.org/10.1016/j.cogbrainres.2005.01.014

Odenbaugh, J., & Alexandrova, A. (2011). Buyer beware: Robustness analyses in economics and biology. *Biology and Philosophy*, 26(5), 757–71. https://doi.org/10.1007/s10539-011-9278-y

Orzack, S. H., & Sober, E. (1993). A critical assessment of Levins's the strategy of model building in population biology (1966). *The Quarterly Review of Biology*, 68(4), 533–546. https://doi.org/10.1086/418301

Palau-Baduell, M., Valls-Santasusana, A., & Salvadó-Salvadó, B. (2011). Autism spectrum disorders and mu rhythm. A new neurophysiological view. *Revista De Neurologia*, 52(Suppl 1), S141–6.

Ramachandran, V. S., & Oberman, L. M. (2006). Broken mirrors. *Scientific American*, 295(5), 62–9.

Rasmussen, N. (2001). Evolving scientific epistemologies and the artifacts of empirical philosophy of science: A reply concerning mesosomes. *Biology and Philosophy*, 16(5), 627–52. https://doi.org/10.1023/A:1012038815107

Raymaekers, R., Wiersema, J. R., & Roeyers, H. (2009). EEG study of the mirror neuron system in children with high functioning autism. *Brain Research*, 1304, 113–21. https://doi.org/10.1016/j.brainres.2009.09.068

Schaffner, K. F. (1993). Theory structure, reduction, and disciplinary integration in biology. *Biology and Philosophy*, 8(3), 319–47. https://doi.org/10.1007/BF00860432

Soler, L., Trizio, E., Nickles, T., & Wimsatt, W. (Eds.). (2012). *Characterizing the Robustness of Science: After the Practice Turn in Philosophy of Science* (Vol. 292). Dordrecht, Netherlands: Springer Science & Business Media.

Spirtes, P., & Scheines, R. (2004). Causal inference of ambiguous manipulations. *Philosophy of Science*, 71(5), 833–45. https://doi.org/10.1086/425058

Stegenga, J. (2009). Robustness, discordance, and relevance. *Philosophy of Science*, 76(5), 650–61. https://doi.org/10.1086/605819

Stegenga, J. (2012). Rerum concordia discors: Robustness and discordant multimodal evidence. *Rerum Concordia Discors: Robustness and Discordant Multimodal Evidence*, 292, 207–26.

Stegenga, J., & Menon, T. (2017). Robustness and independent evidence. *Philosophy of Science*, 84(3), 414–35. https://doi.org/10.1086/692141

Trizio, E. (2012). Achieving robustness to confirm controversial hypotheses: A case study in cell biology. *Achieving Robustness to Confirm Controversial Hypotheses: A Case Study in Cell Biology*, 292, 105–20.

Weichwald, S., & Peters, J. (2021). Causality in cognitive neuroscience: Concepts, challenges, and distributional robustness. *Journal of Cognitive Neuroscience*, 33(2), 226–47. https://doi.org/10.1162/jocn_a_01623

Weisberg, M. (2006). Robustness analysis. *Philosophy of Science*, 73(5), 730–42. https://doi.org/10.1086/518628

Whewell, W., & Butts, R. E. (1968). *William Whewell's Theory of Scientific Method*. Pittsburgh, PA: University of Pittsburgh Press.

Williams, J. H. G., Whiten, A., Suddendorf, T., & Perrett, D. I. (2001). Imitation, mirror neurons and autism. *Neuroscience & Biobehavioral Reviews*, 25(4), 287–95. https://doi.org/10.1016/S0149-7634(01)00014-8

Wimsatt, W. C. (2012). Robustness, reliability, and overdetermination (1981). In L. Soler (ed.) *Characterizing the Robustness of Science* (pp. 61–78). Amsterdam: Springer.

Woodward, J. (2006). Some varieties of robustness. *Journal of Economic Methodology*, 13(2), 219–40. https://doi.org/10.1080/13501780600733376

Yates, L., & Hobson, H. (2020). Continuing to look in the mirror: A review of neuroscientific evidence for the broken mirror hypothesis, EP-M model and STORM model of autism spectrum conditions. *Autism*, 24(8), 1945–59. https://doi.org/10.1177/1362361320936945

9 Prediction, Explanation, and the "Toolbox" Problem

Marco J. Nathan

1 The Once and Future Inference

Once upon a time, in a land far away—well, not *all* that spatially or temporally distant, to tell you the truth, but that's how fairy tales go—there was a small flourishing country: the kingdom of Philosophy of Science. Philosophy of Science was governed by a monarch, King Hempel, who ruled by the covering-law model, a code affectionately referred to as "CLM." King Hempel was a fair, wise, and just leader. He viewed all his subjects as equals. The country was split in two, oft bickering, counties, *Prediction* and *Explanation*. But the law of the land, the CLM, treated both as two sides of the same coin. The entire kingdom lived in unity, simplicity, and harmony. Philosophy of Science, in a nutshell, was thriving and growing by the year.

Alas, nothing lasts forever, not even in fables. One gloomy day, King Hempel was found mysteriously murdered as the rooster crowed the crack of dawn. The assassin had lured the king into a dark alley and mercilessly gored him with a flagpole, before dissolving like a shadow. Things were never quite the same in good ole Philosophy of Science.

After a period of mourning, incredulity, and intellectual turmoil, a new sovereign was finally found. The choice fell upon Sir Thomas McKuhn, who had been coyly plotting a revolution to be appointed Caesar. The paradigm shifted, as logic was no longer heralded as the sole canon of rationality. There was a new sheriff in town, Dr. van der Quine, who promoted a naturalistic attitude, drawing more attention to the details of scientific practice. No more CLM. A new law of the land—the causal-mechanistic model, the notorious "CMM"—was enforced by General DeSalmon. The new leaders brought a breath of fresh air. Mechanism-driven "special" sciences, such as biology, neuroscience, and psychology, were now viewed as inherently distinct from mathematized, law-based, theory-driven physics. The old CLM was soon forgotten and became a relic of a bygone past, confined to dusty textbooks. Stories recounting the glory days of King Hempel were sung around the campfire on chilly nights.

DOI: 10.4324/9781003251392-12

Years lazily went by. People eventually realized that not all that glitters is gold. Incidentally, one also needs a baptismal act and the appropriate atomic essence. The new causal-mechanistic ideal, embodied in the CMM, was far less ecumenical than its predecessor. With the demise of CLM, explanation and prediction were no longer symmetric. War soon broke out.

The playing field was hardly leveled. Causal explanation, led by De-Salmon's troops, swiftly vanquished the enemy. Prediction, outnumbered and deemed dispensable, was banished from the kingdom. It searched for a new home and eventually found one in a neighboring country, the Republic of Natural Science. Planted in fertile soil, prediction quickly grew into a strong, independent research field, with a host of new theoretical and experimental tools.

Meanwhile, in Philosophy of Science, the first cracks began to appear. Galvanized by its initial success, van der Quine, DeSalmon, and their followers were led to believe that the CMM could take care of all business at once. And, at first, this appeared to be so. Explanation became the once and future inference, relegating everything else to the background. But, as it turns out, the mainstream causal-mechanistic approach, with its focus on how things are brought about, is poorly equipped to account for prediction. When forecasts finally started holding their own, this became painfully clear.

The eventual passing of McKuhn and van der Quine left the kingdom in a state of disarray. Civil war ran amok. Some citizens of Philosophy of Science sought refuge in the Realm of Metaphysics, governed by Duke Lewis Kellogg, an old foe of King Hempel. But the old duchy, once thriving, was also in a ruinous state and could barely take care of its own. Others migrated to the larger neighbor, Natural Science, which, in the meantime, had grown bigger and more powerful. Prediction and explanation made amends. Most of them settled in Natural Science. Others returned to Philosophy of Science. But there was finally peace and prosperity. And everyone lived happily ever after—isn't this how any fairy tale worth its salt is supposed to end?

Let's snap out of fiction and back to reality. Our legend is inspired by real events with momentous implications, the subject of this essay. Prediction and explanation, once perceived as symmetrical, have been torn apart and treated independently. The CMM, now dominant in philosophy, captures forecasts indirectly, via causal-mechanistic relations. But prediction, in many areas of the sciences, is rapidly gaining autonomy. Purely predictive inferences, not backed up by causal explanation, are increasingly becoming commonplace, fueled by conceptual and technological advancements. This raises the question of how predictive and explanatory tools can work in unison while remaining distinct. This puzzle, which I dub the "toolbox problem," has a "black-box solution." Prediction and explanation are ultimately grounded in the same causal network. Yet, predictive and explanatory tools require different amounts of mechanistic detail, as well as varying degrees of abstraction and idealization.

Here is the master plan. Section 2 outlines the status quo in contemporary philosophy of science: the methodological hegemony of explanation. Section 3 illustrates the ongoing predictive turn—the emancipation of prediction from explanation—with examples from genomics, molecular medicine, and cognitive neuropsychology. Section 4 raises a philosophical puzzle, namely, how to characterize the interdependence of prediction and explanation while keeping these inferences distinct. Section 5 explores a "black box" solution to our toolbox problem. Section 6 wraps up the discussion with general implications and concluding remarks.

2 The Hegemony of Explanation

There is a recent trend across the natural and social sciences, whereby the epistemic focus is gradually shifting from explanation to prediction. Meanwhile, philosophy of science has been going in the opposite direction, openly privileging explanation above any other kind of inference. The hegemony of explanation is the subject of this section. We'll shift to prediction in the following one.

Traditionally, the three chief goals of science were taken to be *description*, *explanation*, and *prediction*. In the authoritative words of Herbert Feigl (1949, p. 11),

> The aims of the pure (empirical) sciences are then essentially the same throughout the whole field. What the scientists are seeking are descriptions, explanations, and predictions which are as adequate and accurate as possible in the given context of research.

Elaborating on this insight, Feigl notes how "the first aim [description], is basic and indispensable, the second and third [explanation and prediction] (closely related to each other) arise as the most desirable fruits of scientific labors whenever inquiry rises beyond the mere fact-gathering stage" (pp. 10–11). These remarks raise several related questions. Why should science privilege these aims as paramount? What makes description "basic" and "indispensable"? In what sense are prediction and explanation "closely related to each other"? To address these issues, we must focus on how these three goals can be met.

Feigl could safely assert that prediction and explanation are closely related because the covering-law model (CLM), the "official" theory of explanation of logical positivism and logical empiricism—I will not separate these movements here—took care of both endeavors simultaneously. As gestured in Section 1, Hempel and Oppenheim (1948), the main proponents of the CLM, viewed prediction and explanation as two sides of the same coin. Predicting an event is explaining something in the future, yet to be observed. Conversely, explanation is retrodiction: prediction of a happening that occurred in the past. Both prediction and explanation are a matter of logically deriving an event from an explanans consisting of background assumptions and laws of nature. This is where description comes into the picture. A necessary presupposition for predicting or explaining an event is an accurate characterization of initial conditions and underlying nomological regularities. In short, all three basic epistemic aims of science are brought together by the CLM.

This unified picture of scientific inquiry was bound to change with the demise of the CLM, due to the discovery of asymmetries of explanation, and the subsequent emergence of the causal-mechanistic paradigm. Briefly rehashing this familiar story will be helpful to unravel the historical narrative.

Setting complications aside, the hiccup is straightforward. From the standpoint of the CLM, prediction and explanation are structurally analogous. This means that any explanatory inference is thereby predictive and, conversely, any prediction can be treated as an explanation. Whether this symmetry holds water is questionable. Paraphrasing the insights of Scriven (1958) and Bromberger (1966), among others, the length of a shadow cast by a flagpole on a clear day, together with the position of the sun and the basic laws of light refraction, can be used to predict the height of the flagpole. But it is doubtful, to say the least, whether a similar derivation constitutes an explanation of the height of the pole. Along the same lines, reliable symptoms can be used to predict a disease, but they don't explain it.

Unsurprisingly, accounts which supplanted the CLM dropped the alleged symmetry between explanation and prediction. Unificationism, pioneered by Friedman (1974) and Kitcher (1981, 1989), treated explanation as a unifying endeavor, paying little to no attention to forecasting. As well-known as they are, unificationist analyses did not gain much momentum. Hence, in what follows, I shall focus on the framework that has received the lion's share of attention and consensus. This is the *causal-mechanistic* model, or CMM, for short.

What does it mean to approach explanation from a causal-mechanistic perspective? Several influential alternatives have been proposed (Salmon 1984, 1998; Woodward 2003; Strevens 2008). The overarching guiding thought is that explaining an event involves specifying relevant details about what triggers it, that is, how the event in question is brought about and how it would vary under different circumstances. In the words of David Lewis (1986, p. 217, italics omitted), "to explain an event is to provide some information about its causal history." With this core assumption firmly in place, it became clear that grasping complex causal networks requires looking "under the hood" for mechanistic underpinnings. A broad analysis of mechanisms and cognate notions was undertaken, with significant differences in nuance, by Bechtel and Richardson (1993), Machamer et al. (2000), Glennan (2017), and fellow advocates of the so-called "new wave of mechanistic philosophy," which gained full traction at the turn of the millennium.

As explanation became a matter of causes and mechanisms, what happened to prediction? It faded into the background. Allow me to elaborate. Prediction was a hallowed topic in classic philosophy of science, connected to induction and confirmation, long before the CLM. The notorious *problem of induction*—first posed by Hume (2000[1938], 1999 [1748]), rephrased in modern terms by Russell (1912), and revamped by Goodman (1955)—challenges us to justify our belief that the future will resemble the past. Expectations about the future are, at heart, a sort of prediction. The issue of confirmation, as developed by logical empiricists, is, in turn, a de-psychologized form of induction, which focuses on purely logical, probabilistic relations between theory and evidence.

Two remarks. First, the class of inductive inferences, which encompasses all non-deductive forms of reasoning, is broader than the set of predictions *per se*. Second, the problem of induction, conceived as a yet-unresolved philosophical issue, is of marginal significance for practicing scientists who, *pace* Popper, routinely take for granted some principle of induction. As such, the study of confirmation, traditionally part of philosophy of science, was relocated and repackaged in the field of formal epistemology.

Admittedly, a few philosophers of science have devoted attention to prediction. Cartwright (1983, 2007, 2019) has emphasized the gap between causal and predictive knowledge. Spirtes et al. (2000) have sketched a mathematical framework for predictive inferences. In the philosophy of medicine, Broadbent (2013) discusses prediction in epidemiology. And I, for one, have considered the role of predictions in diagnosis and prognosis (Nathan 2016). Nevertheless, to date, no one has undertaken a systematic philosophical analysis of prediction comparable to what has been provided for causal explanation.

Why did philosophers of science trade in prediction for explanation? Could it be that forecasting has little to offer of philosophical value? This seems unlikely. While a clear-cut answer is yet to be found, prediction continues to live in the shadow of its counterpart, in theories of explanation. To be sure, predictive accuracy remains a cardinal theoretical virtue of many scientific models. Across various fields—from climatology to economics, from precision medicine to epidemiology—a simulation able to accurately anticipate the behavior of a complex system is worth its weight in gold. Yet, I surmise that predictive accuracy is often considered a more or less direct consequence of a deep understanding of the system's causal-mechanistic underpinnings. One predicts by dint of explanatory power. Description and explanation remain the true gold standard. This is my best attempt to rationalize the neglect of prediction in philosophy of science. Otherwise, I would find the current situation quite inexplicable.

In sum, with the demise of the CLM, the perceived symmetry of prediction and explanation was lost. Despite a handful of valiant, if relatively isolated attempts, philosophers of science swept prediction under the rug, concentrating quasi-exclusively on description and explanation, construed in causal-mechanistic fashion. Pointing the spotlight on explanation left prediction without a template of its own. To be sure, formal epistemologists, Bayesians in particular, focused on the revision of belief based on new evidence. But this emphasis on confirmation falls short of a full-blown model of prediction. Thus conceived, prediction could no longer be viewed as a self-standing goal of science, but a by-product of explanatory power, a welcome free lunch.

Was neglecting prediction the right move for philosophy of science? For a while, this stance seemed justified by the attitude of the scientific community, which also privileged explanation. Yet, things were bound to change fast. Over the last few decades, many working scientists have begun couching their epistemic aims in terms of predictive accuracy. This is the "predictive turn." It is a trend that has pushed researchers away from explanation and toward purely predictive models. To drive the point home, rather than providing an abstract description, the following section briefly introduces three case studies that illustrate this predictive turn.

3 The Predictive Turn

Section 2 centered on how philosophy of science has come to privilege explanation over prediction. We now shift emphasis to how the predictive turn is reshaping the scientific landscape. Preliminary question: what's the predictive turn? Following Weiskopf (2021), I employ this expression to pinpoint a trend across the natural and social sciences, where the main epistemic focus is gradually shifting from explanation to prediction. I illustrate this movement with three case studies, where tools play a fundamental role, at two distinct levels. First, making sense of the predictive turn presupposes a conceptual "toolbox" that marks off prediction from explanation. Second, and less metaphorically, these inferences require a host of technological innovations that provide fine-grained measurements to ground reliable predictions.

My first example centers on *Genome-Wide Association Studies*, "GWAS" for short. Simply put, GWAS involve an examination of genome-wide sets of genetic variants across a population of reference (Vrieze et al. 2012; van der Sijde et al. 2014; Visscher et al. 2017; Harden 2021). The goal is to employ standard genomic instruments and statistical analysis to determine whether DNA variation can be linked to phenotypic, behavioral, or psychological traits. Is a specific allele correlated with, say, greater height or mathematical aptitude? And is this link explanatory? While GWAS typically look for associations between single-nucleotide polymorphisms and human pathologies, the technique can be applied to genetic properties of any kind, in humans, animals, or plants. GWAS are now popular in neuroscience and neurology, for instance, in autism research (Anney et al. 2017; Torrica et al. 2017; Alonso-Gonzalez et al. 2019).

What kind of knowledge does a GWAS provide? Ideally, by pinpointing markers associated with variation in traits within populations, we should be able to establish a *causal* link between genetic and phenotypic factors, thereby explaining the presence of the latter traits. Unfortunately, this project may be overly optimistic. Starting with Lewontin's (1974) pioneering critique of Analysis of Variance (ANOVA)—a widespread statistical tool—commentators have expressed skepticism regarding the possibility of using GWAS to identify the causes of individual outcomes, thereby causally explaining them, in full or in part. Nevertheless, GWAS have not lost their intended purpose. They remain valuable instruments of prediction. Allow me to elaborate.

Lewontin's original insight has been developed along various lines. Some modestly claim that the link between phenotypes and genes identified by GWAS markers is not a "paradigmatic" cause (Bourrat 2020). Others advance the stronger point that the relation in question cannot be truly causal because the association may be completely spurious (Richardson and Jones 2019), resulting from population structure (Sul et al. 2018), or relying on a pathway that operates via a genotype × environment covariance (Lynch and Bourrat 2017). Adjudicating between these options lies beyond present concerns. The relevant point, for our own purposes, is that a properly conducted GWAS unveils a *correlation* between genotype and phenotype. And a time-worn philosophical adage reminds us that such associations don't necessarily imply causation.

Importantly, the heart of the matter is not merely the truism that genes alone do not causally explain any trait—they never do. The real concern is that the causal relation between genes and phenotypes is often way too indirect to provide an illuminating explanation of individual traits. Hence, when GWAS provide little or no valuable causal-mechanistic information, genetic variation does not explain the trait—or, more modestly, it does not explain it well. Still, genomic analysis comes in handy to *predict* such characteristics. The GWAS framework, in short, is best conceived not as an explanatory tool but, rather, as an instrument of prediction. Witness the predictive turn in full force: the forecasting value of a genomic tool is independent of its explanatory power.

Our second case study is an extension of our reflections on GWAS. As noted, GWAS purport to identify genetic markers associated with phenotypic or behavioral profiles. But genetic markers are a special instance of a much broader phenomenon: *biomarkers*. What is a biomarker?

The *NIH Biomarkers Definitions Working Group* (2001) concisely defines a biomarker as "a characteristic that is objectively measured and evaluated as an indicator of normal biological processes, pathogenic processes, or pharmacological responses to a therapeutic intervention." To paraphrase, a biomarker is a measurable indicator, on any spatial or temporal scale, that can be employed experimentally to evaluate characteristics about its source, regardless of whether such source is a healthy process or a pathological state.

A few examples should help drive the point home. Since 97.7°F–99.5°F body temperature is a normal physiological state for a human being, an approximate value within this range is a biomarker of good health. Similarly, mutated MYH7 increases the probability of hypertrophic cardiopathy, and high prostate-specific antigen (PSA) levels are an indicator of prostate cancer. All three states are biomarkers. From this standpoint, GWAS set out to find genetic biomarkers. Unsurprisingly, the forecasting value of GWAS extends, more generally, to biomarkers of all sorts.

A biomarker, simply put, grounds an informed prediction that a certain condition is or will be present. High PSA levels, under appropriate circumstances, indicate that prostate cancer is the most likely diagnosis for a patient. Yet, PSA levels do not causally explain the presence of the tumorous mass. In general, a biomarker need not, and often does not, causally explain the associated condition. How can a marker offer predictive value without any causal-explanatory insight?

I should make it very clear that one and the same entity can be *both* a cause *and* a biomarker of a certain condition. Mutated MYH7 contributes to hypertrophic cardiopathy and allows us to predict it too. Similarly, the unstable expansion of a CAG repeat within the coding region of the *huntingtin* gene is an indicator—and, unfortunately, a rare instance of a sure-fire marker—of a devastating neurodegenerative disorder, Huntington's Disease, that will develop when the subject reaches their 30s or 40s. Now, it would be a mistake to pinpoint the genetic mutation as the one and only cause of the pathology, as the network in question turns out to be frustratingly complex. Still, the mutation is a recognized cause of the neurological disorder. Having said this, such a condition does not hold generally. A biomarker need not play any causal role. To wit, as far as we know, there is no causal connection between high PSA levels and prostate cancer. And, even when a biomarker does play a causal function, its role as a cause is distinct from its role as a biomarker. A biomarker need only predict, whereas a cause must also contribute to an explanation. In short, biomarkers, *qua* indicators, need not provide any substantial causal or mechanistic knowledge, without affecting their status as biomarkers.

Recent philosophical research at the intersection of causation and medicine has focused on the role of biomarkers in studying the etiology of disease (Russo and Williamson 2012; Illari and Russo 2016; Ghiara and Russo 2019). While the tension between prediction and explanation has not gone unnoticed, once again, it is explanation that has taken the center of the stage.

> On the one hand, biomarkers are not entities, things to which we can attribute some causal power, in the same sense as HPV virus has the power to initiate the onset of cervical cancer. Instead, biomarkers are clues, indicators, *markers* to detect in order to reconstruct the missing link. On the other hand, and related to the previous point, we need to say in which sense, if any, these continuous links, or processes, between exposure and disease are *causal*. This is all the more important because we seek to link *heterogeneous* levels as the macro- and the micro-environment.
>
> (Vineis et al. 2017, p. 4)

In sum, biomarkers provide no causal-mechanistic information about a system. As such, they don't suggest therapies or interventions. Biomarkers, together with all the technological and conceptual instruments required for their detection and analysis, are primarily tools of prediction, not explanation.

My third and final case study illustrating the predictive turn in action comes from the bourgeoning field of *neuroimaging*. Simply put, neuro-imaging encompasses

> a set of new technologies [that] has given us the ability to study how the human brain works in greater detail than ever before. These tools are known as *neuroimaging* methods, because they allow us to create images of the human brain that show us what it is made of (which we refer to as its *structure*) and what it is doing (which we refer to as its *function*).
>
> (Poldrack 2018, p. 1)

Arguably, the most revolutionary tool of all has been *magnetic resonance imaging* (MRI). Now, MRI comes in various forms, and different kinds of MRI scans measure specific aspects of the brain. *Structural* MRI captures aspects of the makeup of neural tissue, such as how much water or fat is present. To determine what the brain is doing, we need *functional* MRI, or "fMRI," which, roughly speaking, detects the shadow of brain activity—engagement in a cognitive task—through its effects on the amount of oxygen in the blood.

Let's focus on so-called *reverse inference*, which basically allows one to infer the engagement of a particular mental process from specific activation patterns or locations in the brain, as opposed to a "forward inference," from mental states to brain processes. Here I provide an admittedly simplified reconstruction of the underlying argument—for a more detailed overview of reverse inference and its limitations, see Nathan and Del Pinal (2017).

Consider a psychological generalization describing how humans typically behave while undertaking a certain cognitive task. For instance, suppose that we perform better on a test when we listen to soothing music. Presumably, there will be various cognitive processes that could explain this tendency. For instance, music may increase our concentration or, alternatively, listening to music may block negative emotions that interfere with cognitive performance. How do we decide which option, if either, is correct? Reverse inference shows how to employ neuroscientific evidence to answer this question. The trick is to find some association between the competing cognitive processes and some underlying areas or patterns of neural activation. For instance, being focused may be associated with a certain kind of brain activity x, whereas blocking emotions could be associated with a different neural pattern y. This being so, we can conduct a neuroimaging scan while subjects are performing the test. If the scan detects type-x activity and not type-y activity, this provides evidence that what explains enhanced performance is focus, as opposed to lack of emotions. To be sure, this constitutes an oversimplification, because most brain regions and patterns of brain activity will be associated with several cognitive tasks—the "lack of selectivity objection." Various strategies have been offered to rule out alternative explanations (Del Pinal and Nathan 2013; Hutzler 2014; Machery 2014). We need not worry about details here.

Once again, the crucial point, for our present purposes, is that the association of a cognitive subprocess with a neural region or pattern need not be a causal one. Indeed, while it is possible that the patterns detected via fMRI are what produce the mental state, this is the exception rather than the rule. All that is required for the argument to go through is an *associative* link, not a bona fide reduction. These associative bridge laws may be conceived as probabilistic and context-sensitive relations that do not identify their relata, either at the type-level or at the token-level (Nathan and Del Pinal 2016). In short, the association between cognitive state and neural pattern can be used to predict ("reverse-infer") the former from the latter or predict ("forward infer") the latter from the former. But neither inference is typically explanatory. To emphasize, such inferences may well be explanatory, if the neural processes in question are causally responsible for the mental state. Nevertheless—and this is the take-home message—they need not be.

In conclusion, reverse and forward inference, alongside the required fMRI technology, are, at heart, instruments of prediction, not explanation. In this respect, they are like GWAS and biomarkers. The moral, of course, isn't that description and explanation are irrelevant in science. What the predictive turn shows is that forecasting may become a goal in and of itself, in the absence of explanation. What philosophical consequences might this have?

4 The Toolbox Problem

The previous section outlined three scientific tools, whose development required a host of technological and conceptual advancements: GWAS, biomarkers, and neuroimaging. All three can be conceived primarily as instruments of prediction, as opposed to explanation. GWAS need not uncover any causal link between genotype and phenotype. As such, they frequently do not explain the presence of the trait under study, without tainting their forecasting value. Biomarkers can increase our confidence in the occurrence of a specific physiological process or reaction, while not offering any insight as to what produces the state at hand. fMRI is grounded in a series of associative bridge laws that reverse-infer the engagement of a cognitive process based on neural activation or, vice versa, forward-infer neural activity based on cognitive engagement. Again, all of this can be effectively done without shedding any light on their causal interplay and, thereby, not warranting any causal-mechanistic explanation. These are clear illustrations of the predictive turn.

Some readers may find none of this strange, concerning, or remotely controversial. As mentioned at the outset, prediction is a traditional goal of science. Why should one be surprised by the emergence of predictive tools?

The development of predictive tools *per se* is hardly shocking. The vexing issue, from a philosophical perspective, is squaring the presence of these instruments—characterized from a purely predictive, as opposed to an explanatory standpoint—with the mainstream causal-mechanistic outlook. I dub this the "toolbox problem" because it challenges us to spell out a framework that captures how prediction and explanation can mutually inform each other without reducing to one and the same. As I will argue in due course, prediction is, indeed, a form of "settling for less," a cheaper version of explanation. But that does not undermine its pivotal role.

In the heyday of logical positivism, the toolbox problem did not occur. The ruling theory of explanation, the CLM, treated prediction and explanation as two sides of the same coin. "[The same logical] schema underlies both explanation and prediction; only the knowledge situation is different. In explanation, the fact Qa [the explanandum] is already known. (...) In prediction, Qa is a fact *not yet known*" (Carnap 1966, p. 17). Hence, a predictive inference is always explanatory and, vice versa, an explanation also has predictive power. The statistical techniques involved in a well-conducted GWAS provide an informed guess as to whether an individual with genotype g will display phenotypic trait t. If this prediction is borne out, we thereby have an explanation of t. The same can be said about biomarkers and neuroimaging. If explanation and prediction are logically equivalent, predictive and explanatory oomph goes hand in hand.

When the CLM was displaced by the CMM, a wedge was drawn between prediction and explanation, which were no longer perceived as symmetrical. So, how are these inferences related? Clearly, they support each other. But how? Explanation is now a matter of causal-mechanistic detail. If prediction is not logically equivalent to explanation, what is the logical structure of a predictive inference? How does predictive value enhance explanatory power and, vice versa, how does explanation contribute to a prediction? This is the toolbox problem.

It is important not to conflate what I call the "toolbox problem" with what has been dubbed the "causal fallacy." The *causal fallacy*, as Broadbent (2013, p. 83) presents it, is the mistake of believing that all explanations have predictive power.

> Proving that X causes Y does not license a good prediction that removing X will lead to a corresponding reduction in the incidence of Y. To put it another way, just because X causes Y, that does not mean that removing X is a sufficient means to removing Y. Just because the frying pan is making you hot does not mean that jumping out of it is a good way to cool down.

Is the causal fallacy really a fallacy? Does all explanation enable prediction? This remains an interesting open question. Still, this issue is tangential to my toolbox problem, which is distinct. It involves explaining how we can have prediction without explanation. How do we get correlational structures underwritten by causal arrows that point in the wrong direction?

As Pearl and Mackenzie (2018, p. 30) quip, "Good predictions need not have good explanations. The owl can be a good hunter without understanding why the rat always goes from point *A* to point *B*." While this seems unassailable, by focusing exclusively on causal-mechanistic relations, one misses the point of the predictive turn. Attentive readers will surely note that there are various ways of answering the toolbox problem. The remainder of this section explores some intuitive options and argues that none of them is ultimately successful. Then, the following section will offer a different "black box" solution to our conundrum.

A first reaction is the timeworn, ostrich-inspired tendency to stick one's head into the sand. From this standpoint, admittedly not especially popular, the toolbox problem is not something we should lose sleep over. Sure, the objection runs, prediction has a role to play in science. And there may well be concepts that predict without explaining. Yet, these are the exception rather than the rule. The issue is not widespread enough to make it worth our while. Better to focus our attention on what really matters for science, namely, mechanistic description and causal explanation.

This initial riposte strikes me as myopic. Our three case studies are but the tip of the iceberg. Predictive inferences of this ilk are ubiquitous. From computer science to climatology, from evolutionary theory to psychology, prediction *sans* explanation is not the exception to the norm. Furthermore, my examples are hardly marginal. GWAS are a central tool in genomics. Biomarkers are the holy grail of precision medicine. And neuroimaging, for better or for worse, has come to dominate cognitive psychology. Hence, dismissing the issue is no more effective than the cognate strategy of sticking your head in the sand in hope that a predator will chase itself away. Better to put our focus elsewhere.

A second, more promising response is to insist that the alleged structural discrepancy between explanation and prediction is merely illusory. The CMM, properly understood and contextualized, is perfectly capable of taking care of both explanation and prediction. Both inferences rely on causal-mechanistic knowledge.

Consider, first, biomarkers and associated conditions, such as the link between high PSA levels and prostate cancer. To the best of my knowledge, high PSA is not among the causes of cancer. Still, there must be something that underlies and explains the reliable correlation between biomarker and pathology. Obviously, it cannot be a cosmic coincidence that high PSA is consistently associated with cancer. There must be some causal connection.

A similar insight applies to neuroimaging. Take, for instance, a computer classifier able to reliably reverse-infer the engagement of cognitive state P from some location or pattern of neural activation N. Now, presumably, P is not completely causally independent of the underlying neural activity N. Clearly, it would be fallacious to infer from this correlation, without further corroborating evidence, that P and N are type-identical, or that N directly causes P. Still, for the association between P and N to be robust, and therefore useful in the context of a reverse inference, there must be some causal connection between the neural substrate and the mental superstrate.

In short, the argument runs, both examples point to the same conclusion. Prediction, just like explanation, is a thoroughly causal-mechanistic endeavor. The CMM can thus take care of both. Toolbox problem solved.

There is something about this second rejoinder that strikes me as correct. Prediction, lest it becomes hocus pocus, must exploit mechanistic links. My own solution, outlined in Section 5, will indeed posit a causal connection between predictor and predicted state. Having said this, as just presented, this reply is too crude. No one should dispute the existence of a mechanistic pathway linking high PSA with cancer or mental states with neural activity. Yet, such a connection does not explain the pathology or mental state. In other words, the causal connection between predictor and prediction is what ensures the *robustness* of the inference (for a discussion of robustness in neuroscience, see Tramacere, this volume). Still—and this is the crucial point—such causal-mechanistic connection need not explain the relevant outcome, that is, the explanandum.

Moving on, a third reaction to the toolbox problem insists that prediction and explanation are fundamentally distinct. Explanation follows the CMM. Prediction does not. Thus, perhaps, the solution consists in retaining the CMM for explanation, while developing an altogether different approach to prediction. From this perspective, two mistakes need mending. First, the CLM wrongly assumed that prediction and explanation are two sides of the same coin. The CMM rectified this by drawing the two inferences apart. Second, the CMM fails to develop an independent account of prediction. That's the missing ingredient.

The predictable follow-up becomes: which model of prediction will do the trick? Many alternatives are on the table, from statistical Bayesian networks approaches, to a purely logical "covering-law model of prediction" that drops any pretense of explaining, to hybrid approaches that purport to combine both insights. All three avenues seem worth pursuing, together with potentially others. Still, I'm skeptical about the prospects of rendering prediction completely independently of explanation. Why? For one thing, it offends the aesthetic taste of those of us who long for some sort of unified scientific methodology. Second, and more to the point, it leaves something out. Prediction and explanation do have something in common, at least intuitively. Making a correct prediction may open the door, even if a slight crack, to providing a corresponding explanation. Conversely, explaining something is an effective strategy to draw an effective prediction. To be sure, we are now back to square one. We still need to address the toolbox problem by characterizing the nature of this connection. True. But throwing in the towel and developing an account of prediction completely severed from explanation throws the baby out with the bath water. I'll advance a better proposal in the following section. First, however, we've got one final option to explore.

A fourth, and final rejoinder would be to return to the CLM. The underlying idea is that we already have a theory that provides a unified treatment of prediction and explanation, namely, the covering-law model. Perhaps the mistake was wandering away from Hempel and Oppenheim's hallowed approach.

This route seems to me to get us out of the frying pan and into the fire. As noted all along, the CMM comes with costs and difficulties of its own. Nevertheless, walking away from the deductive-nomological approach was the right move. The notorious asymmetries are there to remind us that predicting and explaining are not one and the same logical inference. This point was reinforced by our illustrations of the predictive turn. Much explanation requires causation; prediction often does not, settling for correlation. Rehashing the CLM, in other words, is a nostalgic way of reliving the glory days, a past that was abandoned for good reason. We're better off looking to the future, whatever that may be.

Let's take a quick breather. This section introduced the toolbox problem, the issue of showing how prediction and explanation can, intuitively, mutually inform and support each other, without reducing one to the other. There are many ways of addressing this challenge. We explored four possible rejoinders, none of which, I argued, hits the bullseye. Section 5 develops a different, more effective line of argument, a "black-box" solution to our toolbox problem.

5 A Black-Box Solution

The previous section introduced the toolbox problem: the task of characterizing the interplay between prediction and explanation. I explored four rejoinders. First, one can deny that prediction is all that central to science. Second, prediction, like explanation, could be accounted for at a causal-mechanistic level. Third, one may develop a self-standing model that treats prediction independently of explanation. Fourth, the two inferences might be reunited by returning to the old CLM. None of these strategies, I maintained, is ultimately successful. At the same time, there is no need to throw in the towel. This section sketches a "black-box" solution to the toolbox problem and argues that it provides a viable path forward.

Let's begin by emphasizing, once again, that prediction and explanation are *not* structurally identical. Not all successful forecasts are explanatory. Symptoms diagnose diseases without explaining them. Explanation typically requires causation. Prediction, in contrast, only presupposes correlation, that is, robust, reliable association.

Having noted this, the kind of association underlying predictive inference calls for further elucidation. Even if marker B does not explain condition C, there must be *something* responsible for the link between B and C. Symptoms may not explain diseases, but what makes the correlation between symptoms and diseases reliable, robust? In the case of fMRI, specific patterns of neural activation N need not be type- or even token-identical to the associated cognitive state M. (To be clear, M will be token-identical to *some* neural state. But such neural state need not and, typically, will not be the same neural state N that we use in our forward or reverse inferences.) Still, there must be a causal mechanism which explains why engagement in C is reliably accompanied by activation in N. In short, predicting C from B does rely on a causal-mechanistic story. The point is that, as discussed at length, the causal-mechanistic relation in question may well not correspond to a plausible *explanation* of C from B.

These considerations reveal that, while predictive and explanatory inferences do not have the same structure, they are closely related and inform each other. The question becomes what exactly makes them different. And the answer cannot simply lie in causation vs. correlation since, as said, robust correlations are grounded in causal connections of sorts. My proposal is to draw the relevant distinction in the amount and kind of detail provided. To appreciate the point, it will be useful to separate cases where predictions and explanations coincide from cases where they do not.

Consider, first, a scenario where the same trait, property, or condition is both predictive *and* explanatory of a certain state. Here, marker *B* is a cause *C* of effect *E*. For instance, the modified *huntingtin* gene is both a sure-fire predictor that Huntington's Disease (HD) will occur when the patient comes of age and is also one of the driving factors in neural degeneration.

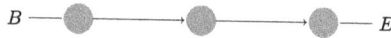

$$B \;—\!\!\!\bullet\!\longrightarrow\!\bullet\!\longrightarrow\!\bullet—\; E$$

What is the difference between using the mutated gene to predict HD and using it to explain it? When we explain HD, specifying some causal-mechanistic details of how the gene induces the pathology will normally deepen and enhance our explanation. To be sure, whether additional information is invariably better, or we eventually reach a threshold where all relevant data has been specified is a hotly debated topic in the specialized literature (Strevens 2016; Craver and Kaplan 2020). Yet, without getting bogged down in tangential complications, understanding and describing how the genetic dysfunction triggers its devastating effects will provide a firmer, more effective explanation of HD. In contrast, these details will not enhance the prediction of HD. An appropriately chosen genetic marker will tell us *that* the condition will appear, or *how likely* it is to appear, without telling us *why*. This why-question, interesting as it surely is, pertains to the purview of explanation, not prediction. Once we establish that condition *E* has an *x*% probability of occurring, motivating this likelihood is not going to improve the forecast in question.

So, for all intents and purposes, we can treat prediction as a mechanism sketch (Craver and Darden 2013) or a black-boxed explanation (Nathan 2021), that is, a placeholder for the causal narrative linking *B* to *E* where most, or even all the relevant causal-mechanistic details have been omitted. Add these causal details back into the model—replace the black box with a "grey" or "transparent" one—and the prediction will, *ipso facto*, turn into an explanation of our explanandum event or data. In short, in this first type of situation, a prediction is just a black-boxed explanation, exactly how some advocates of the CMM suggested, more or less explicitly, all along.

Now, consider the alternative scenario, where a marker is predictive but not explanatory. This could happen for various reasons. I consider two.

In a second possible case, effect *E* is solely or partially causally responsible for biomarker *B*. In such circumstances, we can still use *B* to predict *E*, as the causal link will bolster the association. Yet, as with the flagpole and the shadow, *B* does not explain *E*. If anything, it is *E* that explains *B*. Scriven, Bromberger, and their followers were correct, after all, in their diagnosis that prediction is symmetric while explanation is not. Explanation tends to follow the arrow of causation; prediction does not.

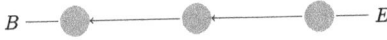

$$B \longleftarrow \bullet \longleftarrow \bullet \longleftarrow \bullet \longrightarrow E$$

A third possibility occurs when E_1 and E_2 are both effects of a common cause *C*. Here, E_1 can be used to predict E_2, just like E_2 could be used to predict E_1. However, E_1 does not explain the occurrence of E_2, just like E_2 does not explain E_1. Both E_1 and E_2 are explained by their common cause *C*. This third scenario is illustrated by the case of high PSA levels and prostate cancer or, to exhume an old example, the relation between stained teeth and lung cancer, both of which are the product of a common cause: smoking.

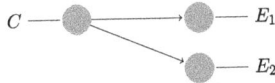

$$C \longrightarrow \bullet \nearrow \bullet E_1 \searrow \bullet E_2$$

In these last two situations, the marker is predictive but not explanatory. Note, once again, that there is an underlying causal-mechanistic connection that ensures the robustness of the association, enabling the prediction. But, unlike our first scenario, adding etiological details will not turn the prediction into an explanation—at least, not an explanation of our explanandum. The shadow predicts the flagpole without explaining it. High PSA levels predict prostate cancer but don't explain it. Both effects are explained by a common cause: genetic predisposition perhaps, although, unfortunately, not much is currently known about this pathology.

Three brief remarks. First, why not use the common cause, as opposed to the correlated marker to predict a condition such as cancer? More generally, could we not use causal explanations to predict effects? Of course, we could. The problem is that causal-mechanistic stories are often quite complex. To wit, not much is currently known about the network of causes of, say, prostate cancer and Huntington's Disease. Thus, having a simple and easy to test marker comes in quite handy for diagnostic purposes.

Second, and relatedly, can a predictive link be explained? Could the causal-mechanistic underpinnings of the relation between PSA levels and cancer not be unveiled, transforming the forecast into a full-blown explanation? Yes, they could. But should they? What exactly is there to be gained? Allow me to elaborate. In some cases, we may want to explain an association to make sure that it is robust enough. When the link between PSA levels and cancer was first observed, researchers could legitimately question the reliability of the marker in detecting a dangerous condition such as prostate cancer. And shedding light on why these conditions tend to correlate may help mitigating legitimate doubts. At the same time, once the robustness of the marker has been established beyond reasonable doubt, an explanation of the marker may be superfluous. What we want to explain is cancer, not PSA levels. When we have substantive evidence that PSA predicts cancer, the explanation of PSA is not all that important—a black box will suffice. It seems better to focus on diagnosing cancer itself and to learn how to cure it.

Third, and finally, what is the relation between prediction and explanation? The CLM treated predictive and explanatory inferences as two sides of the same coin. The CMM drew them apart. Explanation requires specifying the causes underlying a specific phenomenon; prediction does not. These two perspectives can be reconciled by stressing that prediction and explanation pertain to different levels of description, depending on how much mechanistic information is provided. These considerations shed light on ongoing debates concerning the nature of so-called "mathematical" and "causal-dynamical" explanatory models, which include limited causal-mechanistic information (Ross 2015; Green and Jones 2016). Now, whether these explanatory models should be understood as mechanism sketches or as a different type of explanation, or even if they are best conceived from a causal perspective (Woodward 2018; Ross 2021) are questions that I shall not address here. However, our discussion stresses that there is a spectrum of causal models, which vary depending on the amount of abstraction and idealization. On one end of the spectrum, we have detailed "glass box" explanations, where mechanistic components are presented in detail, and the causal link should be as direct as possible. On the opposite side of the spectrum, we have black-boxed predictions, where causal information can be omitted, and the causal link can be much more indirect. In between, there is a continuum of causal models of various sorts. To be sure, spelling out the epistemic norms from these predictive and explanatory inferences, governing the amount of mechanistic detail and the degree of abstraction is a worthwhile project. Yet, this ambitious endeavor lies beyond the scope of the present work.

6 The Moral of the Story

Time to take stock. This essay began, in jest, with a fairy tale. While the tone was humorous, the goal was serious: recounting some momentous episodes in the last 50 years of philosophy of science. While prediction has been neglected in this area of philosophy, some branches of science have witnessed the emergence of a "predictive turn." Admittedly, in fields such as cellular and molecular neuroscience, mechanistic explanation may continue to be the gold standard, at least for now, whereas prediction remains ancillary to understanding. However, GWAS, bio-markers, and fMRI-based inferences show that the situation is quite different in molecular medicine and cognitive neuropsychology, where prediction is rapidly becoming just as important, if not more central than explanation, description, and understanding. And these examples are merely the tip of the iceberg. Hence, if philosophy wants to keep up with methodological advances across the sciences, not merely in se-lected areas, prediction can no longer be relegated to the sidelines. We should devote to it the attention it deserves. This is the only viable strat-egy for appreciating not just the success, but also the limits of scientific explanation.

The second part of the essay discussed various lines of response to what I dubbed the "toolbox problem," that is, the task of providing a unified framework for prediction and explanation, without reducing one to the other. Many intuitive ways of addressing the challenge end up missing the mark. My proposed solution boils down to a "black box" approach. Both prediction and explanation, I suggested, describe the same kinds of entities, laws, and mechanisms. But they do so at very different levels of abstraction and idealization. The structural backbone of these two inferences is the same. Yet, prediction requires not as much causal-mechanistic structure as explanation, and these links may be more or less direct. Effective prediction need not specify the nature of the connection between marker and condition.

Epistemically speaking, explanation is much more demanding, in the sense that it requires a much richer, more detailed characterization of the underlying mechanistic substrate. Still, it would be a mistake to scorn-fully dismiss the focus on prediction as "lazy science." With toy exam-ples, it is easy to brush off the role of correlation. Stained teeth won't be all that useful in the study of cancer, since we know that smoking is the relevant causal variable. But one of the many lessons we learned in the COVID-19 pandemic, is that, when frantically trying to block the spreading of a virus, coughing and sneezing can be valuable predictors. Once again, this is not to downplay the significance of explanation. The point is that our best experimental practice requires a combination of various kinds of inferences.

This black-box strategy has several virtues. In closing, I briefly men-tion two. For one thing, it provides a joint treatment of prediction and explanation, showcasing how these inferences are related albeit distinct. The CLM's mistake was assuming that to explain an event is thereby to predict it. I've argued that there is a substantial discrepancy between these two illocutionary acts, a difference which can be cashed out in terms of the amount of detail required for success. Prediction requires very minimal amounts of mechanistic detail. Explanation, in this re-spect, is much more demanding. Yet, the two inferences are not com-pletely independent. A successful prediction can be an invaluable guide to an explanation and our model shows why: it pinpoints where additional causal-mechanistic structure may be required.

A second advantage of the view outlined here is that it rationalizes the predictive turn, that is, the increasing prominence and growth of instruments of prediction. From our present standpoint, it makes perfect sense why forecasting is often considered the holy grail of science. Prediction is much cheaper than explanation. If all we want to do is figure out whether a specific state is present, a predictive marker is more than enough. Deeper understanding is often desirable, but it is much more expensive and tedious to achieve. From this standpoint, prediction is the first step toward explanation or the final step in some other pursuit. Whether or not we want to take the additional steps demanded by explanation will depend on several contextual features: cost, interest, difficulty, *und so weiter.*

Is the predictive turn something to cherish or bemoan? This remains an open question. Some authors view the current focus on prediction as a way of settling for less. Others see explanation as an expensive luxury, distracting from more urgent and pressing issues—like curing diseases and planning for climate shifts—where prediction is often enough. While these considerations raise deep and important quandaries, this is not the appropriate place to take an explicit position. The significant conclusion drawn in this essay is that, regardless of our stance with respect to prediction, it is high time philosophy gave rightful attention to this prominent kind of inference.

My fairy tale had a happy ending. Prediction and explanation live happily ever after, in peace and harmony. Strictly speaking, this is not a caricatural portrait of the current situation, at least not yet. It's up to us to make sure that dreams turn to reality. But much remains to be done.

Acknowledgments

The author is grateful to Bill Anderson, Janella Baxter, John Bickle, Carl Craver, Guie Del Pinal, Mallory Hrehor, and Antonella Tramacere for constructive comments on various versions of this essay. An early draft was presented on September 28, 2019, at the Tool Development in Experimental Neuroscience workshop in Pensacola Beach, Florida. The audience provided valuable feedback.

References

Alonso-Gonzalez, A. Calaza, C. Rodriguez-Fontenla, and A. Carracedo (2019). "Novel Gene-Based Analysis of ASD GWAS: Insight into the Biological Role of Associated Genes." *Frontiers in Genetics* 10, 733.

Anney, R. J. et al. (2017). "Meta-Analysis of GWAS of Over 16,000 Individuals with Autism Spectrum Disorder Highlights a Novel Locus at 10q24.32 and a Significant Overlap with Schizophrenia." *Molecular*

Autism 8(21). https://molecularautism.biomedcentral.com/articles/10.1186/s13229-017-0137-9#author-information

Bechtel, W. and R. Richardson (1993). *Discovering Complexity: Decomposition and Localization as Strategies in Scientific Research*. Princeton, NJ: Princeton University Press.

Bourrat, P. (2020). "Causation and Single Nucleotide Polymorphism Heritability." *Philosophy of Science* 87(5), 1075–83.

Broadbent, A. (2013). *Philosophy of Epidemiology*. New York: Palgrave MacMillan.

Bromberger, S. (1966). "Why-Questions." In R. Colodny (Ed.), *Mind and Cosmos: Essays in Contemporary Science and Philosophy*, pp. 86–111. Pittsburgh, PA: University of Pittsburgh Press.

Carnap, R. (1966). *An Introduction to the Philosophy of Science*. Mineola, NY: Dover.

Cartwright, N. (1983). *How the Laws of Physics Lie*. Oxford: Clarendon.

Cartwright, N. (2007). *Hunting Causes and Using Them: Approaches in Philosophy and Economics*. Cambridge: Cambridge University Press.

Cartwright, N. (2019). *Nature, the Artful Modeler*. Chicago, IL: Open Court.

Craver, C. F. and L. Darden (2013). *In Search of Mechanisms. Discoveries Across the Life Sciences*. Chicago, IL: University of Chicago Press.

Craver, C. F. and D. M. Kaplan (2020). "Are More Details Better? On the Norms of Completeness for Mechanistic Explanation." *British Journal for the Philosophy of Science* 71(1), 287–319.

Del Pinal, G. and M. J. Nathan (2013). "There and Up Again: On the Uses and Misuses of Neuroimaging in Psychology." *Cognitive Neuropsychology* 30(4), 233–52.

Feigl, H. (1949). "The Scientific Outlook: Naturalism and Humanism." *American Quarterly* 1(2), 135–48.

Friedman, M. (1974). "Explanation and Scientific Understanding." *The Journal of Philosophy* 71(1), 5–19.

Ghiara, V. and F. Russo (2019). "Reconstructing the Mixed Mechanisms of Health: The Role of Bio- and Socio-Markers." *Longitudinal and Life Course Studies* 10, 7–25.

Glennan, S. (2017). *The New Mechanical Philosophy*. Oxford: Oxford University Press.

Goodman, N. (1955). *Fact, Fiction, and Forecast*. Cambridge, MA: Harvard University Press.

Harden, K. P. (2021). "'Reports of My Death Were Greatly Exaggerated': Behavior Genetics in the Postgenomic Era.'" *Annual Review of Psychology* 72, 37–60.

Hempel, C. G. and P. Oppenheim (1948). "Studies in the Logic of Explanation." *Philosophy of Science* 15, 135–75.

Hume, D. (1999 [1748]). *An Enquiry Concerning Human Understanding*. New York: Oxford University Press.

Hume, D. (2000 [1738]). *A Treatise of Human Nature*. New York: Oxford University Press.

Hutzler, F. (2014). "Reverse Inference Is Not a Fallacy Per Se: Cognitive Processes Can Be Inferred from Functional Imaging Data." *Neuroimage* 84, 1061–69.

Illari, P. and F. Russo (2016). "Information Channels and Biomarkers of Disease." *Topoi* 35, 175–90.

Kitcher, P. (1981). "Explanatory Unification." *Philosophy of Science* 48 (4), 507–31.

Kitcher, P. (1989). "Explanatory Unification and the Causal Structure of the World." In P. Kitcher and W. C. Salmon (Eds.), *Scientific Explanation*, pp. 410–505. Minneapolis: University of Minnesota Press.

Lewis, D. K. (1986). "Postscript E to 'Causation'." In *Philosophical Papers*, Volume 2, pp. 193–212. New York: Oxford University Press.

Lewontin, R. (1974). *The Genetic Basis of Evolutionary Change*. New York: Columbia University Press.

Lynch, K. E. and P. Bourrat (2017). "Interpreting Heritability Causally." *Philosophy of Science* 84(1), 14–34.

Machamer, P. K., L. Darden, and C. F. Craver (2000). "Thinking about Mechanisms." *Philosophy of Science* 67, 1–15.

Machery, E. (2014). "In Defense of Reverse Inference." *British Journal for the Philosophy of Science* 65(2), 251–67.

Nathan, M. J. (2016). "Counterfactual Reasoning in Molecular Medicine." In G. Boniolo and M. J. Nathan (Eds.), *Philosophy of Molecular Medicine: Foundational Issues in Research and Practice*, pp. 192–214, New York: Routledge.

Nathan, M. J. (2021). *Black Boxes: How Science Turns Ignorance into Knowledge*. New York: Oxford University Press.

Nathan, M. J. and G. Del Pinal (2016). "Mapping the Mind: Bridge Laws and the Psycho-Neural Interface." *Synthese* 193(2), 637–57.

Nathan, M. J. and G. Del Pinal (2017). "The Future of Cognitive Neuroscience? Reverse Inference in Focus." *Philosophy Compass* 12(7), e12427.

NIH Biomarkers Definitions Working Group. (2001). "Biomarkers and Surrogate Endpoints: Preferred Definitions and Conceptual Framework." *Clinical Pharmacology and Therapeutics* 69, 89–95.

Pearl, J. and D. Mackenzie (2018). *The Book of Why: The New Science of Cause and Effect*. New York: Basic Books.

Poldrack, R. A. (2018). *The New Mind Readers: What Neuroimaging Can and Cannot Reveal about Our Thoughts*. Princeton, NJ: Princeton University Press.

Richardson, K. and M. C. Jones (2019). "Why Genome-Wide Associations with Cognitive Ability Measures are Probably Spurious." *New Ideas in Psychology* 55, 35–41.

Ross, L. N. (2015). "Dynamical Models and Explanation in Neuroscience." *Philosophy of Science* 82(1), 32–54.

Ross, L. N. (2021). "Distinguishing Topological and Causal Explanation." *Synthese* 198, 9803–20.

Russell, B. (1912). *The Problems of Philosophy*. Indianapolis, IN: Hackett.

Russo, F. and J. Williamson (2012). "Envirogenomarkers. The Interplay between Difference-Making and Mechanisms." *Medical Studies* 3, 249–262.

Salmon, W. C. (1984). *Scientific Explanation and the Causal Structure of the World*. Princeton, NJ: Princeton University Press.

Salmon, W. C. (1998). *Causality and Explanation*. New York: Oxford University Press.

Scriven, M. (1958). "Definitions, Explanations, and Theories." In H. Feigl, M. Scriven, and G. Maxwell (Eds.), *Minnesota Studies in the Philosophy of Science*, Volume 2, pp. 99–195. Minneapolis: University of Minnesota Press.

Spirtes, P., C. Glymour, and R. Scheines (2000). *Causation, Prediction, and Search* (2nd ed.). Cambridge and London: MIT Press.

Strevens, M. (2008). *Depth. An Account of Scientific Explanation*. Cambridge, MA: Harvard University Press.

Strevens, M. (2016). "Special-Science Autonomy and the Division of Labor." In M. Couch and J. Pfeifer (Eds.), *The Philosophy of Philip Kitcher*, pp. 153–81. New York: Oxford University Press.

Sul, J., L. Marti, P. Skidmore, A. Cassidy, S. Fairweather-Tait, L. Hooper, and A. A. Roe (2018). "Population Structure in Genetic Studies: Confounding Factors and Mixed Models." *PLoS Genetics* 14(12), e1007309.

Torrica, B., A. G. Chiocchetti, E. Bacchelli, E. Trabetti, A. Hervás, B. Franke, J. K. Buitelaar, N. Rommelse, A. Yousaf, E. Duketis, and C. M. Freitag. (2017). "Lack of Replication of Previous Autism Spectrum Disorder GWAS Hits in European Populations." *Autism Research* 10(2), 202–11.

van der Sijde, M., A. Ng, and J. Fu (2014). "Systems Genetics: From GWAS to Disease Pathways." *Biochimica et Biophysica Acta* 1842(10), 1903–9.

Vineis, P., P. Illari, and F. Russo (2017). "Causality in Cancer Research: A Journey Through Models in Molecular Epidemiology and Their Philosophical Interpretation." *Emerging Themes in Epidemiology* 14, 7.

Visscher, P., N. R. Wray, Q. Zhang, P. Sklar, M. I. McCarthy, J. Brown, A. Matthew, and Yang (2017). "10 Years of GWAS Discovery: Biology, Function, and Translation." *The American Journal of Human Genetics* 101(1), 5–22.

Vrieze, S. I., W. G. Iacono, and M. McGue (2012). "Confluence of Genes, Environment, Development, and Behavior in a Post-GWAS World." *Development and Psychopathology* 24(4), 1195–214.

Weiskopf, D. A. (2021). "Data Mining the Brain to Decode the Mind." In F. Calzavarini and M. Viola (Eds.), *Neural Mechanisms: New Challenges in the Philosophy of Neuroscience*, pp. 85–110. Cham: Springer.

Woodward, J. (2003). *Making Things Happen. A Theory of Causal Explanation*. New York: Oxford University Press.

Woodward, J. (2018). "Some Varieties of Non-Causal Explanation." In A. Reutlinger and J. Saatsi, *Explanation Beyond Causation: Philosophical Perspectives on Non-Causal Explanations*, pp. 117–37. Oxford: Oxford University Press.

Research Tools, Integration, Circuits, and Ontology

10 How Do Tools Obstruct (and Facilitate) Integration in Neuroscience?

David J. Colaço

1 Introduction

For the past decade, philosophers have investigated how the methods, data, and especially the explanatory frameworks of the subfields of neuroscience might be integrated (Craver 2007; Sullivan 2017). This interest is unsurprising, as neuroscientists investigate diverse entities and phenomena at different scales of the brain, which they aim to link via scientific integration. Neuroscientists have developed integrative projects (Shepherd et al. 1998; Markram 2012; Jorgenson et al. 2015; Amunts et al. 2016) to both better understand the brain at different scales and develop treatments for diseases (Markram 2012; Jorgenson et al. 2015).

Given that these integrative projects have been active for a decade, it seems prudent to ask how successful they have been. *Systematic* integrative brain modeling projects, such as the Human Brain Project or Blue Brain, have not fulfilled their ambitious goals (Yong 2019), and the promised therapeutic interventions have yet to be delivered. At the same time, neuroscientists have integrated *locally*, with piecemeal connections made between subfields (Sullivan 2017). This disconnect between desires and reality raises two questions. First, why has integrative neuroscience not matched its expectations? Second, why does it succeed when it does?

In this chapter, I answer these questions by arguing that tools can both obstruct and facilitate scientific integration, where tools are the materials and technologies that researchers use to study brain structure and activity. My argument is built on two premises about popular tools in neuroscience: (1) these tools have different *constraints*, (2) despite these constraints, these tools *productively* generate knowledge. Together, these premises entail that established tools contribute to knowledge production often at the expense of the integration of methods, data, or explanatory frameworks. This fact explains why we can find cases of local integration across neuroscience, but systematic integration remains elusive.

In Section 2, I detail integration in neuroscience. I discuss how different components – methods, data, and explanatory frameworks – might be integrated, and I address the disconnect between desires for integration and its reality. In Section 3, I defend my premises for why tools

DOI: 10.4324/9781003251392-14

obstruct scientific integration. I illustrate them with examples from cognitive neuroscience and molecular and cellular cognition. In Section 4, I explain why some new projects, such as the BRAIN Initiative, prioritize the development of new tools to facilitate integration. I support my claims with a case study of the tool known as CLARITY. This case shows that tools can facilitate integration, explaining why local integration occurs despite as-of-yet unfulfilled desires of systematic integration, given the constraints and productivity of tools.

2   What Kind of Scientific Integration Do Neuroscientists Want?

Neuroscientists claim that integration will elucidate the brain as well as foster treatments for psychiatric disorders. For instance, architects of the tool-focused BRAIN Initiative (Brain Research through Advancing Innovative Neurotechnologies) suggest that integration will inform interventions upon brain systems from cells to circuits, regions, and the whole brain. Integration is needed, the architects argue, because addressing components in isolation has not resulted in viable interventions (Jorgenson et al. 2015, p. 9; see also Bassett and Sporns 2017, p. 355).

2.1 What Is Scientific Integration?

Before evaluating these projects, I first detail what integration is. At its broadest, scientific integration covers "various possible modes of relationship that can be developed between disciplines" (Bechtel 1993, p. 33). This is a start, but it does not explain how subfields link via scientific integration. To clarify the "how" question, O'Malley and Soyer characterize scientific integration as "a multi-faceted dynamic, in which methods, bodies of data and explanations are synthesized in order to understand and intervene more effectively" (2012, p. 59). This characterization captures that we can integrate methods (Mitchell and Gronenborn 2017), data (Leonelli 2016), or explanatory frameworks (Sullivan 2017).

The first mode is methodological integration: "directing a range of methods at a particular biological system or research problem in order to gain a multidimensional understanding of how the system works" (O'Malley and Soyer 2012, p. 60). The BRAIN Initiative aims to integrate methods, given the desire to "facilitate the integration of many multiple approaches into a single experiment" (Jorgenson et al. 2015, p. 5). Thus, researchers want tools that can be used in tandem when they investigate a neural system, so that they can acquire knowledge about different aspects of this system (Kotchoubey et al. 2016).

The second mode is data integration: "the activity of making comparable different data types from a huge variety of inconsistent sources," which "forms a new body of information that can be treated as a unified whole" (O'Malley and Soyer 2012, p. 61). The BRAIN Initiative aims to integrate data: "datasets from different laboratories will cover spatial scales ranging from micrometres to metres... and time scales ranging from milliseconds to minutes, hours or even the lifetime of an organism" (Jorgenson et al. 2015, p. 7). Data integration is an aim of the Human Brain Project, where "unifying computer models" will "integrate all existing data" (Markram 2012, p. 52).

The third mode is explanatory integration: "when combinations of different methods invoke the fusion of explanatory frameworks, commonly in the accommodation of multiple levels of phenomena" (O'Malley and Soyer 2012, p. 61). The BRAIN Initiative aims to integrate explanatory models: "a unified view of the brain will cross spatial and temporal levels, recognizing that the nervous system consists of interacting molecules, cells and circuits" (Jorgenson et al. 2015, p. 9). This mode also is the focal aim of the Human Brain Project (Markram 2012).

This three-part distinction is only one way we can account for scientific integration, but it matches the interests of neuroscientists. Rather than vaguely integrating "disciplines," distinguishing methods, data, and explanatory frameworks also characterizes how subfields of neuroscience can be integrated. This is helpful, as integrating one mode need not entail integrating the others. Further, it explains why integration is conceptually distinct from epistemic aims like generalization. Generalization is inducing or extrapolating about an experimental outcome; integration is about linking methods, data, and frameworks.

We also can distinguish local and systematic integration. While there is no hard separation, local integration is piecemeal both in terms of modes and subfields: two subfields might link their methods, data, or explanatory frameworks. For instance, neurobiology and behavioral neuroscience integrate methods and explanatory frameworks in the study of spatial memory via variants of the Morris water maze (Sullivan 2016, p. 671). This is a case of local integration, which has generated knowledge, predictions, and experimental protocols. By contrast, systematic integration is wholesale. The Human Brain Project and Blue Brain are attempts at systematic data and, more importantly, explanatory integration, as each is intended to develop a brain model that is informed by diverse studies at different scales.

2.2 The Challenge

There is a consensus amongst philosophers and neuroscientists that integration is challenging. Sullivan notes that there are "conceptual and methodological obstacles to integration" in neuroscience (2017, p. 129), while Kotchoubey and colleagues note that there are "methodological and epistemic problems that obstruct the development of human neuroscience" (2016, p. 1). Likewise, the architects of the BRAIN Initiative note that integration is "a particularly daunting challenge" (Jorgenson et al. 2015, p. 7).

The literature on integrative neuroscience suggests that there are challenges for each mode. For methodological integration, there are "methodological gaps" between subfields, which create "problems of integration... when we are trying to connect several disciplinary traditions" (Kotchoubey et al. 2016, p. 5). For data integration, while there is a deluge of data being produced about neural systems (Kotchoubey et al. 2016, p. 1), philosophers like Sullivan argue that "we should not expect that amassing potentially discordant data from many different laboratories under a single common label... will shed light on real divisions in the causal structure of the world" (2017, p. 134). For explanatory integration, there is a worry about what experiments target, which undermines the "connectability" of frameworks that are developed (Sullivan 2016, p. 665). Neuroscientists in different subfields may not investigate the same targets, complicating the synthesis of their explanatory frameworks.

Integrating neuroscience is challenging but not impossible. As already mentioned, cases can be made for local integration. When looking for more systematic integration, network neuroscience adopts an "integrative perspective" when modeling neural systems (Bassett and Sporns 2017, p. 353). Network models are designed to integrate data from different studies performed at different scales, which can be used by researchers to explanatorily integrate models of these scales. So far, scientists have generated models that integrate observations performed on hundreds of neurons with those at higher scales, as "network science tools are perfectly suited to accomplish the important goal of crossing levels or scales of organization, integrating diverse data sets, and bridging existing disparate analyses" (Bassett and Sporns 2017, p. 362).

At the same time, challenges abound in this nascent subfield of neuroscience. Beyond the complaint that these models fail to meet expectations (Yong 2019), network models have yet to integrate explanatory frameworks of most populations of neurons. These limitations reflect that integrative neuroscience has yet to catch up with scientists' desires. More interesting is the fact that network modeling is only part of the puzzle. Researchers need data that support these models (Sporns 2014, p. 653). This fact indicates that there remain issues for integrating data from existing neuroscience studies, which is due to how these studies were performed. This implication, in turn, reveals that network neuroscience (and modeling in neuroscience more generally) is but one part of integrating neuroscience, which can benefit from new experiments.

Thus, there are successful (local) cases of neuroscience integration, but there also is a disconnect between the desires for (especially systematic explanatory) integration and its reality. Why is this the case? I explore an answer that is hinted at by the network neuroscientists: understanding integration requires us to reflect upon the tools of neuroscience. By 'tools,' I mean the materials and technologies that researchers employ when measuring or manipulating brain activity and structure (Bickle 2016). In this chapter, I focus on tools used in the production of data via experimentation and observation.

3 How Do Tools Obstruct Scientific Integration?

The previous section addresses that there is a desire to integrate neuroscience to a greater degree than what has been achieved. One obstacle, it would seem, is the diversity of tools used by neuroscientists. However, why might tools be obstacles?

3.1 Constraints and Productivity

First, all tools *constrain* empirical research. The choice of tools limits what other tools can be used, what domains of systems can be investigated, what aspects of the system can be manipulated or measured, and what data can be produced. Researchers use tools to achieve certain outcomes in an experiment, which requires that they be paired with methods that complement a tool's use. While exploration might lead to discoveries about new ways to use a tool, using a tool beyond its constraints often results in a failure of its ability to produce knowledge.

Colaço describes the "constraining role" of tools by appeal to the preparation and staining techniques used in microscopy: if "one chooses to use a staining technique on a cell to investigate it with microscopy, one will not be able to investigate any components of the cell that are destroyed by the staining process" (2018, p. 38). Thus, tools whose constraints do not overlap are not usable in tandem due to requirements for researchers to prepare or modify the system in distinct ways that accommodate the use of these respective tools. Further, the modifications each tool makes to this target complicate the comparison of instances of the use of tools that each modify but ostensibly measure or manipulate the same target.

Not all constraints result from preparation or modification. Invasive electrophysiological stimulation is constrained inasmuch as it cannot be performed on humans unless cranial intervention is deemed necessary for medical intervention. Other tools are constrained by issues of temporal or spatial scale: magnetic resonance imaging (MRI) cannot image individual neurons. Regardless of the reason for the constraint, if different tools do not overlap in constraints, they cannot be used together to investigate aspects of the same system.

Second, established tools are *productive*. Tools are developed and standardized to be easy and efficient for researchers to reliably produce useful data about the targets whose domain lies within the constraints of the tool. Thus, despite the fact that tools have constraints, they are effective when used within these constraints. These tools can be used to generate knowledge about the systems that researchers want to study. In this sense, tools are "productive" in an epistemic sense. Correspondingly, these researchers also can publish research using these tools, allowing them to be "productive" in the sense that they can achieve prudential aims, such as publishing high-impact work, getting funding, and building one's professional reputation.

The productivity of tools used in existing experimental paradigms is well-supported in the existing literature. For instance, Krohs claims that "many experiments are... done in the way they are actually done, because they are extraordinarily convenient to perform" (2012, p. 53). Tools are easy and efficient means of achieving certain aims in an experiment. However, a tool "strongly channels research," and data that are produced are determined by it (Krohs 2012, p. 53). Likewise, due to their constraints, tools cannot be used in just any experimental design. Thus, when researchers find tools to be productive for the aims that they have, we should expect that researchers will develop protocols that use them as opposed to those that do not.

A consequence of productivity in science rears its head in debates about unification. Harp and Khalifa claim that researchers might sacrifice long-term gains in unifying research for them to achieve short-term gains. Because there remain achievable goals in local research projects, "the utility of an optimal local strategy is sometimes greater than that of an optimal cosmopolitan strategy, even when the value of a local success is lower than that of an unquestionable, and hence cosmopolitan, success" (Harp and Khalifa 2015, p. 441). While these claims address unification, a similar point can be made about integration in neuroscience. So long as existing tools reliably produce useful data about neural systems that researchers want to investigate, then we should expect researchers to continue to use these tools even at the expense of methodological, data, and explanatory integration.

Together, constraints and productivity suggest that researchers can either continue to reliably produce useful data about the systems they investigate, or they can use less productive tools to less reliably produce data that may be less useful for investigating their targets. As long as the established tools continue to produce knowledge about neural systems, using these tools will be a reliable way for researchers to produce this knowledge, regardless of their contribution (or lack thereof) to scientific integration.

3.2 How Do Tools Obstruct Scientific Integration?

Methodological integration is most obviously obstructed by the diversity of tools. Distinct tools have different constraints that are intimately tied to their productivity. If these constraints require the neural system to be prepared or manipulated in incompatible ways, researchers will not be able to direct "a range of methods at a particular biological system" in tandem "in order to gain a multidimensional understanding" of this system. For instance, microscopy often depends on staining and slicing neural tissue in order for researchers to image it, while structural MRI requires the system to be intact and free of metallic stains. These tools cannot be used in tandem without undermining their respective productivity. While sequential uses of some tools, such as Logothetis and colleagues' use of functional MRI (fMRI) and single-cell recording (2001), are possible, this kind of integrative paradigm is challenging to perform and cannot be performed on all brain structures that each tool can be used on individually. These facts are illustrated by how infrequently Logothetis and colleagues' paradigm is reproduced.

By contrast, if tools with distinct constraints are used on different instances of the same neural system, the modifications that must be made to each system for researchers to use the particular tool within its constraints can transform them in inconsistent ways. This inconsistent set of changes, in turn, makes it difficult to relate the effects that each tool has on the neural system under investigation. Along these lines, because tools limit the ability for researchers to efficiently use other tools, the use of a range of methods on a neural system can make a tool less productive. This not only undermines the reliability of the data that any tool can produce when used within its constraints; it also makes it harder to produce these data.

Perhaps readers think that methodological integration is not important in the grand scheme of things. However, data integration is obstructed by tools as well. The data produced from tools reflect their constraints: these data reflect the assumptions, biases, and modifications that must be made about the system in order for researchers to use the tool to produce reliable data about it. This is a problem if we accept that data integration "refers to the process of theorizing and modelling databases," as the theories and models we build of the databases will reflect constraints of particular tools at the expense of those frameworks that are limited by other tools that do not share the same constraints (O'Malley and Soyer 2012, p. 61).

While this problem has its basis in the idea that experiments "can produce highly variable results that are hard to model in any generalizable way," and "combining different data types remains a stubbornly persistent problem" (O'Malley 2013, p. 552), this problem becomes more serious when we consider the effect these procedures have on data production. On one hand, if developing databases requires an appeal to data produced through the use of tools, these datasets will reflect the constraints of these tools. On the other hand, if researchers develop databases based on a framework that is not indebted to the data produced from the use of tools, then these databases may not match the constraints of the diverse tools whose data will plug into these databases.

Either way, the tools complicate "the activity of making comparable different data types," and they therefore can obstruct data integration.

Even with methodological and data integration obstructed, readers might be most interested in explanatory integration. However, explanatory integration is obstructed as well. Explanatory frameworks develop and advance based on data obtained from studies that use tools. As a result, these frameworks reflect the constraints of the tools used to produce these data, and these frameworks also support the subsequent use of these tools to produce data. While it is to be expected that any empirical science's explanatory frameworks will be influenced by the studies that are performed in that discipline, neuroscience, having little in the way of a systematic theory that guides all research, is built on the results of experiment and observation.

The mere fact that different experiments share labels does not generate an integrated explanatory framework. These labels "do not reflect the intra and interdisciplinary consensus as to how to generally define or how to produce, detect and measure the phenomena designated by those labels" (Sullivan 2017, p. 134). This fact, in turn, results from the fact that constructs are differently operationalized in studies that deploy different tools. Because operationalizations capture measurement (Feest 2005), and the constraints of tools must match measures of target phenomena, diverse tools can result in the need to measure targets in distinct ways. At worst, operationalizations can be incompatible, but the larger issue is that how they relate might be poorly understood by researchers, thus undermining explanatory integration.

Neither the constraints nor productivity of tools entails that the three modes of integration cannot occur. Rather, these features of tool use show that the use of tools to generate scientific knowledge can be (and often is) unsympathetic to the aims of scientific integration. In this sense, tools can serve as obstacles to methodological, data, and explanatory integration, leading to an undermining of systematic integration and situational cases of local integration.

3.3 Tools Obstructing Scientific Integration: MCC and Cognitive Neuroscience

An example of how tools obstruct scientific integration between neuroscience subfields can be found when we compare different subfields that study cognition. Take molecular and cellular cognition (MCC), a subfield where molecular and cellular approaches are used to study behavioral and cognitive phenomena. MCC uses tools like "molecular manipulations (e.g., gene targeting, viral vectors, pharmacology), cellular measures and manipulations (neuroanatomy, electrophysiology, optogenetics, cellular and circuit imaging), and a plethora of behavioral assays" in the study of cognition (Silva et al. 2013, p. 8). Researchers use these tools to "intervene into molecular pathways in neurons and attempt to develop explanations that bridge molecules, cells, circuits, and behavior" (Silva et al. 2013, p. 12).

MCC does not readily integrate with other subfields that involve the study of cognition, such as cognitive neuroscience. This lack of integration with cognitive neuroscience is a feature of MCC according to the Molecular and Cellular Cognition Society:

> Unlike Cognitive Neuroscience, which historically has focused on the connection between human brain systems and behavior, the field of Molecular and Cellular Cognition studies how molecular (i.e. receptor, kinase activation), intra-cellular (i.e. dendritic processes), and inter-cellular processes (i.e. synaptic plasticity; network representations such as place fields) modulate animal models of cognitive function.
> (Molecular and Cellular Cognition Society)

Thus, even though these two subfields ostensibly study the same cognitive capacities, they study these capacities with distinct tools. In addition, this quote suggests that MCC researchers perceive their work to be an alternative to cognitive neuroscience, rather than something that is intended to integrate with it.

The differences between MCC and cognitive neuroscience can be illustrated by how memory might be studied in each subfield. To study memory deficits, MCC researchers use tools like electrophysiology and transgenetics to manipulate synaptic and molecular activities in a mouse model organism (Silva 2003). To use these tools on this model organism, the researchers must operationalize memory deficits in a way that can be measured in mice. At this time, tools like electrophysiology and transgenetics have not been used on human subjects due to ethical constraints, leaving open how the mechanistic schemata developed in MCC relate to schemata that represent or explain memory phenomena in other animals (let alone humans).

Cognitive neuroscientists use different tools than those that are used in MCC. When studying human memory phenomena, they often use MRI to correlate brain activity differences between healthy and impaired human subjects (Gabrieli 1998). This tool can be methodologically integrated with other tools like EEG. However, methods like fMRI cannot be concurrently used with electrophysiology in mouse model organisms, due to electromagnetic constraints. This incompatibility obstructs the integration of methods that employ tools with distinct constraints. Further, how memory deficits are operationalized in the two cases is not equivalent, making it difficult to compare the data from humans and mice. This mismatch obstructs data integration from studies whose targets may not be equivalent, even if these targets share the same nomenclature. This fact ultimately obstructs the integration of explanatory frameworks from these subfields. Because the relation between targets is unclear, it also is unclear how the mechanistic schemata in mouse model organisms relate to memory in humans.

This case does not exhaust the tools that are used in MCC or cognitive neuroscience. For instance, cognitive neuroscience can employ more invasive tools in model organisms like the rhesus macaque. Further, cognitive neuroscience has integrated explanatory frameworks from neurobiology (though not MCC) in its history. For instance, neurobiological work on long-term potentiation in the rabbit hippocampus (Colaço 2020) has greatly informed neuroimaging studies on the role of the hippocampus in memory formation and consolidation. Thus, integration between cognitive neuroscience and MCC can occur, but we must be clear about exactly what of these subfields is integrated. This interaction is just one example of a case where the reality fails to meet the desires of the integration of neuroscience, but it highlights what integration is up against. While local methodological, data, and explanatory integration might occur – MCC and cognitive neuroscience have cases of all three – each can be obstructed. Additionally, systematic integration remains elusive and might not be desired by researchers in these respective subfields.

Nonetheless, we must ask how the methods, data, and explanatory frameworks that are used in these subfields might be integrated. Each mode of integration is obstructed. However, MCC and cognitive neuroscience each are individually successful, indebted to the fact that each subfield has productive tools that, when used within their respective constraints, produce useful data about the systems the respective groups of researchers target. These data, in turn, feed into the explanatory frameworks of each subfield, including how the targets are operationalized and how brain activity and structure are understood. Hence, the integration of the methods, data, and explanatory frameworks of these subfields counterbalance with the productivity of those that do not facilitate integration.[1] Further, it is worth speculating whether researchers in either camp want to integrate their methods, data, or explanatory frameworks, even if there were no other obstacles to achieving more systematic integration of these two subfields.

4 What New Tools Change

The previous section explains how tools can obstruct methodological, data, and explanatory integration due to their constraints and productivity. However, my cases show that tools are not an impassible roadblock to scientific integration, despite their propensity in some circumstances to obstruct it. Though systematic integration has failed to meet expectations, I have reviewed successful cases of local integration. What does this fact tell us about integration in neuroscience? To answer this question, I look to the role new tools in neuroscience play in facilitating integration. After all, the project known as the BRAIN Initiative aims "to develop and apply new tools and technologies for revolutionizing our understanding of the brain," which is in contrast to the principally modeling-focused projects of both the Human Brain Project and Blue Brain (Jorgenson et al. 2015, p. 1).

Architects of the BRAIN Initiative note that integration is a "challenge," and Section 2 highlights that the Initiative speaks to issues of integrating methods, data, and explanatory frameworks (Jorgenson et al. 2015, p. 7). Thus, the Initiative is designed to facilitate the integration of methods, data, and ultimately explanatory frameworks regarding research at different "scales" through the development of novel tools. The microscale is the size of cells, molecules, and small circuits, while the macroscale is the size of brain regions or the whole brain (Chang 2015). The mesoscale is everything in-between, encompassing large circuits and small populations of cells (Huang et al. 2018). It is also the least investigated: "one of the greatest current challenges facing neuroscience is that of bridging the gulf that exists between the molecular and the cellular level on one hand and that of brain imaging, cognition and action on the other" (Grillner et al. 2005, pp. 615–616).

4.1 CLARITY

A tool that drove the formation of the BRAIN Initiative is CLARITY, which renders intact tissue transparent and amenable to optical and fluorescent microscopy paradigms (Chung and Deisseroth 2013). This tool is indebted to the Deisseroth laboratory at Stanford. Prior to the development of CLARITY, optical microscopy only could be performed on the microscale, due to the need to slice tissue into thin segments so that light can penetrate them. Indirect macroscale imaging tools – such as MRI – cannot be used by researchers to investigate entities or phenomena at the microscale or mesoscale, due to constraints of the coarseness of indirect imaging. CLARITY solves the problem that some lipids in cellular tissue scatter light. This technique removes these lipids and develops a transparent support structure in the tissue.

The process begins when the tissue is placed in a monomer and linking chemical solution. These chemicals diffuse into the tissue, and they bind to proteins and nucleic acids in this tissue. However, these chemicals do not bind to the lipids that scatter light. Following the binding, the impregnated tissue is heat shocked, which causes the monomer and linking chemicals to bind to one another, forming a "mesh." The biomolecules that bind to the chemicals embed in this mesh as it sets. Following the development of the mesh, detergents are used by researchers to remove the non-embedded molecules like the light-scattering lipids. Because the mesh is in place, the tissue, minus the light-scattering lipids, remains in the configuration it was in at the start of the process.

CLARITY has different constraints when compared to those of microscale slice microscopy or the indirect means of measuring or imaging at the macroscale. Instead of researchers needing to slice tissue into pieces, CLARITY allows researchers to prepare larger dimensions of tissue. Because of its distinct constraints when compared to previous tools, the use of CLARITY produces microscale data about the properties of individual neurons and other cellular material as well as mesoscale data about the structural relations of the population of neurons and other material within the tissue.

Just like any other tool, CLARITY does not lack constraints. The biological system in question is killed by CLARITY, and the hydrogel and detergents used in the process can damage cellular structures in predictable ways. What matters for my discussion of integration in neuroscience is that its constraints are novel when compared to other tools, including the existing optical and indirect imaging methods mentioned above, allowing researchers to produce data that are relevant to the data produced using other tools. Thus, CLARITY overlaps other tools' domains: researchers can use it with existing light and fluorescent microscopy methods to investigate microscopic, mesoscopic, and macroscopic structures.

Unlike many imaging tools of the past, CLARITY is a "multi-scale" tool, with constraints covering the microscale, mesoscale, and macroscale. In this sense, CLARITY crosscuts previous research that used tools with incompatible constraints. This is a direct consequence of CLARITY's comparatively novel set of constraints: the change in constraints affects how the tool informs existing frameworks, helping with methodological, data, and (perhaps most importantly) explanatory integration.

The creators of CLARITY have sought to make this tool productive and easy to incorporate into existing paradigms that deploy other measurement, imaging, and manipulation tools. Beyond publishing works that communicate the theoretical basis and validity of the tool (Chung et al. 2013), these creators developed a "wiki" to communicate the use of the tool, the materials, and the kinds of projects for which CLARITY is useful (CLARITY Resource Center). This "CLARITY resource center" also includes a forum for users of the tool to discuss their uses of CLARITY as well as the issues that they face when they use it. This forum is paired with "boot camps" that train researchers to use CLARITY. These resources provide researchers the opportunity to obtain the first-hand experience of using the tool and second-hand experience from other users. These strategies show that its creators aim to make the use of CLARITY easy, efficient, and reliable.

The point of this section is not to suggest that CLARITY is some kind of "silver bullet" tool that will resolve integration challenges in neuroscience. Rather, it is one tool amongst several that can, and as I will show does, contribute to integration. To put this tool into the broader context of neuroscience inquiry, we must consider some of the limitations of CLARITY. For instance, it takes time and effort for researchers to make a tool productive, and CLARITY is no exception. There remain aspects of its use that make it less productive when compared to other tools. It can take months for researchers to successfully perform CLARITY on neural systems, diminishing its efficiency compared to other imaging tools.

There already have been attempts to reduce the time needed to prepare the tissue and image it (Gradinaru et al. 2018), but the fact that the tool is slow limits its productivity at this time. Likewise, the wiki dedicates a section to troubleshooting the application of the tool, suggesting that it can be difficult to master CLARITY. These troubleshooting tips will likely help ease the use of CLARITY in the future. Nonetheless, their existence reflects the fact that there is a degree of skill required for researchers to use the tool correctly.

4.2 Does CLARITY Facilitate Scientific Integration?

CLARITY is an impressive tool. It can help to generate knowledge about brain structure and integrate with some other methods of neuroscience, and the data produced with CLARITY are designed to be integrated with data resulting from the use of different tools (Gradinaru et al. 2018). Together, these facts support the use of CLARITY by researchers to address brain structures that can be modeled, ultimately contributing to explanatory integration. This is all well and good, but *has* this new tool facilitated integration in neuroscience?

For methodological integration, CLARITY has been integrated into MRI paradigms that allow researchers to advance their understanding of how tissue types, such as lipids and proteins, differentially contribute to imaging results (Leuze et al. 2017). This local integration provides researchers with a better theoretical understanding of how the biological material of the brain relates to their imaging results, with a finding that lipids are the "dominant source of MRI contrast in brain tissue" (Leuze et al. 2017, p. 412). This case shows that the integrative use of multiple tools contributes to knowledge generation about brain tissue and its relation to these tools that could not be achieved through the use of either tool alone. Thus, methodological integration supports both knowledge generation about neural systems and knowledge generation about the theoretical basis of MRI paradigms. The former fosters growth in the theory of the system, while the latter fosters growth in the theory of the technique (Colaço 2018).

For data integration, CLARITY has been paired with diffusion tensor imaging for researchers to collect and model data about white matter microarchitecture (Chang et al. 2017). Though non-invasive, diffusion tensor imaging produces only indirect evidence of white matter structure via the measurement of water diffusion in and around this structure. When paired with CLARITY, researchers can correlate this water movement data with structural data regarding the biological sources of this diffusion. This local integration thus provides researchers a means of combining and relating databases that result from distinct imaging tools, or tools that measure different features of brain structures. Further, it provides data about the relation between datasets, giving researchers an understanding of how data from different tools relate and thus providing them a useful form of "metadata" (Leonelli 2016, p. 97). By understanding the means of integrating these databases, researchers aim to "integrate 3D brain-wide molecular analyses with these large-scale efforts" (Chang et al. 2017, p. 260).

For explanatory integration, CLARITY has been deployed to model prefrontal cortex cell typology, which provides a means of understanding how cell type and population structure correlate with behavior (Ye et al. 2016). Because CLARITY allows for the modeling of intact structures, both phenotyping and cell wiring at the population level can be integrated into a model of the so-called "prefrontal cortex" of mice. This local integration thus provides researchers a means of modeling the rodent prefrontal cortex and its contribution to behavior while also acquiring the cellular and molecular detail of the components of the prefrontal cortex. This explanatory integration is possible because CLARITY can be used by researchers to acquire both microscale and mesoscale data, due to its novel constraints. The ability to generate a detailed, molecularly satisficing, three-dimensional model of a brain area as complex as the prefrontal cortex, even that of mice, also lays the groundwork for producing population-level anatomical models of constructs like memory engrams, facilitated by the integrative use of clarifying tools like CLARITY, labeling techniques, and manipulation tools like optogenetics (Roy et al. 2019).

These cases of the use of CLARITY show how new tools can successfully facilitate all three modes of integration in neuroscience, with the last case involving the facilitation of more than one mode concurrently. What has been achieved in these cases is what the BRAIN Initiative was designed to promote: create and hone a number of new tools that serve as the seeds for integration to concurrently develop across several subfields of neuroscience. By recent accounts, this strategy has been successful, with numerous new tools facilitating local methodological, data, and explanatory integration across a variety of neuroscience subfields (Koroshetz et al. 2018). These cases of integration address issues faced by researchers who have specific aims in certain subfields of neuroscience.

Despite these cases being, by all accounts, successful instances of integration in neuroscience, all of these cases are nonetheless of local integration. Thus, CLARITY, like many other tools affiliated with the BRAIN Initiative, has yet to contribute to the systematic explanatory integration that some researchers desire. For instance, nothing described in this section matches the systematic brain modeling of the Human Brain Project or Blue Brain. This fact puts CLARITY research in the same camp as other cases of integration, such as Sullivan's examples, MCC, and cognitive neuroscience, that I discussed earlier in this chapter. What does this fact tell us?

The success of these CLARITY cases results from the fact that adopting a tool with different constraints has allowed researchers to integrate it with their current protocols and thus maintain a productive level of research, both in terms of generating knowledge and in publishing exciting, high-impact materials. In this sense, tools like CLARITY serve as an evolution or amendment to current, productive practices, rather than a radical revision to these practices. This ability to achieve local integration by changing constraints without sacrificing productivity is the backbone to the BRAIN Initiative's successes. The same cannot be said for attempts at systematic integration that focus on modeling, which have not met their ambitious expectations of systematic data and explanatory integration in the form of a unified model of brain structure and function. The changing of tools has allowed researchers to maintain their research practices in a sympathetic form to their prior research, as opposed to the need to sacrifice their current practices in an effort to achieve their systematic desires. This lack of a comparative compromise mirrors the tradeoff described by Harp and Khalifa: systematic integration does not match with the utility of research practices, which is why it often is not pursued. By contrast, local integration can be matched with the utility of research practices when new productive tools are introduced. Hence, we can find many successful cases of the three modes of local integration, while successful systematic explanatory integration still is elusive.

While I have highlighted an apparent gulf between local and systematic integration, this distinction does not entail that local integration cannot facilitate systematic integration (or vice versa). The BRAIN Initiative's results are compatible with the idea that we ultimately ultimately gain a systematic model of brain structure and function, perhaps through the linking of many cases of local integration. It also is compatible with existing, modeling-focused initiatives for systematic data and explanatory integration. What matters is that tool change can directly and successfully facilitate local methodological, data, and explanatory integration without any direct achievement of systematic integration. Again, this explains why we can find cases of local integration in neuroscience, while systematic integration remains elusive.

Ultimately, the case of CLARITY shows something important about the role of tools in integrative neuroscience: tools can facilitate local integration for the same basic reasons that they can obstruct it. Tools have constraints, which affect how they *can be* used to generate knowledge in a reliable manner. Likewise, tools are productive, which affects how they *likely will be* used to generate knowledge for epistemic and prudential reasons. If tools' constraints do not overlap, it will be a challenge to integrate research practices that respectively deploy them. If they do overlap in a productive manner, which can be achieved by developing new tools with constraints specifically designed to overlap in a productive manner, integration will be facilitated. CLARITY is one example of a new tool that achieves this facilitation of scientific integration.

5 Conclusion

In this chapter, I have shown that resolving the challenges of integration in neuroscience requires us to reflect upon both the constraints and the productivity of the tools that are popular in the discipline. I have explained when tools are obstructions and facilitators of three modes of integration in neuroscience. The fact that productive but constrained tools lead researchers to continue doing research at the expense of engaging in integrative practices is a topic that has not been sufficiently addressed in the philosophy of science, and it is worthwhile to appreciate that this relation is challenging but not impossible for us to overcome.

As I have shown, local integration can be facilitated by new productive tools with novel constraints, even if this does not promote any sort of systematic integration, especially in the short run. This is not a mere possibility; it is actively achieved by projects like the BRAIN Initiative and research with the tool CLARITY. Nonetheless, my premises of constraints and productivity are important to understanding the promise of integration in neuroscience, as they explain why tools both obstruct and facilitate scientific integration.

Note

1 This challenge reflects Bechtel's claims that integration that creates a new subfield such as MCC often results in a great deal of specialization. This specialization, in turn, can result in disintegration between the new subfield and previously established subfields (1993, p. 278).

References

Amunts, K., Ebell, C., Muller, J., Telefont, M., Knoll, A., & Lippert, T. (2016). The human brain project: Creating a European research infrastructure to decode the human brain. *Neuron, 92*(3), 574–581.

Bassett, D. S., & Sporns, O. (2017). Network neuroscience. *Nature Neuroscience, 20*(3), 353–364.

Bechtel, W. (1993). Integrating sciences by creating new disciplines: The case of cell biology. *Biology and Philosophy, 8*(3), 277–299.

Bickle, J. (2016). Revolutions in neuroscience: Tool development. *Frontiers in Systems Neuroscience, 10,* 24.

Chang, E. F. (2015). Towards large-scale, human-based, mesoscopic neurotechnologies. *Neuron, 86*(1), 68–78.

Chang, E. H., Argyelan, M., Aggarwal, M., Chandon, T. S. S., Karlsgodt, K. H., Mori, S., & Malhotra, A. K. (2017). The role of myelination in measures of white matter integrity: Combination of diffusion tensor imaging and two-photon microscopy of CLARITY intact brains. *Neuroimage, 147*, 253–261.

Chung, K., & Deisseroth, K. (2013). CLARITY for mapping the nervous system. *Nature Methods, 10*(6), 508.

Chung, K., Wallace, J., Kim, S. Y., Kalyanasundaram, S., Andalman, A. S., Davidson, T. J.,... & Pak, S. (2013). Structural and molecular interrogation of intact biological systems. *Nature, 497*(7449), 332–337.

CLARITY Resource Center. (2020). http://clarityresourcecenter.org (Accessed June 20th, 2021).

Colaço, D. (2018). Rethinking the role of theory in exploratory experimentation. *Biology and Philosophy, 33*(5–6), 38.

Colaço, D. (2020). Recharacterizing scientific phenomena. *European Journal for Philosophy of Science, 10*(2), 1–19.

Craver, C. F. (2007). *Explaining the brain: Mechanisms and the mosaic unity of neuroscience*. Oxford: Oxford University Press.

Feest, U. (2005). Operationism in psychology: What the debate is about, what the debate should be about. *Journal of the History of the Behavioral Sciences, 41*(2), 131–149.

Gabrieli, J. D. (1998). Cognitive neuroscience of human memory. *Annual Review of Psychology, 49*(1), 87–115.

Gradinaru, V., Treweek, J., Overton, K., & Deisseroth, K. (2018). Hydrogel-tissue chemistry: principles and applications. *Annual Review of Biophysics, 47*, 355–376.

Grillner, S., Kozlov, A., & Kotaleski, J. H. (2005). Integrative neuroscience: Linking levels of analyses. *Current Opinion in Neurobiology, 15*(5), 614–621.

Harp, R., & Khalifa, K. (2015). Why pursue unification?: A social-epistemological puzzle. *THEORIA. Revista de Teoría, Historia y Fundamentos de la Ciencia, 30*(3), 431–447.

Huang, L., Kebschull, J. M., Furth, D., Musall, S., Kaufman, M. T., Churchland, A. K., & Zador, A. M. (2018). High-throughput mapping of mesoscale connectomes in individual mice. *bioRxiv, 422477*. doi: 10.1101/422477

Jorgenson, L. A., Newsome, W. T., Anderson, D. J., Bargmann, C. I., Brown, E. N., Deisseroth, K.,... & Marder, E. (2015). The BRAIN Initiative: Developing technology to catalyse neuroscience discovery. *Philosophical Transactions of the Royal Society B: Biological Sciences, 370*(1668), 20140164.

Koroshetz, W., Gordon, J., Adams, A., Beckel-Mitchener, A., Churchill, J., Farber, G.,... & White, S. (2018). The state of the NIH BRAIN initiative. *Journal of Neuroscience, 38*(29), 6427–6438.

Kotchoubey, B., Tretter, F., Braun, H. A., Buchheim, T., Draguhn, A., Fuchs, T.,... & Rentschler, I. (2016). Methodological problems on the way to integrative human neuroscience. *Frontiers in Integrative Neuroscience, 10*, 41.

Krohs, U. (2012). Convenience experimentation. *Studies in History and Philosophy of Science Part C: Studies in History and Philosophy of Biological and Biomedical Sciences, 43*(1), 52–57.

Leonelli, S. (2016). *Data-centric biology: A philosophical study*. Chicago, IL: University of Chicago Press.

Leuze, C., Aswendt, M., Ferenczi, E., Liu, C. W., Hsueh, B., Goubran, M.,... & McNab, J. A. (2017). The separate effects of lipids and proteins on brain MRI contrast revealed through tissue clearing. *Neuroimage, 156*, 412–422.

Logothetis, N. K., Pauls, J., Augath, M., Trinath, T., & Oeltermann, A. (2001). Neurophysiological investigation of the basis of the fMRI signal. *Nature, 412*(6843), 150–157.

Markram, H. (2012). The human brain project. *Scientific American, 306*(6), 50–55.

Mitchell, S. D., & Gronenborn, A. M. (2017). After fifty years, why are protein X-ray crystallographers still in business? *The British Journal for the Philosophy of Science, 68*(3), 703–723.

Molecular and Cellular Cognition Society. (2021) https://molcellcog.org/about-mccs (Accessed June 20th, 2021).

O'Malley, M. A. (2013). When integration fails: Prokaryote phylogeny and the tree of life. *Studies in History and Philosophy of Science Part C: Studies in History and Philosophy of Biological and Biomedical Sciences, 44*(4), 551–562.

O'Malley, M. A., & Soyer, O. S. (2012). The roles of integration in molecular systems biology. *Studies in History and Philosophy of Science Part C: Studies in History and Philosophy of Biological and Biomedical Sciences, 43*(1), 58–68.

Roy, D. S., Park, Y. G., Ogawa, S. K., Cho, J. H., Choi, H., Kamensky, L.,... & Tonegawa, S. (2019). Brain-wide mapping of contextual fear memory engram ensembles supports the dispersed engram complex hypothesis. *bioRxiv*, 668483. doi: 10.1101/668483

Shepherd, G. M., Mirsky, J. S., Healy, M. D., Singer, M. S., Skoufos, E., Hines, M. S.,... & Miller, P. L. (1998). The human brain project: Neuroinformatics tools for integrating, searching and modeling multidisciplinary neuroscience data. *Trends in Neurosciences, 21*(11), 460–468.

Silva, A. J. (2003). Molecular and cellular cognitive studies of the role of synaptic plasticity in memory. *Journal of Neurobiology, 54*(1), 224–237.

Silva, A. J., Landreth, A., & Bickle, J. (2013). *Engineering the next revolution in neuroscience: The new science of experiment planning*. Oxford: Oxford University Press.

Sporns, O. (2014). Contributions and challenges for network models in cognitive neuroscience. *Nature Neuroscience, 17*(5), 652–660.

Sullivan, J. A. (2016). Construct stabilization and the unity of the mind-brain sciences. *Philosophy of Science, 83*(5), 662–673.

Sullivan, J. A. (2017). Coordinated pluralism as a means to facilitate integrative taxonomies of cognition. *Philosophical Explorations, 20*(2), 129–145.

Ye, L., Allen, W. E., Thompson, K. R., Tian, Q., Hsueh, B., Ramakrishnan, C.,... & Deisseroth, K. (2016). Wiring and molecular features of prefrontal ensembles representing distinct experiences. *Cell, 165*(7), 1776–1788.

Yong, E. (2019). The human brain project hasn't lived up to its promise. *The Atlantic.* https://www.theatlantic.com/science/archive/2019/07/ten-years-human-brain-project-simulation-markram-ted-talk/594493/

11 Understanding Brain Circuits

Do New Experimental Tools Need to Address New Concepts?

David Parker

A primary motive of science is to explain and to translate this insight to practical uses. Neuroscience aims to explain the neural basis of normal and abnormal behaviour and cognition. This is considered one of the biggest open questions in science: although often related to consciousness there is much to do below this level. The human brain consists of billions of interconnected neurons: assuming that each neuron is either active or inactive (a gross simplification), the number of potential brain configurations would exceed the number of elementary particles in the universe (Sagan 1977, p. 66).

Despite this complexity, there are significant claims to understanding, including the cellular mechanisms of memory (Morris 2003) and of the cerebral cortex sufficient for a conscious human brain emulation (always seemingly "within 10 years"; see Miller 2011). There are also claims for translation. An obvious translation is to artificial intelligence and robotics, for example, to address Moravec's paradox, that we can easily simulate higher-level functions (e.g. memory) but not supposedly simpler sensorimotor processes. A less obvious translation is to "improve" the healthy brain (cognitive enhancement), an extension of traditional claims of treatments for neurological and also for psychiatric conditions. The former should face serious caution from the poor history of the latter (Middleton and Moncrieff 2019), which presumably reflects the lack of understanding of what the interventions are actually doing. To illustrate the limited science behind these claims, a 2005 report by the UK Office of Science and Innovation suggested that by 2017 cognitive enhancement may be "part of the knowledge professionals toolkit". This failed prediction reflects its poor scientific basis: one drug, donepezil which reduces the breakdown of acetylcholine, was claimed to *produce* more acetylcholine, allowing the brain to work at a *higher level of efficiency*" (see Howard-Jones 2007), while transcranial current stimulation was claimed to "make areas of the brain work even *harder*" (Thomson 2010; my italics).

These positive claims were contrasted by Torsten Wiesel who said to understand the brain "we need a century, maybe a millennium…we are

DOI: 10.4324/9781003251392-15

at a very early stage of brain science" (cited in Horgan 1999). Gunther Stent (1969) suggested that analysing the physiological processes of behaviour was pointless as they will "degenerate into seemingly ordinary reactions no more and no less fascinating than those occurring in the liver" echoing Charles Sherrington's claim of a remoteness "between the field of neurology and that of mental health ...physiology has not enough to offer about the brain in relation to mind to lend the psychiatrist much help" (Sherrington 1951). There is thus a lack of connection between the components of the nervous system and the outputs they produce. Examining components or behaviours alone is not sufficient: molecular and cellular analyses require knowledge of the behaviour or goal of the system, while top-down behavioural approaches need lower-level insight to constrain potential explanations.

While it seems implicit in neuroscience claims, understanding lacks an accepted definition (de Regt 2013). For example, Bassett and Gazzaniga (2011, p. 6) wrote, "Understanding the brain depends significantly on understanding its emergent properties", while Gregory claimed understanding will remove any appeal to emergence (in Blackmore 2006, p. 105). Bassett and Gazzaniga (p. 8) also say "To understand mind-brain mechanisms it is necessary to characterize relations between multiple levels of the multiscale human brain system, including interactions between temporal scales", while Dennett (1971), Newell (1982), Marr (1982), and Glass et al. (1979), all following Gilbert Ryle's (1949) claim that claim understanding can be obtained at different levels, the computational or behavioural/cognitive, the programme or algorithm, or the physical or implementational level.

Understanding and explanation in biology are claimed to appeal to mechanisms rather than laws (Railton 1981; Machamer et al. 2000). Functional concepts and mechanisms explain how a system and its parts do what they do, while understanding requires that the functional concepts and explanations are both intelligible and correct (Grimm 2006). The phlogiston theory made certain phenomena intelligible and had practical uses, but obviously couldn't be claimed as an understanding of combustion.

In neuroscience, it is easier to say what is not sufficient for understanding. Description is not enough. Claims that more details will explain are illustrated by connectomic approaches (Schroter et al. 2017; Morgan and Lichtman 2013) and that an understanding will follow from recording "from ever more cells over larger brain regions" (Mott et al. 2018). These reflect an "illusion of depth" (Ylikoski 2009) by assuming the more we know the more we will understand. Second, while prediction or the ability to make targeted interventions is important (Woodward 2017), we can predict effects and reliably manipulate systems without explaining how they happen. A classic neurophysiological example is the Jendrassik manoeuvre used clinically for over a century to potentiate reflexes (e.g. the knee-jerk reflex) but which still lacks explanation (Nardone and Schieppati 2008). Lesions provide another example. Spinal cord lesions evoke predictable sensory and motor disturbances that are not explained by the lesion alone, but also reflect diverse functional changes above and below the lesion site. Emphasis on the lesion has focused remedial approaches on regeneration to repair the lesion, but this has failed to translate into a treatment (Steward et al. 2012), presumably because it doesn't properly explain the changes.

Even if we can explain and understand how an effect occurs, this still leaves the question of "why". Sherrington (1899) claimed that neurophysiology can only answer "how" questions: analysing the activity of all the components involved we could understand how we run, but not why (to exercise, compete, escape?). Why questions are teleological and represent the goal or purpose, a final causality replaced in reductionist accounts by the efficient cause, the mechanical account of how an effect occurred. But explaining behaviour requires knowing how and why it occurred. For example, a complete description of "how" may not determine *why* a person exhibits certain psychopathology (a faulty gene or faulty environment?), and thus won't identify the most effective treatment.

Neural circuit analyses, while far from a panacea (Parker 2010), offers a middle-ground between bottom-up and top-down analyses, by considering how components interact to generate outputs. Minimal criteria must for circuit understanding include (Selverston 1980):

1   Characterisation of the circuit output and the associated behaviour. Reductionist analyses physically reduce or constrain systems to varying extents to enable cellular analyses, making direct links between circuit behaviour and behaviour unlikely (Krakauer et al. 2017): spinal cord fictive locomotion provides an example (Parker and Srivastava 2013).
2   The component cells that generate the output must be identified. A circuit neuron is defined as being active when the circuit is active, and its activity influences the circuit output. However, neither criterion unequivocally identifies a neuron as a circuit component (Parker 2010).
3   The connectivity between network neurons must be defined. It is clearly impractical to try to determine all cell-to-cell connections of larger circuits by piecemeal recordings, analyses instead describe connections between cell populations.
4   Identification of circuit neurons and connectivity describes the network structure, but the structure does not determine function. We must also characterise the functional properties of circuit neurons and synapses.

The challenges of reductionist approaches in even simpler systems have been raised, both in terms of their practical and conceptual basis (Selverston 1980; Parker 2010; Krakauer et al. 2017). A practical complication of reductionist explanations is the astronomical number of components to characterise (akin to the "tyranny of numbers" faced by computer engineers before integrated circuits; Warner 2001). Using Bell's number, Koch (2012) claimed that characterising a 1,000 neuron network at exaggerated rates would take 2000 years. Koch's argument is a strawman as he uses non-biological conditions (e.g. all to all connectivity), but the same point was made less theatrically using actual circuit features by Selverston (1980) and Getting (1989).

A circuit approach moves above the level of component cells by analysing how cell populations interact to generate an output. But the output of a circuit is not behaviour (Krakauer et al. 2017). Analogies are often used: Krakauer et al. correctly say we won't understand chess from knowing what the board and the pieces are made of (Krakauer et al. 2017), but circuit analyses are not (or should not be) about the properties of the components, but about how component properties generate outputs. Lateral inhibition in the horseshoe crab retina (Hartline et al. 1956) provides an example of a functional explanation from a component analysis, a building block (Getting 1989) or motif common to diverse sensory systems. In the chess analogy, this would be equivalent to knowing what a rook did rather than what it was made of.

Failure to explain behaviour when we have a wealth of lower-level knowledge is also claimed to illustrate the insufficiency of circuit analyses. *C. elegans* is the prime example (Krakauer et al. 2017), but this can be claimed to reflect the need for more analyses. While we know a lot about the genetics and structure of its nervous system, functional properties, a key criterion for circuit understanding (see above) are poorly understood. Just as proper attention to behaviour is needed (Krakauer et al. 2017), proper attention to cellular data is also important. This requires attention to component and circuit aspects that go beyond a focus on experimentally convenient molecular or anatomical details or large cells or input/output components (Selverston 1980; Parker 2010) to focus on the less tractable and poorly characterised elements (e.g. interneurons). It also requires a proper critique of claims rather than the appeal to authority that seemingly lets hypotheses or assumptions pass as characterisations, explanations, or understanding. *Aplysia* offers an example of a claimed circuit explanation of behaviour (Kandel 2001) from a very detailed experimental focus limited to tractable components that do not logically justify understanding (Glanzman 2010; see Parker 2019). While less notable, but still in receipt of significant personal awards, Grillner's understanding of the lamprey spinal cord locomotor circuit reflects a mass of assumption and extrapolation to cover missing data and conceptual errors (Parker 2006, 2010). Both claims fail, at least from a scientific perspective.

1 Experimental Reductionism

Mechanistic explanations of behaviour in neuroscience typically reduce behaviours to their constituent molecules and cells (Selverston 1980; Getting 1989; Ito 2006; Yuste 2015). Appeals to reductionism include its track record; that by opening "black boxes" it allows greater potential for control and practical use; and that it offers greater generality and simplicity. Reductive explanations relate to a "machine model" (Monod 1972), where interlocking parts combine to move the system from an initial to a goal state, an explanation showing how the component parts and their organisation achieve the system goal (Darden and Craver 2009). Hanahan and Weinberg (2000) claimed, "Two decades from now...it will be possible to lay out the complete integrated circuit of the cell... we will then be able to apply the tools of mathematical analysis to explain". The microprocessor analogy is unfortunate as Jonas and Kording (2017) have shown that current neuroscience approaches are *insufficient* to explain actual microprocessors. Hanahan and Weinberg's 20 years have passed, and features have been identified that negate the circuit-board analogy for even a single cell: a fluid cytoskeleton, "intrinsically disordered proteins", enzymes that affect numerous substrates or perform non-enzymatic functions, pleomorphic molecular assemblies with "probability clouds" of interactions, and stochastic and probabilistic gene expression (see Nicholson 2019).

Apart from clinical case studies, most biological discoveries reflect the use of model organisms with features that make them useful. This relates to Krogh's principle (originally outlined by Claude Bernard in the 19th century; Jørgensen 2001), that for any problem there an animal on which it can be most conveniently studied. Between the 1930s and 1960s a wide range of invertebrate and lower-vertebrate model systems were introduced to determine the general principles of nervous system function (strongly associated with the field of neuroethology). These have relatively simple behaviours and accessible nervous systems containing relatively small numbers of often large cells that allowed circuit characterisations related to behaviours. These natural advantages can be engineered to some extent in more complex (mammalian) systems using early developmental stages or reduced preparations (tissue slices or cultured cells). While we cannot simply extrapolate, the hope is that the conservation of function in simpler or reduced preparations will help us explain more complex or intact systems.

The reductionist approach is illustrated by the field of molecular and cellular cognition, a 'ruthless' reductionism that claims to explain the molecular basis of cognition from genetic manipulations (Bickle 2003). To some extent this link is obvious: if a change in behaviour reliably follows a manipulation, then the manipulation caused the change. But this is a correlation, and useful for that, not an explanation. Molecules don't connect directly like switches to behaviours but work through cells in circuits that form systems that link to behaviour. While we could detail the molecular intervention and the resulting behaviour, explaining the links between them requires knowing how the molecular manipulation worked through different levels.

Two aspects removed by the reductionist neural approach are glial cells and non-wired effects. We now know that glia serve more than the traditional developmental or "housekeeping" role (clearing away released transmitters and extracellular potassium caused by action potential signalling): the tripartite synapse concept sees glia as functional components that receive and send signals to neurons (Araque and Navarrete 2010). Non-wired signals are not passed along axons and synaptic contacts but through the extracellular space and include volume transmission (the diffusion of transmitters up to mm from their point of release; Svensson et al. 2019) and extracellular electrical fields ("ephaptic" signals; Weiss and Faber 2010).

To consider the issue, assume that field effects are important (Figure 1). We know they occur as they are measured in EEGs, but their functional role has received relatively little attention. Field effects are not a component in the conventional sense but reflect the summed activity in cell populations, an example of an emergent biological effect. This generates an extracellular signal that can affect the activity of other cells depending on its magnitude and spread, which are not easy to predict and depend on the specific features of the activity and the extracellular space (Weiss and Faber 2010), which in turn depends on the arrangement of other neurons and the geometry of the extracellular space. Extracellular fields are thus influenced by neuronal activity and neuronal activity by extracellular fields, a circular interaction. Neuronal activity also alters the diameter, and thus resistivity of the extracellular space (Østby et al. 2009) to alter the magnitude and spread of field effects, neuronal activity, and the extracellular space… generating a circular interaction that influences another circular interaction. We could, in principle, understand how this influences an output if we knew the contribution of each cell to the extracellular signal, and how it spreads through the extracellular space to alter neuronal activity and the extracellular space, but this would at best provide a snapshot of constantly evolving dynamic activity. This argument could be negated by begging the question and saying that field effects are an unimportant epiphenomenon. But similar considerations apply to volume transmission and to circular interactions generated by conventional "wired" feedback connections between neurons (Parker 2019; Svensson et al. 2019) which cannot be easily dismissed to appeal to simple accounts. It isn't that we want or need knowledge of the minutiae of wired and non-wired components and connections evolving in real time to explain (Greenberg and Manor 2005, provide a sobering example of the failure to explain when detail exceeds a small limit in a very simple system), but we need to appreciate the role of these effects in any explanation.

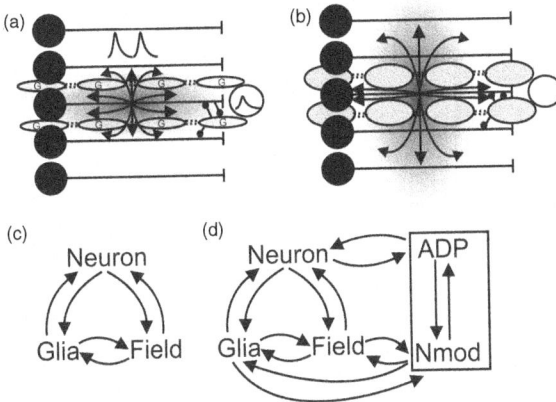

Figure 11.1 Circular interactions along wired and non-wired pathways. (a) Neuronal activity generates extracellular signals (shaded circle), that can alter neuronal excitability. At the synaptic terminal, inputs are evoked in postsynaptic cells and in glial cells (G), and glia can signal back to neurons. Glial cells form a syncytium through gap junction connections (dashed lines), which allows local activity to spread. (b) Neuronal activity can cause swelling of glial cells to 'shrink' the extracellular space and change the extracellular field, neuronal and glial activity, transmitter release and glial cell activity, which alters the extracellular space..., generating multiple circular interactions. (c) These are known features of nervous systems, nothing is exaggerated, and if anything is too simplified. (d) Adding plasticity (both activity-dependent (ADP) and neuromodulator-evoked (NMod), and the interactions between these effects) evokes additional circular interactions. Even if complete ('Laplacian') detail was possible, we would only have snapshots of constantly evolving dynamic activity.

An issue with constitutive reductionism is that each level of a biological system establishes an order that is not necessarily reflected at other levels. Sperry (1980, p. 201) suggested that

> Once generated from neural events, the higher order mental patterns and programs have their own subjective qualities and progress, operate and interact by their own causal laws and principles which are different from and cannot be reduced to those of neurophysiology.

We can stay far below the level of mental events to see this. A sodium channel has atoms and molecules arranged to allow movement of sodium ions underlying an action potential; but an action potential is not reducible to the sodium channel as it reflects multiple ion channels, membrane pumps, and the membrane itself, that together generate the voltage and electrochemical gradients needed for the sodium channel to work.

The reductionist focus on manipulating single system components in isolation is really only possible in decomposable or "nearly decomposable" systems where interactions between parts are minimal, not in systems where the interactions between parts are many and strong ("non-decomposable systems"; Simon 1962). Bassett et al. (2010) refer to Simon (1962) in saying that hierarchical systems are nearly decomposable to claim parts can be examined relatively independently. But Simon didn't say that hierarchical systems are nearly decomposable, just that "At least some kinds of hierarchic systems can be approximated successfully as nearly decomposable systems" (Simon 1969, p. 474). Near-decomposability is an assumption of reductionist approaches, a "fallible" heuristic (Wimsatt 2006), and assumptions need to be considered. Non-decomposability could reflect a temporary failure of experimental or analytical techniques or concepts (e.g. Bechtel 2002) that disappears when we have the correct concepts and details. But is this begging the question to maintain the assumption of near-decomposability, a "promise of jam tomorrow"? It is not enough to inductively claim that many major advances in the life sciences have stemmed from the discovery of ways of decomposing a phenomenon: that there are nearly-decomposable systems in biology does not mean that this applies to all biological systems; we may need to appreciate this to find ways of approaching these systems.

Non-decomposable systems have interactions between components that are many and strong. This seems to define nervous systems where feedforward, feedback and circular interactions are endemic, a heterarchical rather than a hierarchical organisation of component parts performing specific functions in fixed sequences. Heterarchical systems offer challenges to reductionist approaches. Properties examined in reduced preparations or under quiescent conditions can change when the system is active due to the recruitment of wired and non-wired feedback loops or activity-dependent changes in component or system properties. Heterarchical systems also show equifinality (many mechanisms generate the same output) and multifinality (single components influence multiple outputs). Functional imaging has shown that instead of a one-to-one mapping between a region and a function there is a high degree of overlap among regions that are activated by tasks that share no cognitive components (Schroeder and Foxe 2005). A given region can thus influence multiple functions. Price and Friston (2005) claim this will be determined by its connectivity, but this ignores non-wired signals. The lack of obligatory mechanistic sequences means the law of transitivity does not hold in heterarchical systems, complicating the spatial and temporal relations between levels, and meaning that explanations cannot simply build up from lower-level properties. Noble (2012) provides an example from the failure to explain the heart rhythm from lower-level properties.

In non-decomposable systems any manipulation, no matter how "surgical", will also necessarily affect other components through diaschisis (Carrera and Tononi 2014), an acknowledged neurological term that seems less appreciated experimentally. Diaschisis literally means "shocked throughout" to represent the widespread changes in the brain caused by a focal lesion. Any manipulation, no matter how elegant and refined, will necessarily affect downstream (and with feedback, upstream) components. Terms like "specific" or "targeted" imply precision that may be justified from intention (a specific single component was successfully targeted), but not from application (many components will be affected). To offer more than a correlation, and more is often implied, requires knowing how the manipulation alters the system. A manipulation may cause an effect without explaining it.

Reductionist explanations also aim to define individual parameters. For invertebrates, these can be single uniquely identifiable cells but in vertebrates, they are cell populations, characterisation reflecting a population average. Variability is endemic in these populations (Soltesz 2006). Claude Bernard claimed that averages "confuse while aiming to unify, and distort when aiming to simplify" (Bernard 1865, pp. 134–135). An average value may not describe a parameter, especially if the sample size is low, as the average value may not have been seen in any measurement: would this be considered characterisation of a component? Averaging also assumes that the variability is noise, when it may be a signal or reflect the presence within a population or functional sub-groups (Soltesz 2006). Variability does not rule out conventional reductionist approaches but requires larger sample sizes to ensure that we properly characterise components, which for small or inaccessible cells and synaptic connections adds a significant burden.

Finally, reductionism assumes substantivalism, that components are defined by their intrinsic characteristics (e.g. structure, location, or transmitter content), rather than by their relationship to other components. But a transmitter like GABA (or a neuron containing it) is not intrinsically inhibitory, it is defined as such from the receptor it binds to and the receptor's inhibitory effect on the postsynaptic cell. Even then the functional circuit effect could be excitation through disinhibition.

Highlighting these limits of reductionism does not invite the opposite view prevalent with dichotomous thinking, that lower-level details are irrelevant. Regions of the brain show specificity in the types of cells they contain (from the 47 areas in Brodmann's map of a century ago to 98 now; Glasser et al. 2016), the specific anatomy, wiring patterns, and functional properties suggesting that these details are important. If everything could be reduced to Hopfield network representations then the brain would be a collection of identical units that simply process different types of information and relay it to different areas (an argument could be made for this arrangement in the cerebellar cortex). This paradoxically seems to be the view of the Human Brain Project, despite its explicit focus on reductionist detail (Markram et al. 2015), that chaining together multiple simulated cortical columns will produce a fully conscious brain emulation. If we want to understand mechanisms, and for effective and safe translations we should, we need these details.

2 New Tools

Neuroscience tools offer greater control and give more direct results at lower-levels or scales, supporting a reductionist focus (compare the analysis of a protein on a gel with an fMRI scan). In practice, the development of theories and instruments are mutually dependent: we develop tools and techniques to perform specific analyses, and analyses are directed by the available tools. The instruments and their use should be theory-neutral: a measurement obtained with a tool will be the same irrespective of the theory under which it was used. However, how a tool is applied and a measurement interpreted can be affected by a theory. The power of newer technologies to focus on biological details can leave behaviour as an "afterthought" (Krakauer et al. 2017), leading to explanations of behaviour that fail to separate causation from correlation and thus generating erroneous assumptions of links between lower and higher levels.

New techniques are claimed to have caused "revolutions" in neuroscience ("In short: understanding tool development is the key to understanding real revolutions in actual neuroscience"; Bickle 2016). Peter Galison's "Image and Logic" (1997) gives a view of scientific history dominated by tools: steam-engine technology came before thermodynamics and telegraphy and telephony came before information theory. While Einstein, Heisenberg, Schrödinger and Dirac believed that progress in physics would continue through conceptual insight, experimental physics in the mid-20th century focused on new tools. Neuroscience seems to have a similar dichotomy between the need for concepts or techniques and tools.

It is easy to see new tools as revolutionary if a revolution is defined as a fundamental change in the way things are done. This wouldn't fit Thomas Kuhn's (1962) definition of a scientific revolution, "a noncumulative developmental episode in which an older paradigm is replaced in whole or in part by an incompatible new one" (SSR, p. 92). A new technique may revolutionise how or what experiments are done but would only cause a scientific revolution if it led to a paradigm shift, not by increasing precision or allowing novel analyses within a paradigm (this is "normal science"; Kuhn 1962; Parker 2018). The terms scientific revolution and paradigm shift are often used erroneously (e.g. Knafo and Wyart 2015), presumably to emphasise something above "normal science" (seeing this as a pejorative term also misunderstands its meaning; Parker 2018).

The technological aspect of neuroscience is expressed in the aims of the US BRAIN (Brain Research Through Advancing Innovative Neurotechnologies®) project, which promises technology "to produce a revolutionary new dynamic picture of the brain that, for the first time, shows how individual cells and complex neural circuits interact in both time and space", and to find "new ways to treat, cure, and even prevent brain disorders". It doesn't say how it will do this, seemingly beyond examining more components in greater detail. Understanding the nervous system comes from observation, both of brain and behaviour, and the manipulation of its component parts either by accident (injuries or neurological disorders) or experimental design.

Neuroscience research has traditionally been slow but high throughput techniques are accelerating analyses (from automated "behavioural" ethoscopes to high throughput anatomical, molecular and electrophysiological analyses). But while this data gives knowledge, knowledge does not necessarily explain.

In summarising neural circuit analyses, Selverston (1980) said that understanding would be limited to the simplest systems with the techniques then available: these were intracellular and extracellular recording and stimulation, various anatomical approaches combined with cell stains, electron microscopy, the use of physical lesions, pharmacological agents, the ability to kill labelled cells with UV light, and initial attempts at imaging. The range of tools has now increased markedly (see https://www.biomedcentral.com/collections/ntfn). For example:

1   Single-cell transcriptomics allows the classification of cell types beyond classical aspects like location, anatomy or some functional property.
2   Molecular genetic approaches, for example using GAL4 driver lines or the Cre-Lox allow specific cells to be labelled with fluorescent markers under the control of specific promoters; promoter-driven gene knock-outs or knock-ins can modify the function or development of cells (e.g. using genetically encoded toxins like tetanus toxin targeted to specific promoters, or KillerRed which generates conditional toxic products when illuminated); and genetically engineered expression of voltage or calcium reporters using specific promoters to examine certain cell types or a pan-neuronal promoter for whole-brain imaging (e.g. GCaMP, a fusion of calmodulin and GFP), with latest developments offering a combination of both high sensitivity and rapid responses (Zhang et al. 2020).
3   Optogenetics allows the rapid control of excitability by genetically expressing light-sensitive proteins that depolarise or hyperpolarise cells, offering the advantage of rapid loss or gain of function in specific cells depending on the promoter used or region illuminated, while chemogenetics genetically expresses receptors (DREADDS) in cells to allow for their selective control by ligands novel to the system.
4   Connectomics uses high-throughput electron microscopy to characterise cells, axonal processes, and synaptic connections, a "Google

map" of the brain (Morgan and Lichtman 2013). The laborious preparation and photographing of sections have been automated, the bottleneck now being the reconstruction of the tissue. This can be facilitated by expressing fluorescent proteins in cells ("Brainbow" techniques, where Cre-Lox recombination results in a random combination of different fluorescent proteins) to help trace processes through tissue.

5   An aim of the BRAIN project is to examine multiple neurons at the same time (Mott et al. 2018), to overcome the bottleneck of conventional electrophysiology of examining, at best, a handful of neurons at a time. Neuropixel probes allow thousands of neurons to be recorded in cortical and deeper brain structures in intact behaving animals (Steinmetz et al. 2021).

These are all valuable additions to circuit research. But no tool, new or traditional, is without caveats. The neural imaging field shows the importance of highlighting caveats. Imaging was developed in the 1970s (Selverston 1980), but highlighting dissatisfaction with its poor spatial and temporal resolution led to successive improvements in reporters, microscopes, and analyses to the point where signals can now be imaged with millisecond precision in multiple cells (Zhang et al. 2020; although temporal precision falls as the number of cells imaged increases).

Many new tools offer significant control at the molecular and single-cell level, making genetic tractability an advantage of a model system. Genetically tractable models (*Drosophila*, *C. elegans*, zebrafish, mouse) now dominate classical model systems (paradoxically, genetically tractable systems are less amenable to neurophysiological approaches). Instead of the neuroethological approach of using diverse systems suited to addressing specific questions, we may be choosing questions to address in genetically tractable systems, an example of the "law of the instrument". Before molecular genetic approaches, single-cell recording techniques also promoted a reductionist explanatory and analytical focus of invertebrate and vertebrate neural circuits (Selverston 1980; Getting 1989; Ito 2006); the mechanisms of perception, learning and memory (Kandel 2001; Ito 2006; Bliss and Collingridge 2013).

New techniques often claim to overcome the limitations of previous techniques, and they often do, but this doesn't mean that they don't have caveats. Take molecular genetic approaches: positive or negative effects of manipulations using these tools do not unequivocally identify or eliminate a neuron as part of a circuit given the issues of heterarchical systems discussed above (Parker 2019). Interpretation of effects, of both molecular genetic and optogenetic approaches, is complicated by effects on multiple cell types ("leaky" expression; Allen et al. 2015): ideally, a single component at a time is affected so any effect can be related to that component. Claims that molecular genetic approaches could "dissect" neural circuits (Kiehn and Kullander 2004), language that suggests surgical precision, are negated by the promiscuity of supposedly selective targeting: Gosgnach et al. (2006) claimed 'selective ablation' of one class of spinal cord neurons but in the same paragraph say that two other classes were increased and another reduced in number, a poor dissection. If multiple cells are affected then any explanation has to appeal to all effects, not beg the question by dismissing unintended effects using terms like "small increase" or "slight decrease" (Gosgnach et al. 2006). Specific targeting of neuron classes is possible using combinatorial methods, for example using the regulatory elements of two neurally expressed genes (Luan et al. 2020): INTERSECT (intron recombinase sites enabling combinatorial targeting) utilizes multiple recombinases expressed in different cells type to more specifically target cell populations. Optogenetic probes can also be activated by activity-dependent immediate early genes, increasing specificity by limiting targeting to recently active cells (Guru et al. 2015).

There are issues even if a single population of cells is targeted. One issue is that it doesn't consider population variability. A knock-out or optogenetic manipulation will affect all members of the population, essentially averaging the effect. Whether this is acceptable or not depends on the view of variability: if it is considered irrelevant or noise then it doesn't matter, but if variability is functionally relevant then it does. In addition, genetic manipulations can result in adaptive changes within minutes (i.e. not prevented by conditional knock-outs; Frank et al. 2006). Homeostatic plasticity may lead to compensation that results in no apparent phenotype despite a key component being affected, while diaschisis will add to the effect of the intended manipulation and complicate interpretations of what caused a change (Parker 2019). Optogenetic stimulation can also evoke effects in the absence of optogenetic proteins, possibly reflecting light-induced temperature changes (Allen et al. 2015). These artefacts can presumably be controlled for (if they are admitted as caveats; issues are not always highlighted as clearly as in Allen et al. 2015); but diaschisis cannot be removed as it reflects normal features of nervous systems, which means in this case that the potential contribution of these factors to any explanation needs to be considered.

A connectomic map is a very desirable feature, and knowledge of structure is important (ephaptic communication in the escape circuit of goldfish is an example of a structural feature that explained a functional phenomenon; Weiss and Faber 2010). But function must be determined, it doesn't drop out from structure despite claims that structure "may enable predictions of circuit behaviour" (Lichtman and Sanes 2008, p. 349) and that structure "will signify a physiological process without the requirement of repeating the physiological analysis" (Morgan and Lichtman 2013, p. 496). Evidence from many systems over many years suggests a very limited ability to infer function from structure. This is evidenced by *C. elegans*, where a complete connectome has been available for over 30 years but we still lack insight into how the circuit works, and the cerebellar cortex where the organisation has been known for decades without insight into how the cerebellum does what it does, or even what it is doing. This was very elegantly shown by the marked change in output of a circuit of just two neurons depending on the functional properties of the connections between them (Elson et al. 2002).

Although connectomic analyses can be automated, it still requires significant effort. A recent connectome of a portion of the Drosophila brain (around 25,000 neurons) took two years and hundreds of thousands of hours on a paper with around 100 authors (Scheffer et al. 2020). Scaling this up to larger systems may require a disproportionately greater time. Connectomic detail is desirable but given the limited functional insight is the time investment on detailed maps useful (1 mm^3 of visual cortex took six months to obtain the data (Landhuis 2020); considering the volume of the visual cortex is 6 cm^3 the time needed for a complete connectomic map is biblical). A less detailed structure with functional concepts may be a better approach.

3 Conclusion

Technological advances are needed to address the astronomical complexity of even modestly sized networks. But conceptual advances are needed to direct analyses and tool development; we need to know what we need to know, and how to achieve it. Neuroscience has an enormous amount of data on molecular, cellular, synaptic, and developmental mechanisms, and cognition and behaviour, but we lack a coherent framework to link between these aspects. It isn't that we need, or should expect, a unified theory of brain function, just some idea of how to integrate between levels.

Complete reductionist detail of even modest circuits is not possible with current techniques, it may never be, and may not be needed. Various people have highlighted different explanatory levels (Ryle, Newell, Marr, Dennett; see above), the semantic and computational, the programme or algorithmic, and reductionist physical or implementational approaches. Non-reductionist accounts of nervous systems include Lashley's equipotentiality hypothesis, Pribram's holonomic brain theory, and arguably most successfully in linking across levels cybernetic control principles (Pickering 2010). For explanation appeal to a computational or algorithmic level is reasonable, but is it enough for interventions? You may know the 'computations' that a car engine performs, but you would still want a mechanic who knows about the details of engines to fix one. Neuroscience may need to introduce something similar to electromagnetic charge and electromagnetic forces as new fundamental physical properties to explain electromagnetism. While reductionism can appeal to successes, we shouldn't assume its success. A key issue is that although biological components operate according to physical laws, they reflect organisation over various spatial and temporal scales rather than independent parts (field effects may be the obvious example), not forgetting that the nervous system is in a body embedded in an environment.

Critiques of neuroscience reductionist approaches point to its failure to explain, but current failure doesn't necessarily mean that the approach is misguided. The Rosetta Stone was useful before it was decoded (and it wasn't decoded by having more of it or a reductionist analysis of the stone). The same could apply to the relevance of lower-level (or other) properties. For the nervous system, we are still in the early days of understanding a complex system. We can continue to use statistical approaches to explain higher-level phenomena from the mass action of identical parts or abstractions that focus on representations or computations, while also considering the details in the diversity of brain regions, neurons and synapses.

Even techniques that promise to examine multiple components (e.g. the US BRAIN project; Mott et al. 2018) still examine components, and there seems to be a drive to record from ever more cells. A recent review states that we should now shift from considering individual neurons to considering ensembles of neurons as the functional units of the nervous system, and that new technologies will provide a greater understanding of the link between the brain and behaviour (Yuste 2015), without saying what links are needed and how to develop them. We are already data rich but theory light, and assuming more components will give understanding is an illusion (Ylikoski 2009). Analyses at higher levels can generate plausible inferences, but plausible is not necessarily correct.

Neuroscience papers increasingly use multiple methods, 'a methodological decathlon' seemingly to emphasise the importance of the work (Krakauer et al. 2017). Using different methods can produce more robust findings if the results of each are in agreement, and it avoids the danger of being biased towards certain factors and blind to others. But the techniques should genuinely address questions rather than "throw" techniques at a system. The prestige journals seem especially prone to multiple techniques. There is a danger of multiple pieces of neuroscience information seeming to make explanations more satisfying (Weisberg et al. 2008; McCabe and Castel 2008), and thus interfering with proper critique.

Unless halted we may regret the move away from the traditional neurophysiological/neuroethological approaches that explicitly address the neurophysiology of natural behaviours in various model systems (addressing some of the concerns raised in Krakauer et al. 2017): we will not simply lose the insight it can give, but also the insight it has brought. This has always partly reflected a split between invertebrate and vertebrate/mammalian communities (after moving to a vertebrate lab for a post-doc after a PhD on insects I heard that neuroethology was "people doing weird things with insects"), and now reflects the appeal to genetically tractable systems.

Instead of philosophical and scientific competition over the merits of lower-level reductionist or higher-level computational or representative effects, they should be seen as different approaches to the same question, not only as an epistemological diversity but also as an ontological unity. As Simon (1962) said, "In the face of complexity, an in-principle reductionist may be at the same time a pragmatic holist". We can say the same about tools and ideas. The history of neuroscience shows we need both. We need to discuss concepts to identify what we actually need to do and how to use and develop tools to do this. An important, and seemingly relatively simple and non-technologial start is to stop allowing trivial claims to characterisation and understanding by prominent figures (Glanzman 2010; Parker 2006, 2019).

References

Allen, B. D., Singer, A. C., & Boyden, E. S. (2015). Principles of designing interpretable optogenetic behavior experiments. *Learning & Memory, 22,* 232–238.

Araque, A., & Navarrete, M. (2010). Glial cells in neuronal network function. *Philosophical Transactions of the Royal Society London B: Biological Sciences, 365,* 2375–2381.

Bassett, D. S., & Gazzaniga, M. (2011). Understanding complexity in the human brain. *Trends in Cognitive Science, 15,* 200–209.

Bassett, D. S., Greenfield, D. L., Meyer-Lindenberg, A., Weinberger, D. R., Moore, S. W., & Bullmore, E. T. (2010). Efficient physical embedding of topologically complex information processing networks in brains and computer circuits. *PLoS Computational Biology, 6*(4), e1000748.

Bechtel, W. (2002). Decomposing the brain: a long-term pursuit. *Brain and Mind, 3,* 229–242.

Bernard, C. (1865). *An Introduction to the Study of Experimental Medicine* (H. C Greene (1949), Trans.). New York: Henry Schuman Inc.

Bickle, J. (2003). *Philosophy and Neuroscience: A Ruthlessly Reductive Account.* Dordrecht: Springer.

Bickle, J. (2016). Revolutions in neuroscience: tool development. *Frontiers in Systems Neuroscience, 10,* 24.

Blackmore, S. (2006). *Conversations on Consciousness: What the Best Minds Think about the Brain, Free Will, and What It Means to Be Human.* New York: Oxford University Press.

Bliss, T. V., & Collingridge, G. L. (2013). Expression of NMDA receptor-dependent LTP in the hippocampus: bridging the divide. *Molecular Brain, 6,* 5.

Carrera, E., & Tononi, G. (2014). Diaschisis: past, present, future. *Brain, 137,* 2408–2422.

Darden, L., & Craver, C. (2009). Reductionism in biology, *Encyclopedia of Life Sciences.* Chichester: J. Wiley and Sons Ltd.

Dennett, D. C. (1971). Intentional systems. *The Journal of Philosophy*, 68, 87–106.

de Regt, H. W. (2013). Understanding and explanation: living apart together? *Studies in History and Philosophy of Science Part A*, 44(3), 505–509.

Elson, R. C., Selverston, A. I., Abarbanel, H. D. I., & Rabinovich, M. I. (2002). Inhibitory synchronization of bursting in biological neurons: dependence on synaptic time constant. *The Journal of Neurophysiology* 88(3), 1166–1176.

Frank, C., Kennedy, M., Goold, C., Marek, K., & Davis, G. (2006). Mechanisms underlying rapid induction and sustained expression of synaptic homeostasis. *Neuron*, 52, 663–677.

Galison, P. (1997). *Image and Logic: A Material Culture of Microphysics*. Chicago, IL: University of Chicago Press.

Getting, P. (1989). Emerging principles governing the operation of neural networks. *Ann. Rev. Neurosci.*, 12, 185-204.

Glanzman, D. L. (2010). Common mechanisms of synaptic plasticity in vertebrates and invertebrates. *Current Biology*, 20(1), R31–R36.

Glass, A. L., Holyoak, K. J., & Santa, J. L. (1979). *Cognition*. Reading, MA: Addison-Wesley Publishing Company.

Glasser, M. F., Coalson, T. S., Robinson, E. C., Hacker, C. D., Harwell, J., Yacoub, E., Ugurbil, K., Andersson, J., Beckmann, C. F., Jenkinson, M., Smith, S. M., Van Essen, D. C. (2016). A multi-modal parcellation of human cerebral cortex. *Nature*, 536, 171–178.

Gosgnach, S., Lanuza, G. M., Butt, S. J. B., Saueressig, H., Zhang, Y., Velasquez, T., Riethmacher, D., Callaway, E. M., Kiehn, O., & Goulding, M. (2006). V1 spinal neurons regulate the speed of vertebrate locomotor outputs. *Nature*, 440, 215–219.

Greenberg, I., & Manor, Y. (2005). Synaptic depression in conjunction with A-current channels promote phase constancy in a rhythmic network. *The Journal of Neurophysiology*, 93, 656–677.

Grimm, S. R. (2006). Is understanding a species of knowledge? *The British Journal for the Philosophy of Science*, 57, 515–535.

Guru, A., Post, R. J., Ho, Y.-Y., & Warden, M. R. (2015). Making sense of optogenetics. *The International Journal of Neuropsychopharmacology*, 18, pyv079.

Hanahan, D., & Weinberg R. A. (2000). The hallmarks of cancer. *Cell*, 100, 57–70.

Hartline, H. K., Wagner, H. G., & Ratliff, F. (1956). Inhibition in the eye of limulus. *The Journal of General Physiology*, 39, 651–673.

Horgan, J. (1999). *The Undiscovered Mind*. London: Widenfeld and Nicholson.

Howard-Jones, P. A. (2007) *Neuroscience and Education: Issues and Opportunities, TLRP Commentary*. London: Teaching and Learning Research Programme.

Ito, M. (2006). Cerebellar circuitry as a neuronal machine. *Progress in Neurobiology*, 78(3), 272–303.

Jonas, E., & Kording, K. P. (2017). Could a neuroscientist understand a microprocessor? *PLoS Computational Biology*, 13(1), e1005268.

Jørgensen, C. B. (2001). August Krogh and Claude Bernard on basic principles in experimental physiology. *BioScience*, 51(1), 59–61.

Kandel, E. (2001). The molecular biology of memory storage: a dialogue between genes and synapses. *Science, 294*, 1030–1038.

Kiehn, O., & Kullander, K. (2004). Central pattern generators deciphered by molecular genetics. *Neuron, 41*, 317–321.

Koch, C. (2012). Modular biological complexity. *Science, 337*, 531–532.

Knafo, S., & Wyart, C. (2015). Optogenetic neuromodulation: new tools for monitoring and breaking neural circuits. *Annals of Physical and Rehabilitation Medicine, 58*, 259–264.

Krakauer, J. W., Ghazanfar, A. A., Gomez-Marin, A., MacIver, M. A., & Poeppel, D. (2017). Neuroscience needs behavior: correcting a reductionist bias. *Neuron, 93*(3), 480–490.

Kuhn, T. (1962). *The Structure of Scientific Revolutions*, 1st edn. Chicago, IL: University of Chicago Press.

Landhuis, E. (2020). Probing fine-scale connections in the brain. *Nature, 586*, 631–633.

Lichtman, J., & Sanes, J. (2008). Ome sweet ome: what can the genome tell us about the connectome? *Current Opinion in Neurobiology, 18*, 346–353.

Luan, H., Kuzin, A., Odenwald, W. F., & White, B. H. (2020). Cre-assisted fine-mapping of neural circuits using orthogonal split inteins. *eLife, 9*, e53041.

Machamer, P., Darden, L., & Craver, C. F. (2000). Thinking about mechanisms. *Philosophy of Science, 67*, 1–25.

Markram, H., Muller, E., Ramaswamy, S., Reimann, M. W., Abdellah, M., Sanchez, C. A., ... & Schurmann, F. (2015). Reconstruction and simulation of neocortical microcircuitry. *Cell, 163*, 456–492.

Marr, D. (1982). *Vision: A Computational Investigation into the Human Representation of Visual Information*. New York: W.H. Freeman & Company.

McCabe, D. P., & Castel, A. D. (2008). Seeing is believing: the effect of brain images on judgments of scientific reasoning. *Cognition, 107*(1), 343–352.

Middleton, H., & Moncrieff, J. (2019). Critical psychiatry: a brief overview. *BJ Psychiatry Advances, 25*, 47–54.

Miller, G. (2011). Blue brain founder responds to critics, clarifies his goals. *Science, 334*, 748–749.

Monod, J. (1972). *Chance and Necessity: An Essay on the Natural Philosophy of Modern Biology*. New York: Vintage.

Morgan, J. L., & Lichtman, J. W. (2013). Why not connectomics? *Nature Methods, 10*, 494–500.

Morris, R. G. M. (2003). Long-term potentiation and memory. *Philosophical Transactions of the Royal Society of London. Series B: Biological Sciences, 358*(1432), 643–647.

Mott, M. C., Gordon, J. A., & Koroshetz, W. J. (2018). The NIH BRAIN initiative: advancing neurotechnologies, integrating disciplines. *PLoS Biology, 16*(11), e3000066.

Nardone, A., & Schieppati, M. (2008). Inhibitory effect of the Jendrassik maneuver on the stretch reflex. *Neuroscience, 156*(3), 607–617.

Newell, A. (1982). The knowledge level. *Artificial Intelligence, 18*, 87–127.

Nicholson, D. J. (2019). Is the cell really a machine? *The Journal of Theoretical Biology, 477*, 108–126.

Noble, D. (2012). A theory of biological relativity: no privileged level of causation. *Interface Focus, 2*, 55–64.

Østby, I., Øehaug, L., Einevoll, G., Nagelhus, E., Plahte, E., Zeuthen, T., Lloyd, C., Ottersen, O., & Omholt, S. (2009). Astrocytic mechanisms explaining neural-activity-induced shrinkage of extraneuronal space. *PLoS Computational Biology, 5*, e1000272.

Parker, D. (2006). Complexities and uncertainties of neuronal network function. *Philosophical Transactions of the Royal Society B: Biological Sciences, 361*, 81–99.

Parker, D. (2010). Neuronal network analyses: premises, promises and uncertainties. *Philosophical Transactions of the Royal Society London B: Biological Sciences, 365*, 2315–2328.

Parker, D. (2018). Kuhnian revolutions in neuroscience: the role of tool development. *Biology and Philosophy, 33*, 17.

Parker, D. (2019). Psychoneural reduction: a perspective from neural circuits. *Biology & Philosophy, 34*(4), 44. doi:10.1007/s10539-019-9697-8.

Parker, D., & Srivastava, V. (2013). Dynamic systems approaches and levels of analysis in the nervous system. *Frontiers in Physiology, 4*, 15.

Pickering, A. (2010). *The Cybernetic Brain: Sketches of Another Future*. Chicago, IL: University of Chicago.

Price, C. J., & Friston, K. J. (2005). Functional ontologies for cognition: the systematic definition of structure and function. *Cognitive Neuropsychology, 22*, 262–275.

Railton, P. (1981). Probability, explanation, and information. *Synthese, 48*, 233–256.

Ryle, G. (1949). *The Concept of Mind*. Chicago, IL: University of Chicago Press.

Sagan, C. (1977). *Dragons of Eden: Speculations on the Evolution of Human Intelligence*. New York: Random House.

Scheffer, L. K., Xu, C. S., Januszewski, M., Lu, Z., Takemura, S.-Y., Hayworth, K. J., Huang, G. B., ... & Plaza, S. M. (2020). A connectome and analysis of the adult Drosophila central brain. *eLife, 9*, e57443 C57441.

Schroeder, C., & Foxe, J. (2005). Multisensory contributions to low-level, 'unisensory' processing. *Curr Opin Neurobiol, 4*, 454-458.

Schroter, M., Paulsen, O., & Bullmore, E. T. (2017). Micro-connectomics: probing the organization of neuronal networks at the cellular scale. *Nature Reviews Neuroscience, 18*, 131.

Selverston, A. (1980). Are central pattern generators understandable? *Behavioral Brain Sciences, 3*, 535–571.

Sherrington, C. S. (1899). On the relation between structure and function as examined in the arm. *Transactions of the Liverpool Biological Society, 13*, 1–20.

Sherrington, C. S. (1951). *Man on His Nature: The Gifford Lectures, Edinburgh, 1937–8*. Cambridge: Cambridge University Press.

Simon, H. (1962). The architecture of complexity. *Proceedings of the American Philosophical Society, 106*, 467–482.

Simon, H. (1969). *The Sciences of the Artificial, Third Edition.*: The MIT Press.

Soltesz, I. (2006). *Diversity in the Neuronal Machine*. New York: Oxford University Press.

Sperry, R. W. (1980). Mind-brain interaction: mentalism, yes; dualism, no. *Neuroscience. 5*, 195–206.

Steinmetz, N. A., Aydin, C., Lebedeva, A., Okun, M., Pachitariu, M., Bauza, M., Beau, M., ... & Harris, T. D. (2021). Neuropixels 2.0: a miniaturized high-density probe for stable, long-term brain recordings. *Science*, 372, eabf4588.

Stent, G. (1969). *The Coming of the Golden Age*. Garden City, NY: Natural History Press.

Steward, O., Popovich, P. G., Dietrich, W. D., & Kleitman, N. (2012). Replication and reproducibility in spinal cord injury research. *Experimental Neurology*, 233(2), 597–605.

Svensson, E., Aspergis-Schoute, J., Burnstock, G., Nusbaum, M., Parker, D., & Schioth, H. (2019). General principles of neuronal co-transmission: insights from multiple model systems. *Frontiers in Neural Circuits*, 12, 117.

Thomson, H. (2010). Mental muscle: six ways to boost your brain. https://www.newscientist.com/article/mg20827801-300-mental-muscle-six-ways-to-boost-your-brain/#ixzz67nP7rZgk.

Warner, R. (2001). Microelectronics: its unusual origin and personality. *IEEE Transactions on Electron Devices*, 48, 2457–2467.

Weisberg, D., Keil, F., Goodstein, J., Rawson, E., & Gray, J. (2008). The seductive allure of neuroscience explanations. *The Journal of Cognitive Neuroscience*, 20, 470–477.

Weiss, S., & Faber, D. (2010). Field effects in the CNS play a functional role. *Frontiers in Neural Circuits*, 4, 1–10.

Wimsatt, W. C. (2006). Reductionism and its heuristics: making methodological reductionism honest. *Synthese*, 151, 445–475.

Woodward, J. (2017). Explanation in Neurobiology: An Interventionist Perspective. In D. Kaplan (Ed.), *Explanation and Integration in Mind and Brain Science* (pp. 70–100). Oxford: Oxford University Press.

Zhang, Y., Rózsa, M., Bushey, D., Zheng, J., Reep, D., Liang, Y., Brousaard, G. J., ... & Looger, L. L. (2020). *jGCaMP8 Fast Genetically Encoded Calcium Indicators*. Janelia Research Campus. Online resource. doi:10.25378/janelia.13148243.v4

Ylikoski, P. K. (2009). The Illusion of Depth of Understanding in Science. In H. W. de Regt, S. Leonelli, & K. Eigner (Eds.), *Scientific Understanding: Philosophical Perspectives* (pp. 100–119). Pittsburgh, PA: University of Pittsburgh Press.

Yuste, R. (2015). From the neuron doctrine to neural networks. *Nature Reviews Neuroscience*, 16, 487–497.

12 Cognitive Ontologies, Task Ontologies, and Explanation in Cognitive Neuroscience

Daniel C. Burnston

1 Introduction

The development of new scientific tools provides opportunities for progress, but also gives scientists reason to reinvestigate, reconsider, and maybe revise their assumptions about the domain under investigation. In cognitive neuroscience, this has manifested in the debate over "cognitive ontology" – that is, the set of mental functions or faculties investigated by the neurosciences. Psychology comes equipped with a series of intuitive mental categories – perception, cognition, memory, imagination, verbal reasoning, emotion, etc. Cognitive neuroscience has traditionally proceeded under the assumption that these, or some suitably explicated set of these, will be realized in the processes that neuroscientists investigate. For better or worse, however, this assumption sits poorly with the current evidence, which indicates the massive multifunctionality of individual parts of the brain, the wide distribution of activity corresponding to intuitive mental categories, and the importance of global network and ecological context in determining what an individual part of the brain does. These data stress, and perhaps break, the "new phrenological" (Uttal, 2001) approach to cognitive and systems neuroscience, invalidating cherished means of analysis such as subtractive methodology and reverse inference.

One powerful thought in the field is that part of the problem is our intuitive conception of psychology. Indeed, Poldrack once said that "*the fundamental problem is our stone age psychological ontology*" (Bunzl, Hanson, & Poldrack, 2010, p. 54). Perhaps the standard mentalistic categories used in the psychological sciences are just too simple, too general, and too crude to capture how the brain implements behavior. Perhaps those categories need to be revised, refined, or even abandoned to understand brain function. A host of questions immediately arises, however, surrounding how committed we should remain to our standard list of cognitive kinds. Do they successfully describe brain function, only at a network level? Could we discover discrete implementations of kinds if they are suitably amended, for instance by subdividing them into more specific kinds? Or should they just be gotten rid of, resulting in a view

DOI: 10.4324/9781003251392-16

of the brain on which it is "unanalyzable" (Uttal, 2001) into distinct functions, where its function is "protean" and lacking generalizability (Hutto, Peeters, & Segundo-Ortin, 2017)?

Theorists interested in cognitive ontology are thus facing a conundrum that is both methodological and ontological. What cognitive categories are realized in the brain cannot be determined independently of our methods of investigation. But in cognitive neuroscience, those methods traditionally employ those categories as basic assumptions – i.e., they are what *is being investigated*, and thereby constrain the interpretation of otherwise inscrutable brain data. Theorists have begun to use formal tools from databasing, machine learning, and meta-analysis as a way of addressing this problem. The hope is that the use of these tools can turn the issue of cognitive ontology into a problem for data science, rather than metaphysics. By analyzing large amounts of studies using an agreed-upon, publicly shareable taxonomy of cognitive function, neuroscientists hope to be able to *discover* the ways in which cognitive categories relate to brain activation, and thereby provide a groundwork for the substantiation, revision, or abandonment of those categories.

I refer to these projects collectively as "databasing and brain mapping" projects, and in this paper, I assess their status and prospects. Ultimately, I will argue that the problem is not so much with our intuitive mental ontology *per se*, but with the standard explanatory framework assumed by the cognitive neurosciences. The standard framework assumes that categories of mental function are *explanatory* kinds, and that cognitive neuroscience proceeds by showing how these explanatory categories are *instantiated* in brain activity. As such, the standard framework is committed to there being an ultimate taxonomy of distinct and discretely realized cognitive kinds, whose instantiation in the brain causally explains behavior. I will argue that databasing and brain-mapping projects, rather than substantiating this standard framework, should inspire us to abandon it. Instead, I advocate an alternative view of neuroscientific explanation on which what explains are ways in which brain systems organize to implement the informational demands of a particular task or context (Burnston, 2016, 2021). On this alternative, the best reading of the role of psychological constructs is as *heuristics* for investigation, rather than as explanatory kinds (cf. Feest, 2010).

My aims are both descriptive and normative. I both believe that this is what successful neuroscientific explanation *does* look like, and that it is how we *should* think about it. This comes along with a variety of methodological prescriptions, including a plea for increased focus on *task*, rather than *cognitive* ontologies. I hope to clarify the potential advantages and pitfalls of using formal analytical tools in the cognitive ontology debate along the way.

I proceed as follows. In Section 2, I introduce the standard explanatory framework of cognitive neuroscience, articulate its commitments, and discuss methodological and empirical problems for the framework present in the literature. Then, in Section 3, I outline some of the formal tools that have been applied to the problem, and in Section 4 show that no clear consensus has emerged on how results employing these methods are supposed to relate to the standard framework. In Section 5 I outline my preferred approach to understanding the role of psychological constructs in neuroscientific explanation, and in Section 6 show how this approach offers distinct normative prescriptions than the standard framework. Section 7 concludes.

2 The Standard Explanatory Framework of Cognitive Neuroscience

As I understand it, the standard explanatory framework in cognitive neuroscience is as follows. First, psychological kinds are explanatory. Behavior is explained by citing mental functions such as memory, attention, language processing, action planning, etc. Second, explanation is *causal* explanation. It is the realization of psychological kinds in neural processes that explains behavior. To take one philosophical gloss on the issue, consider Piccinini and Craver's (2011) account of the role of psychological theories in cognitive neuroscience. Psychology, on their view, provides *mechanism sketches* of cognitive phenomena. They outline a causal sequence of mental functions that can explain the phenomena of interest. A full *mechanism schema*, on the other hand, will show how this abstract functional organization is realized in lower-level causal interactions in the brain, eventually bottoming out in the electrical and chemical processes of individual cells. This can be read as a way of combining Cummins' (1983) functional decomposition approach to psychological explanation with the explanatory goals of cognitive neuroscience.

This kind of view is very influential (Boone & Piccinini, 2016), describes the traditional explanatory practices of cognitive neuroscientists well, and comes with a number of advantages. First, it gives a metaphysically appealing picture of mental causation, wherein psychological states cause behavior via their realization relation to the physical processes of the brain. Second, it explains the importance of *operationalization* and *localization* in cognitive neuroscience. 'Memory' is not something we can study directly; we can only study behavior. On the standard story, behavioral tasks are designed to dissociate the different components of putative cognitive processes. The brain is then studied to show how those functional differences are causally realized in distinct parts of the brain. These changes can be measured either through differences in activation – the traditional "subtraction" methodology in fMRI research – or through intervention, by studying artificially induced or naturally occurring brain injuries. By finding different localizations of distinct functions, one explains the causal differences between, for example, a

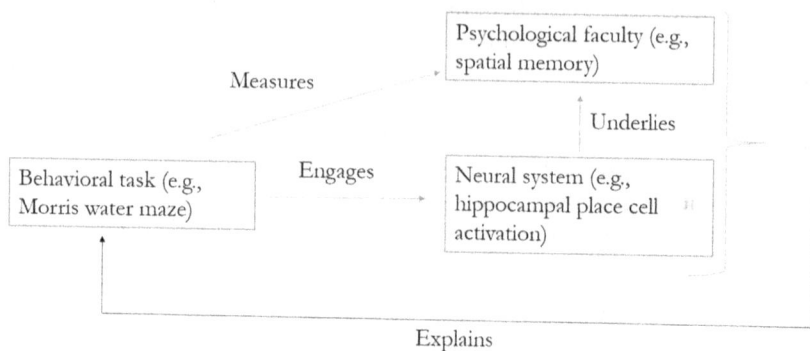

Figure 12.1 The standard explanatory framework.

memory process and an attentional process. A diagram of the standard framework is provided above (Figure 12.1).

Despite its appeal, the standard framework faces a large class of problems, which we can generally refer to as *individuation* problems. Individuation problems are the result of the realism about psychological kinds inherent in the standard framework, along with the complexity of causal processes in the brain. Basically, different *explanantia* need to be distinct. The standard framework is committed, in each instance, to establishing exactly what psychological functions are explaining a behavior, how they interact, and how the behavior arises as a result of that interaction. Individuation problems lead us to question whether this commitment is in fact met in cognitive neuroscience – they suggest that, very frequently, we have not, and even *cannot*, establish exactly which psychological faculties are at work and the pattern of their interaction.

There are two kinds of individuation problems that have seen extensive discussion in the literature. The first is an individuation problem with *operationalization* and *measurement*. The question here is whether tasks individuate particular mental faculties. Sullivan (2010), for instance, questions whether the Morris water maze, a famous task in neuroscience, can be taken as a specific measurement of "spatial memory," the cognitive kind with which it is generally associated, rather than measuring learning, the change of representational capacities, or just ability to find a platform under the surface of some water. Sullivan (2014) also applies the argument to tasks such as Stroop tasks. While standardly thought of as measuring attention, Sullivan persuasively argues that elements of attention, memory, language processing, and perceptual processing are all indexed in the standard versions of Stroop tasks.

The second version of individuation problem applies to the kinds themselves. The worry is that psychological kinds are simply not distinct from one another. So, perhaps memory is not distinct, metaphysically speaking, from action planning or imagination (De Brigard, 2014; Schacter, Benoit, De Brigard, & Szpunar, 2015; but cf. Robins, 2016). Perhaps "basic" emotions (Griffiths, 2002), or "concepts" (Machery, 2009), or psychiatric categories such as "schizophrenia" (Tekin, 2016) do not correspond to natural kinds. Recently, these worries have been extended to core cognitive capacities like working memory (Gomez-Lavin, 2020).

I am moved by these considerations, but will not focus on them here. What I will assess in detail is the last variety of individuation problem, which occurs in the purported *realization* of cognitive kinds. The traditional approach to cognitive neuroscience hopes to specify *the* function of each part of the brain. This "atomistic" (Burnston, 2021) approach is motivated by the goal of causal decomposition in the brain. If we can specify the function of each part, then we can understand any given behavior as the result of causal interaction between these functions. A one-to-one mapping between the mental ontology and the neuroscientific ontology would occasion a particularly powerful form of mechanistic explanation.

Current data, however, sits uneasily with individuating atomic mappings between functions and brain activation. Widespread data from many distinct parts of the brain suggest the *multifunctionality* of individual brain parts, *overlap* between instantiations of distinct mental categories, and *distribution* of brain activation corresponding to distinct kinds. Multifunctionality of particular parts of the brain undermines the ability to say, given activation in a particular part, what function that part is performing, and hence how it is causally interacting with other parts. This is part of the problem with the traditional subtractive methodology and reverse inference. *Overlap* and *distribution* of function undermine the ability to distinguish between the causal contribution of distinct kinds at the neural level.

It is worth considering further why this is. Suppose we are observing a behavior, and activation in a number of parts of the brain. If one can decompose the behavior into distinct psychological processes, and localize each of those processes, then one can theorize about the causal interactions between them. But significant distribution and overlap of instantiation muddy the division between localization and interaction. This is because they allow for too much inferential freedom in how one interprets the instantiation relation. Suppose two putatively distinct faculties overlap in their instantiation. Is this due to the fact that they share some common functional core and other elements that differ? Is it because we have not explicated them sufficiently relative to each other? Or is it because they are not, in fact, distinct after all? Similarly, given wide distribution corresponding to a given function, is that distribution an indication that the construct ranges over multiple distinct sub-functions that interact? Or that our experiments in fact index multiple distinct functions? Or, again, that the construct does not describe the mechanistic functioning of the brain?

In most cases of mental faculties, this is the situation that actually obtains – the data suggests multifunctionality, distribution, and overlap. But the standard framework requires that distinct explanantia be distinct, including in their instantiations. So, the current data conflicts with the standard framework. Given this conflict, one can either attempt further work to substantiate the standard framework, or one can abandon it. To substantiate the framework, one would have to either try to further differentiate the instantiation relations between distinct kinds, or revise the ontology so that more specific mappings emerge. One could, of course, pursue some combination. If abandoning the framework, one would have to specify what kind of explanation results from that abandonment.

The idea of revision of the cognitive ontology is appealing, and it is often suggested in mechanistic contexts that higher-level kinds will have to be split or revised in light of causal explanation at a lower level (Bechtel, 2008; Bickle, 2003). Similarly, it is often suggested that databasing and brain-mapping techniques can help us revise our ontology. I will consider these claims in detail in the next section. But it is worth noting that the ontology revision proposal is less anodyne than is normally supposed. Attempting to fine-grain our taxonomy does not guarantee that distinct functions will be discovered – Feest (2010), for instance, nicely explains how continuous attempts to distinguish implicit memory from other forms of memory are what eventuated in the conclusion that implicit memory may not be distinct from perceptual association. And even a successful distinction may not be mechanistically useful – attempts to distinguish face perception, body perception, and place perception, for instance, do not show clearly distinct realizers but interdigitated "archipelagoes" of voxels with a statistical preference for one kind of information over another (Kanwisher, 2010). This is not a discovery of clearly distinct parts with causal interactions between them.

In the next two sections, I introduce databasing and brain mapping techniques in more detail, and argue that, while proponents of these techniques are generally *realist* about psychological kinds, they do not clearly opt for either substantiation, revision, or abandonment of the standard framework, instead vacillating between these options. I also raise doubts that the databasing and brain mapping techniques on offer can perform any of these functions. This motivates my own take on the issue, which I will pursue in Section 5.

3 Databasing and Brain Mapping

There are two main aspects to the databasing and brain-mapping projects I will discuss. The first is the collection of compendious amounts of neural data from across studies. The shareability of scientific data, as well as the best means to collect it, disseminate it, and use it, are problems across the biological sciences (see, e.g., Bechtel, 2017; Darden et al., 2018; Leonelli, 2012), and neuroscience is no different. One reaction to the massive amount of research using, for instance, fMRI methodology, is to try to systematize and understand this expansive dataset as a whole. So, collection of the information is the first step. Several open-access databases have been created in cognitive neuroscience to play this role, including the Brain Map (Fox & Lancaster, 2002), Neurosynth (Yarkoni et al., 2011), The Cognitive Atlas (Poldrack et al., 2011), the Experiment Factory (Sochat et al., 2016), and The Cognitive Paradigm Ontology (Turner & Laird, 2012).

While these projects differ in their precise focus, they all share a number of aspects. First, the idea is to collect activation data in a theoretically unbiased way. What is archived is the raw activation data from a set of fMRI studies. One can then ask questions about this data. Second, one of the questions that everyone wants to ask about this data is how, whether, and in what sense patterns in the data correspond to psychological concepts. This is done in a number of ways. In the Cognitive Atlas, each study, in addition to the data, is categorized according to the type of tasks manipulated. Each task type is then defined, and the psychological concepts that it is supposed to measure are listed. So, one can look for the ways in which the same concepts are realized similarly or differently across different tasks, or one can look at how different tasks/concepts diverge or overlap. In Neurosynth, the *text* of papers is archived along with the raw fMRI data, so one can look for ways in which *usage* of key mental terms by scientists varies along with changes in brain activation, and vice-versa. Finally, the hope across these projects is that the search for patterns can be *automated*. Given the scale of the data set, automated data analysis is used in the attempt to find meaningful patterns.

The analytical techniques applied to this collected data range from traditional meta-analyses to statistical classifiers to generative, probabilistic models, each with their associated benefits and detractions. Meta-analytic techniques take already reported correlations between cognitive concepts and activation patterns, and attempt to identify, generalize, and summarize the relationships discovered in the literature. Statistical decoders train models to predict, given the presence of brain activation, what cognitive concepts are being assessed in the range of studies (or vice versa, see below). While there are a range of generative models, one popular technique is *Latent Dirichlet Allocation* (LDA), which is a Bayesian algorithm that models the text in a corpus of words (in this case, the text from fMRI studies) as being generated by a grouping of topics, themselves construed as probabilistic groupings of individual words. One can then attempt to correlate greater influence (or "loadings") of those topics with brain activation.

There are a range of attitudes taken by brain mappers to their projects, which I will discuss in detail below. In general, however, I think there are two fundamental assumptions they share. First, they are *realists* about mental faculties. Second, and relatedly, they are committed to the *measurement* relation between tasks and those faculties. For instance, Hastings et al. (2014) describe the project as one on which "ontological realism is a foundation" (p. 4). Lenartowicz et al. (2010) suggest that "the elements of the mental ontology are not directly accessible but rather must be accessed through experimental manipulations and measurements (i.e., tasks)" (p. 680).

In these quotes, theorists are committing to the idea that mental functions are real entities, and that tasks are measurements of them. This is reflected in much of the databasing work. In the Cognitive Atlas and Brain Map, for instance, tasks are explicitly categorized according to the mental constructs they are supposed to measure. While Neurosynth collects a range of textual data, the preprocessing of that data indicates a realist commitment. Generally, LDA models using Neurosynth focus on the abstracts of paper, and specifically on the cognitive terms contained therein. In attempting to map these uses to the brain, then, these projects assume that, at least at an abstract level, the concepts we employ in thinking about the mind correspond to physical categories within the brain.

As I will show below, this set of commitments interacts in complicated ways with the standard framework. For now, I want to discuss a few early results from these frameworks to show that, far from solving individuation problems, brain mapping projects tended to illustrate them. The question will then be what attitudes brain mappers take to these results.

In a meta-analysis of fMRI research, Anderson, Kinnison, and Pessoa (2013) compared different patterns of activation according to the cognitive categories listed in Brain Map. They were interested in a number of properties, including the range of cognitive concepts associated with each area's activation, the distribution of activation corresponding to those concepts, and the degree to which distinct brain areas were likely to be active in studies measuring the same mental concepts. What they showed was that individual parts of the brain exhibit a range of "diversity profiles," but that most areas' activation corresponded with significantly more than one cognitive concept. Moreover, areas within previously identified functional-connectivity networks tended to be highly "assortative," meaning they tended to be active for similar cognitive concepts, suggesting both the distribution of individual functions and the overlap in neural activation between functions. Importantly, taking functional networks such as the "fronto-parietal" network and the "ventral attention" network, as basic units to correlate with cognitive concepts showed a similar pattern of results.

Poldrack, Halchenko, and Hanson (2009) performed a decoding analysis of the results from eight different fMRI studies investigating a range of cognitive constructs. They began with statistical maps of the entire brain – i.e., z-scored activation coordinates from every condition in the eight studies. The question was then whether one could train a decoder to predict which tasks and/or cognitive concepts were named in the studies, such as "risk-taking". They trained a support vector machine to predict, on the basis of a given brain-wide activation, what task and what cognitive concept was being measured in a case and showed that the classifier could successfully classify both with 80%–90% accuracy. They further trained a neural network with six hidden nodes to match the predictive accuracy of the support vector machine. Importantly, however, the nodes operated over a widely distributed set of voxels. When analyzed as a six-dimensional system (one for each hidden node), each cognitive concept was shown to be related to a combination of each dimension, and each dimension was associated with a range of cognitive concepts.

Poldrack et al. (2012) performed a topic modeling analysis with the following structure. First, they took the results and text from over 5,000 papers in the *Neurosynth* database. They began by exploring the topic structure in the text. They then selected topics that corresponded to mental concepts in the Cognitive Atlas and measured how the topic loadings on these topics correlated with brain activity. Here, however, they also show multifunctionality and distribution in the results. For instance, they report:

> topic 43 (with terms related to visual attention) was associated with activity in the bilateral lateral occipital cortex, parietal cortex, and frontal cortex. Topic 86 (with terms related to decision making and choice) was associated with regions in the ventral striatum, medial, orbital, and dorsolateral prefrontal cortex. Topic 93 (with terms related to emotion) was associated with bilateral activity in the amygdala, orbitofrontal cortex, and medial prefrontal cortex.
>
> (2012, p. e1002707)

These results are perfectly interesting in their own right, in that they quantify the "specificity" with which our intuitive cognitive concepts interact with brain activation. It is just that, on their face, they are in conflict with the standard model because they show multifunctionality and distribution rather than univocal relationships between psychological constructs and activation. The question is what to do in response to these results with regard to the standard framework.

Let me stress that I am reconstructing positions here – I think each of the options I am about to articulate is present, to some degree, across papers and theorists within the field. As far as I can tell, there are three options with regard to the standard framework. First, one could attempt to substantiate the framework by pursuing more fine-grained analyses in an attempt to discover more and more specific activation patterns for particular cognitive concepts, perhaps further leading to decomposition and causal explanation. Second, one could attempt to use the analyses to *revise* our cognitive ontology. On this view, it might be the case that the standard framework can be maintained, but only after the appropriate revisions to the ontology. Third, one might use these results as motivation to *abandon* the standard framework altogether and opt for some other kind of project. In the next section, I outline each of these perspectives, along with examples from the literature which might suggest them, and give reasons to question them. This will motivate my own proposal about psychological constructs in Section 5.

4   Three Options with Regard to the Standard Framework

4.1 Substantiate?

One view one could take towards the standard framework is that it is basically right, *and* our ontology is basically right, but that the results of multifunctionality and distribution are due to insufficiently fine-grained measurement. The solution, if this is one's perspective, would be to re-fine analyses so that the "true" and univocal associations between psychological constructs and brain activation can be uncovered.

I think that this is the position that is least strongly considered in the literature, but there are a few trends that suggest it. Indeed, one direction in which the literature has gone over the last few years is in the direction of more fine-grained analysis and the search for increased specificity. Poldrack and Yarkoni (2016) thus describe the project as one of "quantifying the true specificity of hypothesized structure-function associations" (p. 589). This, one assumes, means that they indeed take there *to be* relations there to be discovered, further indicating realism about psychological kinds. Moreover, recent projects take the goal of brain mapping projects to be enabling both *forward* and *reverse* inference – that is, the predictive ability of brain mapping models between constructs and activation patterns should be bidirectional. This, to me at least, further suggests a belief in the importance of the instantiation relation. Finally, there is how these projects are qualitatively described. For instance, Varoquaux et al. (2018) suggest that one of the goals of mapping projects is "precisely describing the function of any given brain region" (2018, p. 1).

Varoquaux et al. performed a decoding analysis using a hierarchical general linear model (GLM) framework. In particular, their reverse inference required multiple layers of linear regressions on activity in the brain. The first layer was tuned to individual oppositions between task conditions. Then, a second layer used another regression that compared each cognitive term to all others, predicting which term was overall most relevant. They compared the results of this decoder to other approaches, showing that it resulted in sharper divisions between distinct functions.

There are a few things to be said here, however. First, this study measured terms in the Cognitive Paradigm Ontology rather than the Brain Map or the Cognitive Atlas, and these terms more directly describe task conditions (e.g. "response with left hand") than psychological constructs (e.g., "motor control"). Second, they focused primarily on perceptual and motor areas for which there are already more-or-less well-understood general function ascriptions. Finally, even *these* results showed distributed and interdigitated functional populations, with, for instance, "face" and "place" areas being more or less separated, but each involving multiple subpopulations distinct from each other.

Another recent approach to bidirectional decoding is from Rubin et al. (2017), which employs LDA on over 11,000 articles from Neurosynth. They start by noting that previous studies show mainly wide patterns of activation for particular constructs, and thus are no help in finding "relatively simple, well-defined functional-anatomical atoms." To overcome this, they performed an LDA analysis constrained *both* by the semantics of the terms and by groupings in spatial coordinates. They report that, not only were they able to uncover topics with relatively clear functional upshot, (e.g., topics related to "emotion"), but that each topic "is associated with a single brain region." At first, this sounds a lot like the explanatory aim of the standard framework – i.e., to find a constrained localization corresponding to each psychological function.

A closer reading questions this analysis, however. As the researchers note, the probabilistic nature of the model suggests that the decoding analysis uncovers the construct *most likely* associated with a given area, but not the only one. This is further illustrated by the fact that individual topics were allowed to spatially overlap in the model, and many multifunctional areas did indeed show significant overlap between related topics. Further specifying to individual topics in many cases required conditioning further on more spatial coordinates, hence suggesting, again, distribution of function. So, while the results in this model are *predictive* at a very specific construct-spatial level, it is not clear that this reflects the reality of the system. And this is noted explicitly by the researchers. It is worth quoting them in full:

While the topics produced by the model generally have parsimonious interpretations that accord well with previous findings, they should be treated as a useful, human-comprehensible approximation of the true nomological network of neurocognition, and not as a direct window into reality. For the sake of analytical tractability, our model assumes a one-to-one mapping between semantic representations and brain regions, whereas the underlying reality almost certainly involves enormously complex many-to-many mappings. Similarly, rerunning the GC-LDA model on different input data, with different spatial priors, a different number of topics, or with different analysis parameters would necessarily produce somewhat different results.

(Rubin et al., 2017, p. 14)

So, while one trend in the literature is to look for increasingly specific relationships between extant psychological constructs and patterns of activation, it is not clear that even successful results in this endeavor substantiate, or should be read as attempting to substantiate, the standard framework.

4.2 Revise?

The idea that the databasing and brain mapping project can help us revise our cognitive ontology is extremely common. For example, Poldrack and Yarkoni (2016) suggest that "formal cognitive ontologies [are useful] in helping to clarify, refine, and test theories of brain and cognitive function" (p. 587), and that "biological discoveries can and should inform the continual revision of psychological theories" (p. 599).

These quotes suggest that, ultimately, the role of the databasing and brain mapping project will be in helping us to explicate our mental ontology. Sometimes, this is pitched in terms of a discovery science – we should let the brain tell us what its functional categories are, and revise our ontology accordingly (Poldrack et al., 2012). In this section, I suggest two related problems for this view. The first is the *interpretability* problem, and the second is the *seeding* problem. In general, however, the issue is this: without a *rubric* for how and when to revise our mental categories in light of brain mapping data, we lack the ability to use results from brain mapping to revise the ontology in any specific way. This suggests that metaphysical commitments about the nature of mental states *precede*, rather than being compelled by, brain mapping data.

The interpretability problem is akin to a problem discussed by Carlson et al. (2018; cf. Ritchie, Kaplan, & Klein, 2016; Weiskopf, 2021) for uncovering neural *representations* via machine learning techniques. They argue that, given a particular ability to decode some stimulus from neural activity, it is unclear how to interpret that result in terms of representational content. The worry, I take it, is that the ability to decode a stimulus from an activation does not mean that the activity represents the stimulus under anything like the way we would describe it. The analog problem here is that simply showing that a pattern of activity in the brain is specific to, say, decision-making (or to a high topic loading on a topic that happens to comprise words we associate with decision-making), doesn't give us any indication of whether the pattern of activity is in fact performing something we would call "decision-making." The more distribution and overlap uncovered in the analysis, the more exacerbated this problem becomes, because of the inferential freedom discussed in Section 2.

So, given the association of a pattern of activity with a mental construct, should we take that construct as substantiated, as in need of explication, or what? What degree of correlation/predictability, or what degree of specificity, is required to count the kind as substantiated, and at what point should we consider it in need of revision? The brain mapping results themselves provide no rubric for how to make these decisions.

The seeding problem is related to the interpretation problem and is based on the fact that even *constructing the analyses* requires adhering, to an unspecified degree, to our extant cognitive constructs. In an analysis based on Brain Map or the Cognitive Atlas, one only *considers* concepts that are a current part of our mental ontology. This presumes that the basic structure of the brain corresponds closely enough to those categories in order for them to be useful in understanding the brain. But what justifies this assumption? In principle, a specific-enough correlation between mental constructs and brain activity might justify the assumption, but it is precisely a *lack* of specificity of this type that prompts the idea of ontology revision.

In topic-modeling analyses, the topics that are often focused upon are the ones that one can intuitively or statistically pair with an already-known mental construct. Varoquaux et al., for example, advertise that 100 of the 200 topics in the model correspond to well-understood mental constructs. What about the other ones, however? Even given a substantiation of some of our mental categories, what the analysis would suggest is that our ontology is at least impoverished, and it does not come with any prescriptions for what to say in these other cases.

Again, the point of this is not to discount the analysis. The point of if it is just to deny that the analysis on its own offers us any principled way of revising our cognitive ontology. Put differently, the principles for ontology revision cannot be uncovered bottom-up from these analyses. Metaphysical commitments must be undertaken in constructing and interpreting the analyses themselves. Again, theorists in the field recognize this problem. Poldrack and Yarkoni (2016), for instance, note that there is "no algorithmic way" to approach ontology revision in light of specific mapping results. They seem to suggest, however, that more analysis and case-by-case thinking will allow for sufficient explication. The individuation and seeding problems should raise concerns for that approach.

4.3 Abandonment?

One also finds more-or-less explicit discussion of the explanatory ideals of the standard framework in the literature. The clearest cases of these are Yarkoni and Westfall (2017) and Anderson (2014). Yarkoni suggests explicitly that results from databasing and brain-mapping projects suggest abandoning *explanation* altogether, in favor of a purely predictive neuroscience. Anderson's view does not cite prediction per se, but does suggest that we need to change to a *dispositional* approach to brain organization, wherein we do not understand a part of the brain as contributing a specific causal influence at a specific time, but instead as exhibiting dispositions to contribute to a range of functions.

I lack the space to assess these proposals in detail, but for my purposes, it suffices to note that they both, more-or-less-explicitly, move away from the mechanistic kind of explanation inherent to the standard framework. Much has been said about the relative merits of mechanistic explanation versus prediction in explanation (Craver, 2006), and now is not the time to re-adjudicate these issues. What I want to argue for in the remainder of the paper is that abandoning the standard framework is not itself equivalent to abandoning mechanistic explanation. Instead, we can abandon the standard framework by abandoning the central explanatory role it affords to mentalistic constructs.

5 An Alternative View

5.1 Mental Constructs as Heuristics

My proposal is based on the following negative claim: *posits of psychological faculties do not explain behavior*. Individuation problems arise from the notion that posits of psychological faculties are explanatory. That is why they must be distinct from each other; that is why they must be discretely realized; and that is why causal interactions between them need to be established. Get rid of their explanatory status, and all of those problems go away – it's not particularly worrisome of psychological kinds are not clearly distinct from each other, if specific behavioral tasks don't measure only one of them at the expense of others, or even if they massively "crosscut" the causal patterns we measure in the brain (Hochstein, 2016; Weskopf, 2011).

This leaves us with two questions. First, what does explain behavior? And second, do psychological posits play any role in understanding it? These questions can be asked within the context of brain mapping projects as well. What sort of explanation should these projects be seen as working towards? And should mental concepts play any role as they seek them?

My answers are as follows. First, information processing in the brain explains behavior directly, and not in virtue of instantiating some particular mental function. As I will attempt to show, this proposal is compatible with each brain area being multifunctional, and with function generally being distributed (Burnston, 2016, 2021). Second, mentalistic concepts are best understood as playing a *heuristic* role (cf. Feest, 2010).

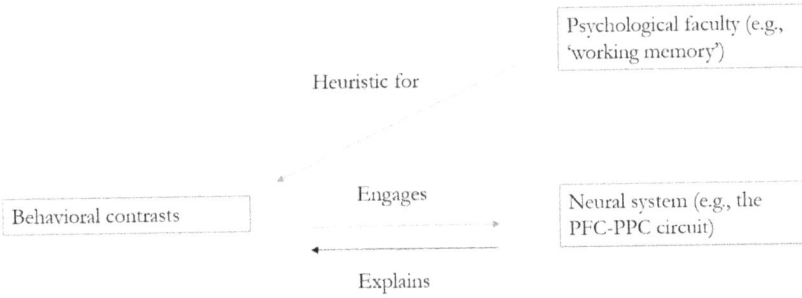

Figure 12.2 The heuristic approach to mental constructs.

Rather than serving as explanantia, we should view mental categories as helping us parse behaviors into rough, and revisable, similarity classes. They provide traction on an otherwise impossibly complex space of behavioral abilities and guide the search for important distinctions between types of behaviors, so that we can *then* investigate how the brain implements those differences. Importantly, they can play this role even if *there is no fact of the matter* about which neural processes implement which psychological constructs. Hence, no individuation problems are faced (Figure 12.2).

5.2 An Exemplar

The heuristic view makes a number of invocations about successful explanations in neuroscience. First, overlap between mental constructs across tasks and contexts should be just as important as separation between them. Second, understanding the differences in structure between tasks is paramount for understanding neural function. Third, assuming spatial decomposition between distinct purported mental faculties would *limit*, rather than enabling, understanding of how the system works.

I will discuss one example in detail. Murray, Jaramillo, and Wang (2017) pursued a modeling study of the interaction between the prefrontal cortex (PFC) and the posterior parietal cortex (PPC). The initiating motivation for their study is that both the PFC and the PPC have been shown physiologically to be involved across a wide range of both working memory (WM) and decision-making (DM) tasks. The question, then, is what their distinct contributions are.

Murray et al.'s approach was as follows. They modeled each area as a fully recurrent neural network, and each area had distinct subpopulations selective for distinct perceptual stimuli. The PFC and PPC networks were bi-directionally connected via long-range projections. The main difference between the two populations was a difference in local structure. In particular, the PFC population was modeled as having a higher degree of internal influence – both in self-excitation of each subpopulation, and in inhibitory connections between them, than the PPC. Given this network structure, the investigators could model the dynamics of the system in a range of task types, and think about how the network responded in each.

Murray et al. posited that one key factor involved in working memory tasks is *multi-stability*. That is, the network can represent a range of possible stimuli, but given that it has already represented one, it must maintain that information across a delay, perhaps in the presence of distractors. So, they modeled the presentation of a stimulus and whether its representation could be maintained in the network even as other modeled stimuli were presented. What they showed is that a particular dynamics occurred during "successful" working memory trials, in which both PFC and PPC populations represented the stimulus during presentation. During delay, presentation of a distractor would "switch" the PPC representation to representing the distractor, but PFC would not switch. After the distractor was removed, the PFC → PPC long-range connections would enforce the PPC populations to "switch back" to representing the remembered stimulus. This model predicted a range of physiological results found in PFC and PPC during these kinds of tasks, as well as predicting types and durations of distractor-presentation that would cause errors. Importantly, this explanation relied on the degree of internal connection in each area, and the feedback connections from the PFC to the PPC. For instance, if the internal connections within the PFC were not sufficiently strong, then it would not maintain the representation during distractor presentation.

For decision tasks, the investigators asked whether the network could produce an evidence-accumulation-to-threshold kind of process. These processes have been shown to be important for a range of decision-making processes including perceptual decisions and multi-attribute choices (Teodorescu & Usher, 2013). Murray et al. modeled a perceptual decision-making task, in which one out of a range of possible perceptual outcomes must be decided on in the presence of a noisy signal. They showed that the network could implement an evidence-accumulation process, in which buildup of evidence occurred primarily in the PPC population and selection of outcome in the PFC population. Intriguingly, these dynamics also were dependent on the degree of internal structure in the populations. Specifically, if the PFC population had a lesser degree of internal recurrent influence, the network would evolve towards a decision more slowly, whereas if it was strongly internally connected it would evolve very quickly. As predicted, at a higher degree of internal influence the network "decided" faster, which in turn contributed to more errors when the stimulus was noisier, and more time to integrate evidence would have been helpful.

So, the *very same* network could implement both the kind of information processing required in a WM task, and the kind required in a perceptual DM task. One of the most intriguing results, however, is that these two kinds of information processing *trade-off* in a network. Greater resistance to distraction in the PFC network required a high degree of internal influence in that module. But a high degree of internal influence also shortened the timeline over which perceptual evidence could be accumulated. They posited that the particular structure of the PFC-PPC circuit helps ameliorate this tradeoff. In particular, if one removed the recurrent connections from the PFC to the PPC, then high performance in the decision-making task would result in lower performance in the working memory task.

I suggest that this kind of modeling project results in a mechanistic understanding of the network, but only by exhibiting the three properties I discussed above. First, the understanding of the circuit developed in the study *starts out* from the data point that both working memory and decision employ overlapping circuits. Second, understanding the informational requirements that are in common and differ across tasks is central to the explanation. In particular, there is something in common between working memory and decision-making tasks, namely that it is useful to have both a population that is multiple in its responses paired with a more categorically responding population. The difference in internal structure between the PFC and the PPC leads to the former having more univocal responses, which lead to both its robustness in WM contexts and its thresholding behavior in DM contexts. However, the *differences* between the tasks are also vitally important, because they illustrate the tradeoff in the network. WM contexts benefit from stronger interconnection, since it increases resistance to distractors. But DM contexts benefit from weaker interconnection, since it allows for an increase in evidence-gathering. This in turn leads to a mechanistic hypothesis, namely that the distinction between the PFC and PPC circuits in their degree of self-influence, and the feedback connection from the former to the latter, help ameliorate this tradeoff.

Importantly, because the explanation takes this form, it would be a *mistake* to attempt to spatially map WM and DM to distinct brain systems. There is not one part "doing" working memory and another part "doing" decision-making, and therefore there is not a causal relationship between so-individuated parts. There is one distributed circuit underlying those intuitively distinct functions. Given this, I submit, there is no metaphysically important distinction between working memory and perceptual decision-making. What there are are *distinct task demands*, and the ways in which those demands are implemented by a distributed system.

The heuristic view, unlike the standard view, simply doesn't assume that there is a fact of the matter about (i) whether WM is *really* distinct from DM, (ii) which tasks measure one versus the other, or (iii) whether a brain part really performs one rather than the other. What it suggests, as seems to be the case, is that there are deep commonalities in the brain systems performing these functions. The explanation also does not require that there be any firm division between the ultimate set of tasks that are WM, versus those that are DM, tasks. There are simply tasks with different informational requirements that are implemented differently in the network.

This is compatible with working memory and decision-making having played important heuristic roles in the understanding of this system. It was not, perhaps, initially obvious what the relationship between WM and DM might be. The concepts were operationalized differently. However, the persistent discovery of overlapping involvement in each of these tasks by the distributed PFC/PPC circuit led to the question of exactly how these functions are implemented. This led to a modeling project which uncovered both the commonalities and the differences between the informational requirements of, and the neural processing instantiating, tasks that correspond more-or-less closely to each of these categories.

I have only discussed one example, but I take this to be an exemplar of how multifunctional distributed circuits might be decomposed. I discuss a variety of other examples in other venues (Burnston, 2020, 2021). If this case *is* exemplary, however, then it stresses the normative bit of the heuristic approach, as opposed to that of the standard framework.

6 Normative Upshot

6.1 For Ontologies

Whether each process instantiates attention, some form of memory, or something else, I contend, is not as important for explaining how the brain implements the informational demands of the particular task. The normative upshot for databasing projects is that more explicit attention needs to be paid to the kinds of behavioral paradigms at work and the way that they tend to vary (Figdor, 2011; Sullivan et al., 2021).

This is not to say that databasing projects have not paid attention to tasks. Projects such as the "Cognitive Paradigm Ontology" (Turner & Laird, 2012) are specifically intended to index the different types of behavioral experiments involved in studying cognition, and Sochat and colleagues (2016) have recently argued that standardization and publicity of experimental design are vital for coordinating the study of cognition between laboratories. But the particular way in which tasks are approached in the field tends to strongly mirror the standard framework. For instance, Sochat et al. (2016) argue that the Cognitive Atlas should be "integrated" with a task ontology, by which they mean that each type of behavioral experiment should be categorized according to the kind of psychological function it is used to study. Standardization is important so that neuroscientists can "select paradigms based on the specific cognitive functions that they are thought to measure" (2016, p. 7).

The heuristic approach views the situation differently. While an investigator may "base" their search for behaviors to study on associations with cognitive functions that interest them, this basis is a heuristic one and not an instance of measurement. That is, a neuroscientist interested in "working memory," broadly speaking, should not pursue particular behavioral paradigms because they *measure* that explanatory construct, but instead as a way of looking for behavioral distinctions that may make a difference in how the brain processes information.

This has important upshot for how databases are constructed. In Neurosynth and the Cognitive Atlas, behavioral tasks are given abstract definitions, the assumption being that their role is to measure cognitive functions rather than themselves serving as explananda. In the Cognitive Paradigm Ontology and Brain Map, importantly, there are entries for experimental manipulations such as epoch, stimulus, and response, but as far as I can tell these categories have not been standardized, organized for comparative analysis, or as rigorously codified as the mental constructs have been.

From the standpoint of the heuristic approach, this is generally insufficient. In the exemplars above, what makes a difference for explanation is understanding how the brain responds differentially to variations in task demands, from the presentation of the stimulus, often through a delay or across learning, to an eventual behavior. Differential responses to *these* variations are what explain how the brain implements the behavior. Other subfields of neuroscience employ different variations – for instance, other areas of decision-neuroscience specifically vary reward types and regimes in conjunction with changes in stimuli and behavioral requirements. But entries in ontologies almost never contain detailed information of this sort, or at least that information is not standardized and codified.

Now, given the potentially infinite ways that behavior can be varied, codifying the kinds of behavioral and stimulus changes, the duration of temporal epochs and how they relate, etc., will be both a significant and a difficult task. But it is exactly the *point* of databasing projects to codify large amounts of data and make it accessible across individuals trying to explain things in a field. The normative bite of the heuristic view is that this project is more important than trying to find the "true specificity" between abstract mental constructs and brain activity.

This is not to *deny* that psychological concepts should be included in databasing projects. What it does suggest though is that the current state of the situation, on which most tasks are associated with a range of cognitive concepts, is neither surprising nor problematic. If the goal of these concepts is to serve as heuristics in the search for behavioral paradigms that index behavioral differences, then it is not surprising that these constructs should overlap both with each other and in the brain, and there is no need to try to theorize that overlap away.

So, suppose a neuroscientist is interested in 'working memory' or 'decision'. They approach a databasing tool in trying to devise research questions and develop experiments. What they find is that their construct of interest overlaps with other related constructs, and they find a huge number of extant behavioral distinctions that have been shown to make a difference in how the brain operates in, broadly, those cognitive contexts. This allows them to understand the behavioral distinctions that have been done, where brain activity has been measured in these conditions, etc. If they are interested in a particular part of the brain, they may find related behavioral measures that might clarify its function. If they are interested primarily in a construct, they may find a range of areas and distinctions that they could investigate, or use in the backdrop of forming new ones. The use of the psychological construct is a *heuristic for investigation*, rather than an explanatory claim.

This is, of course, an ideal, but I think it is an ideal that is importantly distinct from the current focus in databasing and brain-mapping projects.

6.2 For Functional Connectivity Analyses

An exciting series of recent functional connectivity studies have begun the attempt to uncover dynamic principles for the entire brain during the course of behavior. Functional connectivity measures the co-activation of brain regions, with the assumption being that co-active regions are coordinating in producing the relevant behavior. One can track changes in functional connectivity with changes in the task or even across temporal epochs of the same task. One can then ask a variety of questions about the functional principles underlying these changes.

Here are just a few examples. Shine et al. (2016) hypothesized that network interconnectivity scales with *task complexity*. So, they measured functional connectivity in a range of tasks and compared the overall degree of connectivity in the brain during each. They showed that "language" tasks or "working memory" (in this case, N-back) tasks resulted in higher levels of connectivity than more "simple" motor tasks.

Other studies have attempted to spatially decompose the brain into parts that help *organize* its dynamic changes across tasks, versus those that are in charge of performing those tasks. So, Shine et al. (2018) took whole-brain data across a range of tasks and applied principal components analyses to both the *spatial* and *temporal* data. They showed that the first principal component in the temporal domain correlated with activity in the spatial regions associated with the "rich club" network, and hypothesized that these regions underlie an across-task organizing function, whereas regions more closely responding to the other components were more task-specific.

This is cutting-edge work, and I do not wish to speculate too much on its eventual upshot. What I want to suggest, however, is that the heuristic approach offers distinct normative prescriptions than the standard framework for how to pursue further investigation. The standard framework suggests that these dynamical processes must be divided up, both spatially and temporally, according to distinct psychological faculties, and the causal relationship between those faculties explained. The heuristic view denies this necessity. Instead, it invocates the need to understand the structure of the tasks further – what distinctions in stimuli or behavioral requirements drive the different dynamic shifts, and what about the function of the brain networks involved enables them to enact those requirements specifically?

The authors of these studies seem to view them, at least in part, as stepping beyond the standard framework. As Shine and Poldrack note: "these results shifted the focus from where in the brain a particular function resides to how the coordinated recruitment of segregated specialist neural regions works together to accomplish the challenges associated with complex behavioral tasks" (2017, p. 396).

But it is important to note that, at least as of now, the invocations of the heuristic approach have not been followed. For instance, there is no analysis of what "complexity" of tasks amounts to in the Shine et al. (2016) paper. The notion is left intuitive. Nor is there any analysis of what exactly makes tasks "language" tasks versus "memory" tasks in the other studies. This is a lacuna in these projects, according to the heuristic approach.

7 Conclusions

A number of years ago, it was common for textbooks in the philosophy of mind to teach the following: either our intuitive conception of the mind, with its commitments to intentional attitudes, etc., is true, or behaviorism is. I hope this strikes the modern reader as almost charmingly anachronistic. One can find newer versions of the dichotomy, however. Uttal (2001), in his famous criticism of fMRI research, argues that the alternative to discovering discrete localizations for distinct cognitive faculties is to view the mind as "unanalyzable," by which he means indivisible into distinct parts. More recently, Hutto et al. (2017) have suggested that the way to react to the "protean" – by which they mean dynamically reconfigurable – functionality of the brain is to embrace enactivist views of cognition, with their attendant rejection of mental representation and computation (Anderson, 2014; Silberstein & Chemero, 2013).

I have tried to argue that one can abandon the standard explanatory framework of cognitive neuroscience, and its attendant commitments about psychological constructs, without abandoning mechanistic explanation in the brain. And, while I haven't argued for it here, I claim elsewhere (Burnston, 2020) that this general approach extends to representational explanation as well. The heuristic approach to cognitive ontology is a *very* different stance on explanation than is currently assumed in the literature, and I believe it deserves to be taken as a realistic option in this emerging field.

References

Anderson, M. L. (2014). *After phrenology: Neural reuse and the interactive brain.* Cambridge: MIT Press.

Anderson, M. L., Kinnison, J., & Pessoa, L. (2013). Describing functional diversity of brain regions and brain networks. *Neuroimage, 73,* 50–58.

Bechtel, W. (2008). *Mental mechanisms: Philosophical perspectives on cognitive neuroscience.* New York: Routledge.

Bechtel, W. (2017). Using the hierarchy of biological ontologies to identify mechanisms in flat networks. *Biology & Philosophy.* doi:10.1007/s10539-017-9579-x

Bickle, J. (2003). *Philosophy and neuroscience: A ruthlessly reductive account* (Vol. 2). Dordrecht: Springer Science & Business Media.

Boone, W., & Piccinini, G. (2016). The cognitive neuroscience revolution. *Synthese, 193*(5), 1509–1534.

Bunzl, M., Hanson, S. J., & Poldrack, R. A. (2010). An exchange about localism. In Hanson and Bunzl (Eds.), *Foundational issues in human brain mapping* (pp. 49–54). Cambridge: MIT Press.

Burnston, D. C. (2016). A contextualist approach to functional localization in the brain. *Biology & Philosophy, 31*(4), 527-550.

Burnston, D. C. (2020). Contents, vehicles, and complex data analysis in neuroscience. *Synthese.* doi:10.1007/s11229-020-02831-9

Burnston, D. C. (2021). Getting over Atomism: Functional Decomposition in Complex Neural Systems. *The British Journal for the Philosophy of Science, 72*(3), 743-772. doi:10.1093/bjps/axz039

Carlson, T., Goddard, E., Kaplan, D. M., Klein, C., & Ritchie, J. B. (2018). Ghosts in machine learning for cognitive neuroscience: Moving from data to theory. *Neuroimage, 180,* 88–100.

Craver, C. F. (2006). When mechanistic models explain. *Synthese, 153*(3), 355–376. Retrieved from http://rd.springer.com/article/10.1007/s11229-006-9097-x

Cummins, R. C. (1983). *The nature of psychological explanation.* Cambridge: Bradford/MIT Press.

Darden, L., Pal, L. R., Kundu, K., & Moult, J. (2018). The product guides the process: Discovering disease mechanisms. In E. Ippoliti & D. Danks (Eds.), *Building theories* (pp. 101–117). Dordrecht: Springer.

De Brigard, F. (2014). Is memory for remembering? Recollection as a form of episodic hypothetical thinking. *Synthese, 191*(2), 155–185.

Feest, U. (2010). Concepts as tools in the experimental generation of knowledge in cognitive neuropsychology. *Spontaneous Generations: A Journal for the History and Philosophy of Science, 4*(1), 173–190.

Figdor, C. (2011). Semantics and metaphysics in informatics: Toward an ontology of tasks. *Topics in Cognitive Science, 3*(2), 222–226.

Fox, P. T., & Lancaster, J. L. (2002). Mapping context and content: the Brain-Map model. *Nature Reviews Neuroscience, 3,* 319. doi:10.1038/nrn789

Gomez-Lavin, J. (2020). Working memory is not a natural kind and cannot explain central cognition. *Review of Philosophy and Psychology.* doi:10.1007/s13164-020-00507-4

Griffiths, P. (2002). Is emotion a natural kind? In R. C. Solomon (Eds.), *Thinking about feeling* (pp. 233–249). Oxford & New York: Oxford University Press.

Hastings, J., Frishkoff, G. A., Smith, B., Jensen, M., Poldrack, R. A., Lomax, J., ... Martone, M. E. (2014). Interdisciplinary perspectives on the development, integration, and application of cognitive ontologies. *Frontiers in Neuroinformatics, 8,* 62.

Hutto, D. D., Peeters, A., & Segundo-Ortin, M. (2017). Cognitive ontology in flux: The possibility of protean brains. *Philosophical Explorations, 20*(2), 209–223.

Kanwisher, N. (2010). Functional specificity in the human brain: a window into the functional architecture of the mind. *Proceedings of the National Academy of Sciences of the United States of America, 107*(25), 11163–11170. doi:10.1073/pnas.1005062107

Lenartowicz, A., Kalar, D. J., Congdon, E., & Poldrack, R. A. (2010). Towards an ontology of cognitive control. *Topics in Cognitive Science, 2*(4), 678–692.

Leonelli, S. (2012). Classificatory theory in data-intensive science: The case of open biomedical ontologies. *International Studies in the Philosophy of Science, 26*(1), 47–65.

Machery, E. (2009). *Doing without concepts*: Oxford University Press.

Murray, J. D., Jaramillo, J., & Wang, X. J. (2017). Working Memory and Decision-Making in a Frontoparietal Circuit Model. *Journal of Neuroscience, 37*(50), 12167–12186. doi:10.1523/JNEUROSCI.0343-17.2017

Piccinini, G., & Craver, C. (2011). Integrating psychology and neuroscience: Functional analyses as mechanism sketches. *Synthese, 183*(3), 283–311. doi:10.1007/s11229-011-9898-4

Poldrack, R. A., Kittur, A., Kalar, D., Miller, E., Seppa, C., Gil, Y., ... Bilder, R. M. (2011). The cognitive atlas: Toward a knowledge foundation for cognitive neuroscience. *Frontiers in Neuroinformatics, 5,* 17. doi:10.3389/fninf.2011.00017

Poldrack, R. A., Mumford, J. A., Schonberg, T., Kalar, D., Barman, B., & Yarkoni, T. (2012). Discovering relations between mind, brain, and mental disorders using topic mapping. *PLoS Computational Biology, 8*(10), e1002707. doi:10.1371/journal.pcbi.1002707

Poldrack, R. A., & Yarkoni, T. (2016). From brain maps to cognitive ontologies: Informatics and the search for mental structure. *Annual Review of Psychology, 67,* 587–612.

Ritchie, J. B., Kaplan, D. M., & Klein, C. (2016). Decoding the brain: Neural representation and the limits of multivariate pattern analysis in cognitive neuroscience. *The British Journal for the Philosophy of Science, 70*(2), 581–607.

Robins, S. K. (2016). Optogenetics and the mechanism of false memory. *Synthese, 193*(5), 1561–1583.

Rubin, T. N., Koyejo, O., Gorgolewski, K. J., Jones, M. N., Poldrack, R. A., & Yarkoni, T. (2017). Decoding brain activity using a large-scale probabilistic functional-anatomical atlas of human cognition. *PLoS Computational Biology, 13*(10), e1005649. doi:10.1371/journal.pcbi.1005649

Schacter, D. L., Benoit, R. G., De Brigard, F., & Szpunar, K. K. (2015). Episodic future thinking and episodic counterfactual thinking: Intersections between memory and decisions. *Neurobiology of learning and memory, 117*, 14–21. doi:10.1016/j.nlm.2013.12.008

Shine, J. M., Bissett, P. G., Bell, P. T., Koyejo, O., Balsters, J. H., Gorgolewski, K. J., . . . Poldrack, R. A. (2016). The dynamics of functional brain networks: Integrated network states during cognitive task performance. *Neuron, 92*(2), 544–554. doi:10.1016/j.neuron.2016.09.018

Shine, J. M., Breakspear, M., Bell, P. T., Martens, K. E., Shine, R., Koyejo, O., . . . Poldrack, R. A. (2018). The low dimensional dynamic and integrative core of cognition in the human brain. *bioRxiv, 266635*. doi:10.1101/266635

Shine, J. M., & Poldrack, R. A. (2017). Principles of dynamic network reconfiguration across diverse brain states. *Neuroimage*. doi:10.1016/j.neuroimage.2017.08.010

Silberstein, M., & Chemero, T. (2013). Constraints on localization and decomposition as explanatory strategies in the biological sciences. *Philosophy of Science, 80*(5), 958–970.

Sochat, V. V., Eisenberg, I. W., Enkavi, A. Z., Li, J., Bissett, P. G., & Poldrack, R. A. (2016). The experiment factory: Standardizing behavioral experiments. *Frontiers in Psychology, 7*, 610. doi:10.3389/fpsyg.2016.00610

Sullivan, J. A. (2010). Reconsidering 'spatial memory' and the Morris water maze. *Synthese, 177*(2), 261–283. Retrieved from http://rd.springer.com/article/10.1007/s11229-010-9849-5

Sullivan, J. A. (2014). Stabilizing mental disorders: prospects and problems. In H. Kincaid & J. A. Sullivan (Eds.), *Classifying Psychopathology: Mental Kinds and Natural Kinds* (pp. 257 - 281). Cambridge, MA: MIT Press.

Sullivan, J. A., Dumont, J. R., Memar, S., Skirzewski, M., Wan, J., Mofrad, M. H., . . . Prado, V. F. (2021). New frontiers in translational research: Touchscreens, open science, and the mouse translational research accelerator platform. *Genes, Brain and Behavior, 20*(1), e12705.

Tekin, Ş. (2016). Are mental disorders natural kinds?: A plea for a new approach to intervention in psychiatry. *Philosophy, Psychiatry, & Psychology, 23*(2), 147–163.

Teodorescu, A. R., & Usher, M. (2013). Disentangling decision models: From independence to competition. *Psychological review, 120*(1), 1.

Turner, J. A., & Laird, A. R. (2012). The cognitive paradigm ontology: Design and application. *Neuroinformatics, 10*(1), 57–66. doi:10.1007/s12021-011-9126-x

Uttal, W. R. (2001). *The new phrenology: The limits of localizing cognitive processes in the brain.* Cambridge: The MIT Press.

Varoquaux, G., Schwartz, Y., Poldrack, R. A., Gauthier, B., Bzdok, D., Poline, J. B., & Thirion, B. (2018). Atlases of cognition with large-scale human brain mapping. *PLoS Computational Biology, 14*(11), e1006565. doi:10.1371/journal.pcbi.1006565

Yarkoni, T., Poldrack, R. A., Nichols, T. E., Van Essen, D. C., & Wager, T. D. (2011). Large-scale automated synthesis of human functional neuroimaging data. *Nature methods, 8*(8), 665.

Yarkoni, T., & Westfall, J. (2017). Choosing prediction over explanation in psychology: Lessons from machine learning. *Perspectives on Psychological Science, 12*(6), 1100–1122. doi:10.1177/1745691617693393

Section 4
Tools and Integrative Pluralism

13 "It Takes Two to Make a Thing Go Right"

The Coevolution of Technological and Mathematical Tools in Neuroscience

Luis H. Favela

> It takes two to make a thing go right.
>
> Rob Base and DJ E-Z Rock, *It takes two* (Ginyard, 1988)

1 Introduction

There should be no doubt that technological developments have played significant roles throughout the history of scientific discoveries and progress. This is as true in the physical sciences (e.g., particle accelerators in physics) as in the life sciences (e.g., microscopes in biology). What is less apparent is the role mathematical developments have played in facilitating and supporting many of those discoveries. Mathematical tools for analyzing data may not be at the forefront of discoveries centering on the physical structure of investigative targets of interest (e.g., cells); but they certainly are crucial in research focused on the dynamics of phenomena (e.g., planetary motion). Consequently, for science to progress, research on the movement and temporal aspects of phenomena often requires the coevolution of technological *and* mathematical tools.

Recently, it has been increasingly argued by some philosophers of neuroscience that experimental tools are not just important but are fundamental to neuroscience research (e.g., Barwich, 2020; Bickle, 2016; Silva, Landreth, & Bickle, 2014). Put in its sharpest terms, the line of thought goes like this: From Golgi's staining technique to functional magnetic resonance imaging, and from deep brain stimulation to optogenetics, the history of neuroscience is principally *a history of tool development*. Moreover, it has been argued that this history is best characterized as one that exhibits reductionist (Bickle, 2006, 2016) and mechanistic explanations (Craver, 2002, 2005). Across these claims, little to no mention of data analysis methods are mentioned nor the underlying assumptions of those techniques. Here, I argue that the mathematical

DOI: 10.4324/9781003251392-18

assumptions of applied data analyses have played crucial—though often underappreciated—roles in the history of neuroscience. First, I present the Hodgkin and Huxley model of action potentials as an example of research constrained by technological and mathematical limitations of its time. Second, I draw attention to a feature of neurons that is overlooked by the Hodgkin-Huxley model: scale-invariant dynamics. After describing scale-invariant dynamics, I then point out consequences scale-invariant neuronal dynamics have for explanatory approaches in neuroscience that rely on—what can be broadly described as—decomposition strategies of neuronal activity. I conclude by emphasizing the necessity of mathematical developments in providing more appropriate and encompassing explanations of neural phenomena in toto.

2 Single Neuron Models

The canonical Hodgkin and Huxley (1952) model of action potentials in the squid giant axon is considered not just "the single most successful quantitative model in neuroscience" (Koch, 1999, p. 171), but also "one of the great success stories in biology" (Häusser, 2000, p. 1165). Many of the details of the model are not essential for my current aims (Figure 1a). For detailed explanations of this model see Gerstner, Kistler, Naud, and Paninski (2014), as well as Koch (1999) for discussion and further references. For now, it is important to understand that this model treats the action potential as an "all-or-none" event (e.g., Bear, Connors, & Paradiso, 2016; Churchland & Sejnowski, 1992/2017; Eagleman & Downar, 2016). The action potential is treated as a binary event that occurs within distinctly defined timescales (Figure 1b). Moreover, those timescales have a lower boundary, specifically, 10 milliseconds (ms) in the canonical Hodgkin-Huxley model (Hodgkin & Huxley, 1952, p. 528; Koch, 1999, p. 334; Marom, 2010, p. 23). What that means is that the action potential of a neuron (i.e., its "spike" of activity) is treated within the Hodgkin-Huxley model as occurring at least 10 ms from initiation to termination of all involved processes (Marom, 2010, p. 22).

As was known then and now (e.g., Marom, 2010), although there were empirically justifiable reasons at the time (e.g., Adrian & Zotterman, 1926), defining the action potential as a 10 ms event was due to investigator observational preferences in combination with technological limitations. Observational preferences were constrained by the limits of the recording technology, namely, the voltage clamp. Although the voltage clamp was instrumental in providing the data that lead to the development of the Hodgkin-Huxley model, it was limited in its ability to record the full range of ion channels, charged particles, and other physiologically relevant features of neuronal activity (Schwiening, 2012). This resulted in the need to sum across molecular activity (Gerstner et al., 2014)—certainly a necessity when calculating at the molecular

(a)

$$I = C_M \frac{dV}{dt} + \bar{g}_K n^4 (V - V_K) + \bar{g}_{Na} m^3 h (V - V_{Na}) + \bar{g}_l (V - V_l)$$

> I = Total membrane current (function of time and voltage)
> C_M = Cell membrane capacity per unit
> dV = Change of membrane potential from resting value
> dt = Time
> g's = Sodium (Na), potassium (K), and leak (l)

(b)

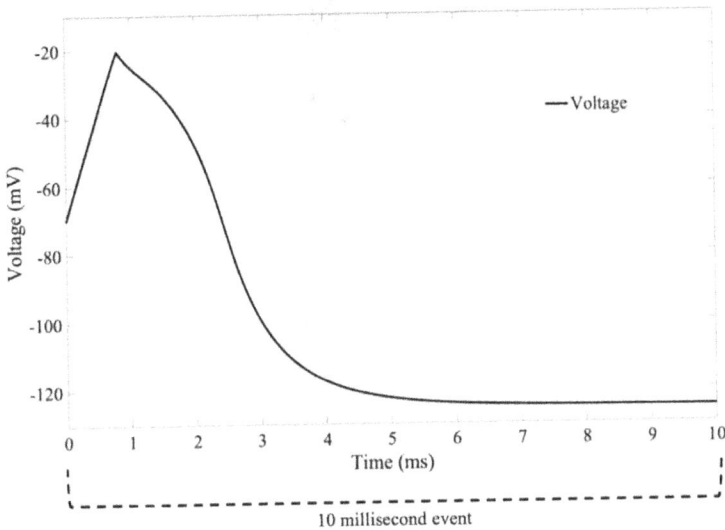

Figure 1 Hodgkin-Huxley model. (a) The canonical Hodgkin and Huxley (1952) model of action potentials in the squid giant axon. Definitions of key model variables (box). (b) The basic shape of an action potential as produced by the Hodgkin-Huxley model (created with MATLAB [MathWorks®, Natick, MA] script based on Kothawala, 2015). The x-axis captures the entire range of time in which an action potential occurs. According to the model, the lower temporal boundary of an action potential is 10 ms. This means that the entire event, from start to finish, occurs within that time frame.

scale—and collapse other physiological features into imprecise "leak" terms, a sort of "catch all" variable used in models that have causally relevant features that have not been precisely measured. Other limitations involved the manner in which the data was calculated. Hodgkin and Huxley calculated data from the voltage clamp via hand calculators (Koch, 1999, p. 160). Specifically, Hodgkin and Huxley utilized a

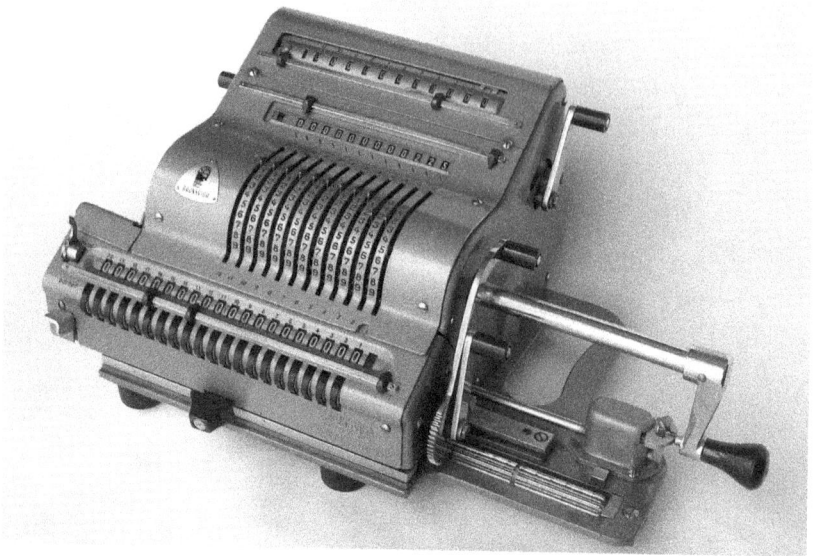

Figure 2 The Brunsviga 20, "one of the most popular mechanical calculators. It was produced up to the early 1970s and marketed with the slogan 'Brains of Steel'" (Schwiening, 2012). (Reprinted with permission from Wikipedia. CC BY-SA 2.0 DE.)

mechanical calculator, the Brunsviga 20 (Figure 2), which required them to spend a few weeks and many thousands of rotations of the machine's crank in order to carry out the calculations (Schwiening, 2012).

Although the canonical Hodgkin-Huxley model is described by some as being linear in nature (e.g., Gerstner et al., 2014; Hodgkin & Huxley, 1952, pp. 538–540), there is debate about whether or not it is able to capture the relevant types of nonlinearities exhibited by feedback that are now established as occurring during action potentials (e.g., Marom, 2010; Schwiening, 2012).[1] Regardless of whether or not the canonical Hodgkin-Huxley model is linear or nonlinear, or can capture particular forms of feedback, it is clear now that even single neurons are appropriately understood as nonlinear systems (e.g., Izhikevich, 2007).

Advancements in recording technologies have facilitated the ability of neuroscientists to obtain more detailed data on neuronal activity (e.g., multielectrode arrays [MEA]; Gross, 2011), making it possible to record more detailed and accurate data from longer timescales of neuron activity. As a result, it is becoming increasingly evident that the relevant timescales for explaining even "basic" single-neuron activity can require looking far below and above that 10 ms window presumed to characterize single neuron spikes. Action potentials do not appear to have strictly defined windows of activity, specifically, nonlinearities in the forms of feedback and hysteresis significantly contribute to the event.[2] Instead of viewing action potentials as having clear startup and finish conditions (Figure 1b), it is more accurate to view action potentials as continuous, nonlinear cycles. This is clearly depicted in models as early as the FitzHugh-Nagumo model (FitzHugh, 1961; Nagumo, Arimoto, & Yoshizawa, 1962; Figure 3a) and more recent models, such as the Izhikevich model (Izhikevich, 2007; Figure 3b).

3 Scale-Invariant Neuronal Dynamics

As mentioned in the previous section, there is debate as to the degree or not that the canonical Hodgkin-Huxley model accounts for a wide range of nonlinear features of action potentials, such as hysteresis. I am not entering that debate here. The primary purpose for presenting the Hodgkin-Huxley model was to provide an example of an achievement in neuroscience that was constrained by the technology and related mathematical techniques of its time (e.g., Brunsviga 20; Figure 2). Additionally, I also mentioned that some earlier models of single-neuron activity, like the FitzHugh-Nagumo model, were able to explicitly account for certain forms of nonlinearity (FitzHugh, 1961; Nagumo et al., 1962; Figure 3a). In this section, I focus on scale invariance in neuronal activity, which is a more recent finding in neuroscience. Scale invariance was discovered in large part due to both improved technologies (e.g., recording techniques) and mathematical techniques (e.g., fractal analysis; more on that below).

At its most general, a phenomenon is "scale invariant" when its structure (i.e., spatial and/or temporal) is self-similar from various points of observation (Bak, 1996; Gisiger, 2001). Scale invariance can be abstract or statistical. Many illustrative examples of abstract scale-invariant spatial structures are found in fractal geometry (Mandelbrot, 1983; Figure 4). The Koch curve (i.e., Koch snowflake, Koch triangle)—like the Cantor and Mandelbrot sets—exhibits a topology that is perfectly recreated at each iteration or scale of observation. That is to say, the overall "curved, triangle-like" shape appears at one spatial dimension (Figure 1a), is repeated at a higher dimension (Figure 1b), and again at another dimension (Figure 1c). Scale invariance need not be perfectly precise as in abstract fractals like the Koch curve. Scale invariance can be defined in statistical terms. A phenomenon is *statistically* scale invariant when certain properties are repeated at various scales. This is the type of scale invariance found in natural structures such as bronchial tubes, coastlines, and unfurling ferns.

In recent years, an illustrative example of increased research on scale invariance are the now well-known scale-invariant properties prevalent

(a)

$$\dot{V} = V - \frac{V^3}{3} - W + I$$

$$\dot{W} = 0.08(V + 0.7 - 0.8W)$$

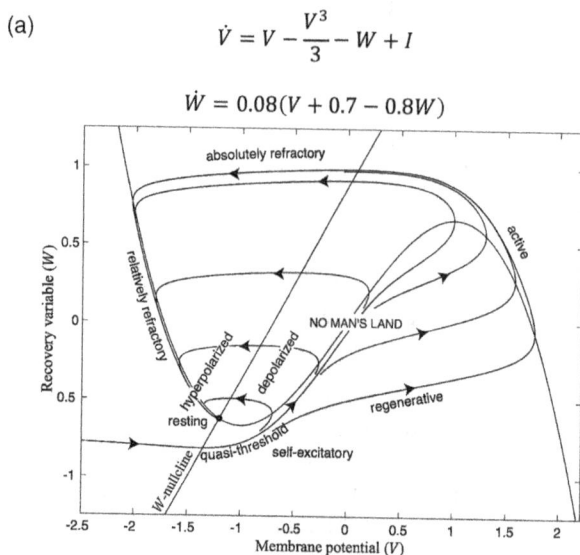

(b)

$$v' = 0.04v^2 + 5v + 140 - u + I$$

$$u' = a(bv - u)$$

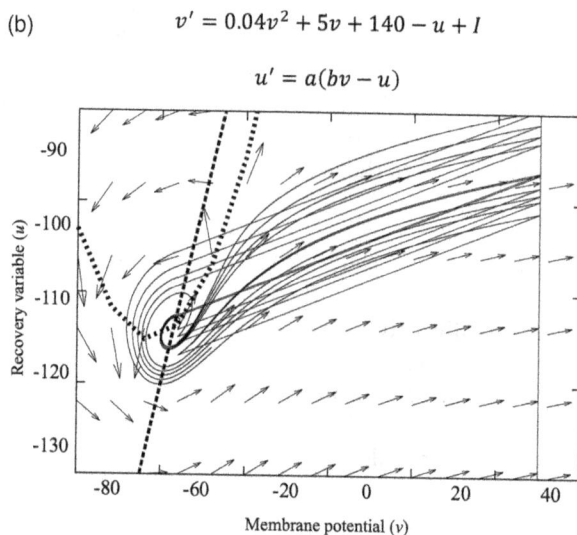

Figure 3 Models of nonlinear single-neuron activity. (a) FitzHugh-Nagumo model and phase space portrait. (Modified and reprinted with permission from Scholarpedia. CC BY-NC-SA 3.0.). (b) Izhikevich model and phase space portrait. Note that the phase space portrait depicts a strange attractor as the Izhikevich model parameters are set to depict chaotic time evolution. The FitzHugh-Nagumo model is not able to depict chaotic neuronal behavior no matter how the parameters are tuned. (Modified and reprinted with permission from Nobukawa, Nishimura, Yamanishi, & Liu, 2015.)

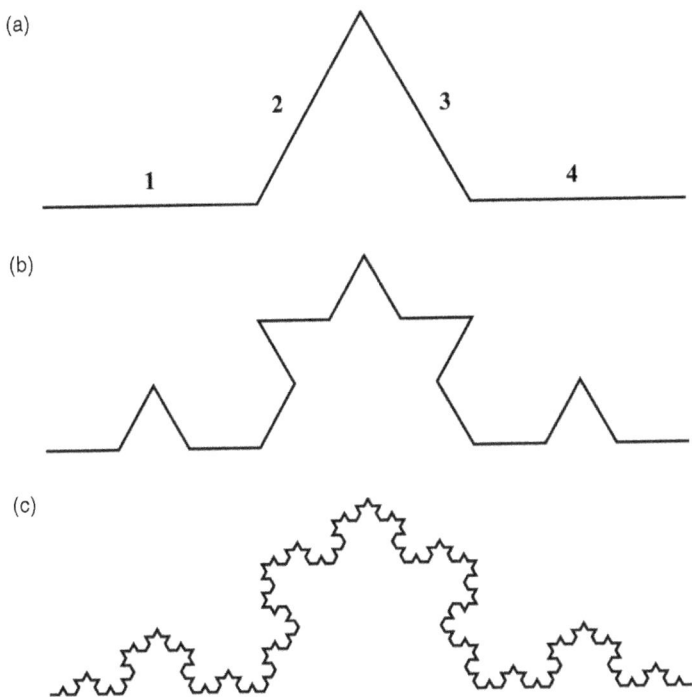

Figure 4 The Koch curve is an example of an abstract spatial fractal. Here, three iterations of self-similarity are depicted (a, b, and c). (Modified and reprinted with permission from Wikipedia. CC BY-SA 3.0.)

in network structures. Scale-invariant networks have few nodes with many connections and many nodes with few connections (Figure 5b). Consequently, such networks have no specific or *average* number of connections that characterize the entire system. Since such networks resist being properly characterized by standard statistical means (e.g., averages), scale-invariant networks are more accurately described in terms of power-law distributions (He, 2014). It has become commonly accepted that many phenomena and systems of diverse composition are scale invariant in this way, for example, cellular metabolism, Hollywood actors that have worked together, sexual relationships, and the World Wide Web (Barabási & Bonabeau, 2003). There is increasing evidence that neural systems exhibit scale invariance (e.g., Boonstra, He, & Daffertshofer, 2013; Di Ieva, 2016; He, 2014; Poli, Pastore, & Massobrio, 2015), such as neuron branching patterns and neuronal network connections (Figure 5d). For current purposes, I focus on the scale invariance exhibited by neuronal dynamics (for a wide range of examples see Boonstra et al., 2013). In short, neuronal dynamics are considered scale

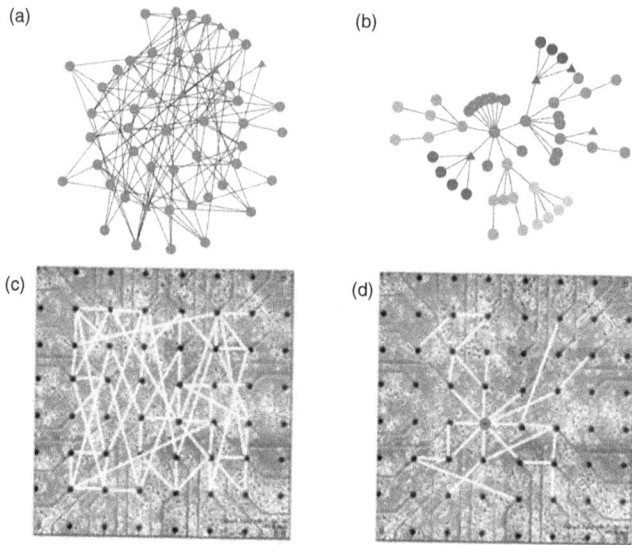

Figure 5 Random networks and scale-invariant networks. (a) Abstract random network illustrating that most nodes have a comparable number of connections. (b) Abstract scale-invariant network illustrating many nodes with a small number of connections and few nodes with a high number of connections. Dissociated neurons developing *in vitro* and coupled to multielectrode array (MEA), exhibiting (c) random network connectivity and (d) scale-invariant connectivity, with a highly connected unit (center), or hub. (Modified and reprinted with permission from Josserand et al., 2021 and Poli et al., 2015. CC BY.)

invariant when there is no single or average time scale that properly characterizes its activity, which includes attempting to define an event as occurring within specific windows of time. There are several consequences that result from the fact that many neural systems exhibit scale-invariant spatial and/or temporal structures. In the next section, I explore one such consequence, specifically, the inability of investigative and explanatory approaches in neuroscience that rely on decomposition strategies to properly account for scale-invariant neuronal dynamics.

4 Consequences of Scale-Invariant Dynamics for Explanations in Neuroscience

In a recent paper, Bechtel (2015) argues against the claim that scale-invariant biological phenomena cannot be explained mechanistically.[3] He rejects the following argument, which I summarize as follows:

1   Mechanistic explanations require that the phenomena being explained have well-defined boundaries, such as a temporal boundary.

2 Many biological phenomena exhibit scale-invariant features.
3 Scale-invariant phenomena have no well-defined temporal boundaries.
4 Therefore, scale-invariant biological phenomena cannot be explained mechanistically.

Marom (2010) presents such an argument and serves as one of Bechtel's targets. Marom argues that there is empirical evidence suggesting that neuronal activity is scale invariant and, thus, is just the type of biological phenomenon that cannot be explained mechanistically. Marom's argument includes discussion of the Hodgkin-Huxley model, which leads him to conclude:

> Indeed, the lesson from our journey across levels of organization, from behavior through neural assemblies to single neurons and proteins, suggests that dreams on all-encompassing microscopic timescale-based descriptions, aimed at explaining the temporal richness of macroscopic levels, should be abandoned. Other approaches are called for.
>
> (2010, p. 23)

In short, Marom claims that there are no uniquely defined timescales that could justify defining action potentials as events that have a lower boundary of 10 ms. Consequently, macroscale neuronal activities that appear as scale invariant are not merely the result of additive or linear combinations of microscale contributions. Instead, they are truly scale invariant: the micro timescales contribute to and constrain the macro timescales, but so too does the macro contribute to and constrain the micro, such that no single scale serves a more fundamental explanatory role than the others.

Bechtel's reply to Marom is that scale-invariant phenomena can still be explained mechanistically. But to do so requires that we appreciate the role of mechanisms in scientific practice. According to Bechtel, scientists often posit "bounded mechanisms" for the purposes of testing hypotheses (2015, pp. 84–85). A scientist can understand that a phenomenon is interconnected (e.g., networks) and still pursue a mechanistic account of that phenomenon by drawing boundaries around that organism. Those bounded mechanisms are not abstractions, however. "Abstractions," according to Bechtel, leave information out. Instead, those bounded mechanisms are idealizations. Idealizations, according to Bechtel, are models with *simplifying* falsehoods (2015, p. 85). For example, if phenomenon X is understood to be highly interconnected, an explanation of X that assumes that it is not affected by all its connections would be an abstraction. But to localize X to, for example, its nearest neighbors is to provide a *"first approximation"* (2015, p. 85; italics in original) that appreciates the practical challenges of accounting for all the actual connections. Such an explanation would be both an idealization and a mechanism.

Although he accepts that neuronal dynamics can be scale invariant, Bechtel remains committed to providing mechanistic explanations of those dynamics. Accordingly, Bechtel remains committed to mechanisms being bounded, on the further stipulation that such bounded mechanisms are idealizations and not abstractions. For example, the action potential is a "bounded mechanism" that occurs within 10 ms windows. Such an idealization is purported to be acceptable because it makes the timescales of that phenomenon tractable to investigators' cognitive limitations (2015, p. 92)—and I would add technological limitations. Thus, the Hodgkin-Huxley model can be understood as an idealization of action potentials, with the 10 ms feature being a simplifying falsehood—though not an abstraction that leaves out relevant features. This is a very streamlined presentation of Bechtel's argument, for example, he makes a further claim that such idealized mechanisms can point out areas for further investigation in a mechanistic explanation. What matters for my current purposes is Bechtel's attempt to make room within mechanistic accounts to explain the scale-invariant activity.

There is a lot in Bechtel's reply to Marom to agree with, for example, the fact that scientists are epistemically limited creatures who need to simplify some phenomena in order to get an intellectual grip on them. However, I think Bechtel's reply overlooks a central issue raised by Marom. If mechanisms are, by definition, *bounded*, then scale-invariant phenomena (e.g., flicker noise, power laws; Gisiger, 2001) are, by definition, *not* mechanisms. In the case of action potentials, the canonical Hodgkin-Huxley model sets a lower boundary on the phenomenon at 10 ms. In other words, it treats action potentials as starting and finishing within windows of time of at least 10 ms (Figure 1a). As discussed above, such a claim was justified as being consistent with the best science of the time (e.g., Adrian & Zotterman, 1926). With that said, it was constrained by technological (i.e., voltage clamp) and mathematical (i.e., the type of calculations that could be conducted on a Brunsviga 20 calculator; Figure 2) limitations. Technological advancements have certainly played a role in revealing scale-invariant dynamics, both within single neurons and across neuronal populations (e.g., MEA; Gross, 2011). However, data produced by advanced equipment alone does not provide a substantial reason to justify the existence of scale-invariant dynamics in neuronal systems. The other part needed for the right account—remember, "it takes two to make a thing go right"—is the pairing of data from suitable technology *with* the appropriate mathematical tools.

In the case of single-neuron activity, the right mathematical tools are those from nonlinear dynamical systems theory (NDST; e.g., Favela, 2020a, 2020b, 2020c; Izhikevich, 2007; Liebovitch & Toth, 1990). NDST methods are crucial to assessing scale-invariant structures and can contribute to establishing whether a phenomenon is *justifiably* defined as scale-invariant or not and, if so, what kind of scale-invariant characteristics it has. What is more, applying NDST methods to complex and nonlinear phenomena typically requires powerful computers. For example, generating phase portraits of relatively simple two-dimensional dynamical systems was often not practical before computers. Hodgkin and Huxley's "Brains of Steel" mechanical calculator was certainly not up to the task (Figure 2). In view of that, the Izhikevich model of single-neuron activity required both the appropriate processing power (i.e., modern computers) *and* data analysis methods (i.e., NDST) to provide qualitative and quantitative accounts of that phenomenon's nonlinear dynamics. Additionally, considerable computational processing power is needed to analyze and model the more complex and nonlinear features of neurons like chaotic dynamics (Figure 3b).

As mentioned above, nonlinear dynamics are not my central topic; scale-invariant dynamics are. Scale-invariant properties are a particularly unique set of phenomena with regard to the need for coevolving technological and mathematical tools. Many aspects of mammalian biological phenomena exhibit scale-invariant structures, such as eye saccades, heart beats, neuronal networks, and postural sway. Accordingly, different mathematical tools are needed to properly determine the ways they are scale invariant. For example, detrended fluctuation analysis (Peng et al., 1994) can assess structural self-similarity in a signal; but it will not necessarily make it clear if the structure results from linear or nonlinear processes (Bryce & Sprague, 2012). In the case of appropriate mathematical methods for assessing the scale-invariant dynamics of action potentials, if such activity is, for example, fractal, then it would not have been possible to accurately analyze such data, regardless of technological advancements, until the 1980s. The reason is because the concept "fractals" and related data analytic methods were not introduced to the broader scientific community until then (Mandelbrot, 1983).

In order to identify self-similar features of scale-invariant structures, whether resulting from linear or nonlinear processes, the concept "fractals" and their measurement must be part of an investigator's toolbox. Fractals, such as the Koch curve (Figure 4) are paradigmatic examples of scale invariance: the overall structure of the system is maintained at each level of observation. Such phenomena are thus not appropriately explained in terms that, for example, treat them as having an average value. Instead, as Mandelbrot pointed out, such phenomena are appropriately characterized via a *fractal dimension*. The fractal dimension provides a quantitative means of characterizing scale invariance that accounts for all of its scales. The equation for calculating the fractal dimension is:

$$n = \frac{1}{s^d} \tag{1}$$

It is helpful to explain this equation via the Koch curve. For demonstration purposes, we will look at a four-lined Koch curve (Figure 4a). Here n is the number of line segments at a particular scale of observation;

in this case, it is 4. Next, S is the scale factor, or the size reduction at each iteration; here it is 1/3. Our equation is now: $4 = 1/(1/3)^d$, or $4 = 3^d$. We want to figure out d, or the fractal dimension. To do so, we take the log of both sides: $d = \log 4/\log 3$, which gives us a fractal dimension $d = 1.26$. In English, this means that the fractal dimension of the Koch curve is 1.26, which means it is not a straight line ($d = 1$) or a square ($d = 2$), but closer to being a straight line than a square ($d = 1.26$). There are various other methods for mathematically assessing fractals and multifractals (Lopes & Betrouni, 2009).

The point of this example is to demonstrate that before Mandelbrot's invention—or, perhaps, discovery—of fractal geometry, it was not possible to appropriately account for scale-invariant phenomena, for example, via more standard statistical tools such as calculating the arithmetic mean. The consequence for neuronal activity is that it was not until the 1990s (e.g., Liebovitch & Toth, 1990) that scale-invariant dynamics could be properly identified. Before then, such properties were misidentified via other statistical methods. Since scale-invariant structures have no primary scale or average scale, they have no specific window to identify as the start and finish boundary. Such a view of neuronal activity is further evidenced by other NDST-based work, such as the Izhikevich model (2007; Figure 3b), which treats action potentials as continuous cycles and not binary, "all-or-none" events (cf. Figure 1b). If true, that is, if action potentials are not bounded within discrete windows of time, then action potentials cannot be accounted for via decomposition strategies, such as those common to mechanistic approaches in actual scientific practice.[4]

In concluding this section, an important clarification needs to be made in order to address a significant critique of the current line of argument. The critique centers on the notion of "bounded" in regard to natural phenomena. As discussed above, the currently relevant aspect of the Bechtel/Marom debate centers on the idea that mechanistic explanations treat targets of investigation as bounded, namely, as having delineated borders, which can be spatial or temporal. The Hodgkin-Huxley model of action potentials and its 10 ms event window were presented as an example of such a bounded mechanism. Scale-invariant neuronal dynamics was presented as an unbounded natural phenomenon, which means it is not accessible to mechanistic explanation (i.e., if "mechanistic explanations" include the stipulation of boundedness; see Bechtel, 2015; Marom, 2010). The critique of this line of argument centers on the point that even scale-invariant neuronal dynamics are "bounded" in a number of ways, for example, there *is* a window of time in which they occur (e.g., they do not last for months, years, or centuries) and they *are* spatially confined (e.g., they occur in an area of the brain, and not across the whole brain, let alone body and world). This is an understandably compelling critique. However, it does not concern the way in which scale-invariant dynamics are "unbounded."

The way in which scale-invariant dynamics are unbounded involves the inability of single, bounded values to *characterize* the phenomenon. A time series (Figure 6) need not be infinite nor recorded from an event that has no measurable spatial location in order to be scale invariant. A scale-invariant time series exhibits the same pattern among windows of various lengths of time. For example, if a heartbeat shows a pattern of activity over 60 minutes, then, to be considered scale invariant, that (statistically) same pattern should be shown in each of two 30-minute windows of time, at each of four 15-minute windows, and so on. In that way, the time series is not properly understood as "bounded" in that there is no single length of time that characterizes the entire signal. That is to say, it is not correct to treat the event as a bounded 60-minute event, or a 30-minute event, and so on; but in terms of the structure of the patterns across various scales. It is in that sense that Marom argues that neuronal dynamics do not have timescales, and it is in that sense that they are unbounded, and, thus, not properly explained mechanistically.

5 Conclusion

It is highly unlikely to find disagreement among the scientific research community that technological advancements have paved the way for some of the greatest advances and discoveries. What is less often acknowledged—especially in neuroscience—is the necessity of coevolving our mathematical tools with technological advances, and vice versa. Consequently, technological advancements that produce more detailed and accurate data recording will not alone necessarily provide proper explanations of biological phenomena. Mathematical tools like those provided by NDST are needed as well in order to properly characterize data. The Hodgkin-Huxley model was informed and constrained by the available technological (i.e., voltage clamp) and mathematical (i.e., Brunsviga 20 calculator) tools of the time. Since then, more advanced technology (e.g., multielectrode arrays) and mathematics (e.g., fractal analysis) have highlighted some of the limitations of the Hodgkin-Huxley model as a comprehensive model of action potentials across temporal scales. Scale-invariant neuronal activity provides a rich example of this. In order to identify scale-invariant activity, researchers needed more accurate measurements (e.g., MEA), data analyses (e.g., detrended fluctuation analysis), and—in this case—new concepts altogether. In order to properly account for scale-invariant activity, a new concept—namely, fractals and the fractal dimension—was needed, as was accompanying innovative mathematical analyses. One consequence of the existence of scale-invariant neuronal activity discussed here involves the limitations of research approaches centered on decomposition strategies—i.e., "mechanistic" approaches understood in terms of actual scientific practice—to account for phenomena that are without discrete (i.e., "bounded") temporal

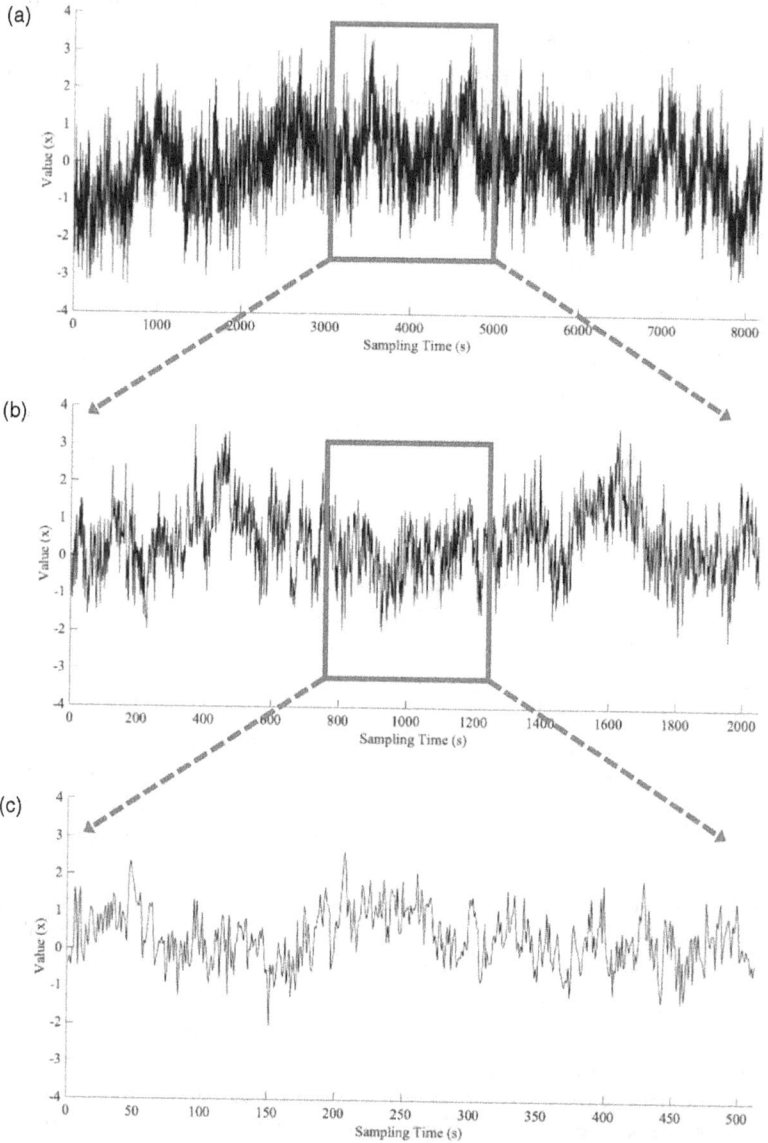

Figure 6 Time series exhibiting statistical scale invariance at multiple windows of time. Data obtained from the spontaneous activity of single neurons (i.e., mitral cells) in the rat main olfactory bulb are shown (Stakic, Suchanek, Ziegler, & Griff, 2011). Synthetic time series reproduced from results of detrended fluctuation analysis (Favela, Coey, Griff, & Richardson, 2016). Statistical scale invariance demonstrated in windows based on power of two: (a) 8,192 seconds, (b) 2,048 seconds, and (c) 1,024 seconds. The overall structure of the time series is repeated within each window of time. As a result, the time series is not properly characterized via a single value (e.g., mean) or window of time.

boundaries. In conclusion, an attempt has been made here to motivate the claim that progress in neuroscience takes two things to make it go right, namely, technological *and* mathematical advancements.

Acknowledgments

I would like to thank Ann-Sophie Barwich, John Bickle, and Carl Craver for their interest in this project. Thanks to John Beggs for many conversations about several aspects of this material; I've learned a great deal from him. Thanks to Mary Jean Amon for assistance with creating Figure 6. Various stages and versions of this paper have benefited from constructive feedback by audiences at the Tool Development in Experimental Neuroscience: A Science-in-Practice Workshop & the 57th Annual Meeting of the Alabama Philosophical Society (2019, September), the Center for Philosophy of Science at the University of Pittsburgh (2019, October), NeuroTech: An Interdisciplinary Early Career Workshop on Tools and Technology in Neuroscience (2020, January), and the Neuroscience Alliance at the University of Central Florida (2020, February).

Notes

1 "Linearity" can be understood as a mathematical relationship among data (e.g., time series), in that each successive data point is additively related to its previous point. Such phenomena exhibit outputs that are proportional to inputs (Lam, 1998). "Nonlinearity" can also be understood as a mathematical relationship among data. But here, each successive data point can observe a variety of relationships to previous points, such as exponential or multiplicative (Lam, 1998; May, 1976; Stam, 2005). Other, more interesting, forms of nonlinearity found in biological systems include patterned dynamics (e.g., fractals; Di Ieva, 2016) and phase transitions (e.g., catastrophe theory; Isnard & Zeeman, 1976/2013).

2 Hysteresis is a nonlinear phenomenon. There are multiple forms of hysteresis that can be exhibited by both biological and nonbiological systems. All forms are characterized by their being constrained by historical variation, that is, when a system's current state is strongly dependent on its history (Haken, 1983). Ferromagnetic materials (e.g., common magnets that hold up pictures on your refrigerator) provide clear illustrations of strong historical dependence characteristic of hysteresis effects (Dris, 2016). If a material such as iron is magnetized, once it is demagnetized, then it will require different magnetic fields to re-magnetize it. The reason the same magnetic field will not magnetize the piece of iron again is because the "system" (i.e., its atomic composition) "remembers" its previous state, that is, is constrained by states it has been in before. Thus, the current state of the system depends on its previous state such that magnetization does not occur at absolute, context-free values.

3 Bechtel's (2015) use of "scale free" and the current of "scale invariant" refer to the same phenomenon. The terms are commonly used interchangeably in the relevant literatures (e.g., Barabási, 2016; Broido & Clauset, 2019; Serafino et al., 2021). For that reason, when discussing Bechtel's argument, I will switch out "scale invariance" for "scale free" for consistency of terminology in the current work.

4 It is extremely challenging to define "mechanism" or "mechanistic explanation" in a way satisfactory to most philosophers of science. In the current work, I limit my application of the concept of "mechanism" to ways consistent with actual scientific practice, that is, in the sense discussed by Bechtel (2015). For that reason, I emphasize *decomposition* as common to the ways scientists investigate and define "mechanisms" (e.g., Andersen, 2014; Illari & Williamson, 2012; Khambhati, Mattar, Wymbs, Grafton, & Bassett, 2018). That is to say, scientists commonly aim to *decompose*—or "break apart"—a target of investigation in order to understand it in terms of its parts, namely, the constitution, contribution, and interaction of those parts.

References

Adrian, E. D., & Zotterman, Y. (1926). The impulses produced by sensory nerve endings. Part 3. Impulses set up by touch and pressure. *The Journal of Physiology, 61*(4), 465–483.

Andersen, H. (2014). A field guide to mechanisms: Part I. *Philosophy Compass, 9*(4), 274–283.

Bak, P. (1996). *How nature works: The science of self-organized criticality.* New York, NY: Springer-Verlag.

Barabási, A.-L. (2016). *Network science.* Cambridge University Press. Retrieved July 7, 2021 from http://networksciencebook.com

Barabási, A.-L., & Bonabeau, E. (2003). Scale-free networks. *Scientific American, 288*(5), 60–69.

Barwich, A. S. (2020). What makes a discovery successful? The story of Linda Buck and the olfactory receptors. *Cell, 181*(4), 749–753. doi:10.1016/j.cell.2020.04.040

Bear, M. F., Connors, B. W., & Paradiso, M. A. (2016). *Neuroscience: Exploring the brain* (4th ed.). New York, NY: Wolters Kluwer.

Bechtel, W. (2015). Can mechanistic explanation be reconciled with scale-free constitution and dynamics? *Studies in History and Philosophy of Biological and Biomedical Sciences, 53,* 84–93.

Bickle, J. (2006). Reducing mind to molecular pathways: Explicating the reductionism implicit in current cellular and molecular neuroscience. *Synthese, 151,* 411–434.

Bickle, J. (2016). Revolutions in neuroscience: Tool development. *Frontiers in Systems Neuroscience, 10*(24). doi:10.3389/fnsys.2016.00024

Boonstra, T. W., He, B. J., & Daffertshofer, A. (2013). Scale-free dynamics and critical phenomena in cortical activity. *Frontiers in Physiology: Fractal and Network Physiology, 4*(79). doi:10.3389/fphys.2013.00079

Broido, A. D., & Clauset, A. (2019). Scale-free networks are rare. *Nature Communications, 10*(1017), 1–10. doi:10.1038/s41467-019-08746-5

Bryce, R. M., & Sprague, K. B. (2012). Revisiting detrended fluctuation analysis. *Scientific Reports, 2*(315), 1–6. doi:10.1038/srep00315

Churchland, P. S., & Sejnowski, T. J. (1992/2017). *The computational brain* (25th anniversary ed.). Cambridge: The MIT Press.

Craver, C. F. (2002). Interlevel experiments and multilevel mechanisms in the neuroscience of memory. *Philosophy of Science, 69*(S3), S83-S97.

Craver, C. F. (2005). Beyond reduction: Mechanisms, multifield integration and the unity of neuroscience. *Studies in History and Philosophy of Science Part*

C: *Studies in History and Philosophy of Biological and Biomedical Sciences*, 36(2), 373–395.

Di Ieva, A. (Ed.). (2016). *The fractal geometry of the brain*. New York: Springer.

Dris, S. (2016). Magnetic hysteresis. *LibreTexts*. Retrieved July 7, 2021, from https://eng.libretexts.org/@go/page/333

Eagleman, D., & Downar, J. (2016). *Brain and behavior: A cognitive neuroscience perspective*. New York, NY: Oxford University Press.

Favela, L. H. (2020a). Cognitive science as complexity science. *Wiley Interdisciplinary Reviews: Cognitive Science*, 11(4), e1525, 1–24. doi:10.1002/WCS.1525

Favela, L. H. (2020b). Dynamical systems theory in cognitive science and neuroscience. *Philosophy Compass*, 15(8), e12695, 1–16. doi:10.1111/phc3.12695

Favela, L. H. (2020c). The dynamical renaissance in neuroscience. *Synthese*. doi:10.1007/s11229-020-02874-y

Favela, L. H., Coey, C. A., Griff, E. R., & Richardson, M. J. (2016). Fractal analysis reveals subclasses of neurons and suggests an explanation of their spontaneous activity. *Neuroscience Letters*, 626, 54–58. doi:10.1016/j.neulet.2016.05.017

FitzHugh, R. (1961). Impulses and physiological states in theoretical models of nerve membrane. *Biophysical Journal*, 1(6), 445–466.

Gerstner, W., Kistler, W. M., Naud, R., & Paninski, L. (2014). *Neuronal dynamics: From single neurons to networks and models of cognition*. Cambridge: Cambridge University Press.

Ginyard, R. (1988). *It takes two* [Recorded by R. Ginyard (Rob Base) and R. Bryce (DJ E-Z Rock)]. On *It takes two* [Vinyl]. Englewood, NJ: Profile Records.

Gisiger, T. (2001). Scale invariance in biology: Coincidence or footprint of a universal mechanism? *Biological Reviews*, 76, 161–209.

Gross, G. W. (2011). Multielectrode arrays. *Scholarpedia*, 6(3), 5749. doi:10.4249/scholarpedia.5749

Haken, H. (1983). *Synergetics: An introduction* (3rd ed.). Berlin: Springer-Verlag.

Häusser, M. (2000). The Hodgkin-Huxley theory of the action potential. *Nature Neuroscience*, 3(11), 1165. doi:10.1038/81426

He, B. J. (2014). Scale-free brain activity: Past, present, and future. *Trends in Cognitive Sciences*, 18(9), 480–487.

Hodgkin, A. L., & Huxley, A. F. (1952). A quantitative description of membrane current and its application to conduction and excitation in nerve. *The Journal of Physiology*, 117(4), 500–544.

Illari, P. M., & Williamson, J. (2012). What is a mechanism? Thinking about mechanisms across the sciences. *European Journal for Philosophy of Science*, 2(1), 119–135.

Isnard, C. A., & Zeeman, E. C. (1976/2013). Some models from catastrophe theory in the social sciences. In L. Collins (Ed.), *The use of models in the social sciences* (pp. 44–100). Chicago, IL: Routledge.

Izhikevich, E. (2007). *Dynamical systems in neuroscience: The geometry of excitability and bursting*. Cambridge: MIT Press.

Josserand, M., Allassonnière-Tang, M., Pellegrino, F., & Dediu, D. (2021). Interindividual variation refuses to go away: A Bayesian computer model of language change in communicative networks. *Frontiers in Psychology: Language Science*, 12(626118). doi:10.3389/fpsyg.2021.626118

Khambhati, A. N., Mattar, M. G., Wymbs, N. F., Grafton, S. T., & Bassett, D. S. (2018). Beyond modularity: Fine-scale mechanisms and rules for brain network reconfiguration. *NeuroImage*, 166, 385–399.

Koch, C. (1999). *Biophysics of computation: Information processing in single neurons.* New York, NY: Oxford University Press.

Kothawala, A. (2015). Simulation of nerve action potential using Hodgkin Huxley model [MATLAB script]. *MATLAB Central File Exchange.* Retrieved July 7, 2021 from https://www.mathworks.com/matlabcentral/fileexchange/53659-simulation-of-nerve-action-potential-using-hodgkin-huxley-model

Lam, L. (1998). *Nonlinear physics for beginners: Fractals, chaos, solitons, pattern formation, cellular automata and complex systems.* Singapore: World Scientific.

Liebovitch, L. S., & Toth, T. I. (1990). Using fractals to understand the opening and closing of ion channels. *Annals of Biomedical Engineering, 18,* 177–194.

Lopes, R., & Betrouni, N. (2009). Fractal and multifractal analysis: A review. *Medical Image Analysis, 13*(4), 634–649.

Mandelbrot, B. B. (1983). *The fractal geometry of nature.* New York, NY: W. H. Freeman and Company.

Marom, S. (2010). Neural timescales or lack thereof. *Progress in Neurobiology, 90,* 16–28.

May, R. M. (1976). Simple mathematical models with very complicated dynamics. *Nature, 261,* 459–467.

Nagumo, J., Arimoto, S., & Yoshizawa, S. (1962). An active pulse transmission line simulating nerve axon. *Proceedings of the IRE, 50*(10), 2061–2070.

Nobukawa, S., Nishimura, H., Yamanishi, T., & Liu, J. Q. (2015). Analysis of chaotic resonance in Izhikevich neuron model. *PloS One, 10*(9), e0138919. doi:10.1371/journal.pone.0138919

Peng, C. K., Buldyrev, S. V., Havlin, S., Simons, M., Stanley, H. E., & Goldberger, A. L. (1994). Mosaic organization of DNA nucleotides. *Physical Review E, 49*(2), 1685–1689.

Poli, D., Pastore, V. P., & Massobrio, P. (2015). Functional connectivity in *in vitro* neuronal assemblies. *Frontiers in Neural Circuits, 9*(57). doi:10.3389/fncir.2015.00057

Schwiening, C. J. (2012). A brief historical perspective: Hodgkin and Huxley. *The Journal of Physiology, 590*(11), 2571–2575.

Serafino, M., Cimini, G., Maritan, A., Rinaldo, A., Suweis, S., Banavar, J. R., & Caldarelli, G. (2021). True scale-free networks hidden by finite size effects. *Proceedings of the National Academy of Sciences, 118*(2), 1–11. doi:10.1073/pnas.2013825118

Silva, A. J., Landreth, A., & Bickle, J. (2014). *Engineering the next revolution in neuroscience: The new science of experiment planning.* New York, NY: Oxford University Press.

Stakic, J., Suchanek, J. M., Ziegler, G. P., & Griff, E. R. (2011). The source of spontaneous activity in the main olfactory bulb of the rat. *PLoS One, 6*(8), e23990. doi:10.1371/journal.pone.0023990

Stam, C. J. (2005). Nonlinear dynamical analysis of EEG and MEG: Review of an emerging field. *Clinical Neurophysiology, 116*(10), 2266–2301.

14 Hybrid Brains
Interfacing Living Neurons and Circuits with Computational Models

Astrid A. Prinz

1 Beyond the Connectome – Dynamics Matter

One of the core tenets of neuroscience is that in order to understand how the brain processes information, we must understand the 'connectome', meaning the structural layout of the nervous system – who connects to whom, at scales ranging from individual neurons to entire brain regions (Sporns 2010). For the unique model system that is *Caenorhabditis elegans*, a nematode, the complete connectome of its 302 neurons has been mapped (Cook et al. 2019), yet we are far from fully understanding how its brain functions. Knowing the connectome of a brain may be a necessary, but not a sufficient prerequisite to understanding nervous system function. It is equally important to understand the temporal dynamics of neuronal activity (Koppell et al. 2014).

Over the past decades, technological advances in several areas have greatly increased our ability to monitor and manipulate neuronal activity. These areas include multi-electrode neural interfaces, imaging of brain activity with genetically encoded or externally applied optical probes sensitive to neuronal membrane potential or calcium signals, and selective stimulation of neuron populations with optogenetics. Nonetheless, many aspects of and factors in neuronal signaling remain beyond the reach of experimental monitoring and manipulation, especially on the functionally relevant time scale of neuronal communication, which is in the range of milliseconds.

Computational modeling of neurons and neuronal circuits can help fill this gap and provide an increasingly useful complement to experimental investigation and manipulation of neuronal activity. In the following sections, I discuss strengths and potential pitfalls of modeling as a tool to study neuronal circuit function and describe how 'wet lab' experiments can be combined with computational modeling into hybrid circuits in real-time through the dynamic clamp, in a 'best of both worlds' scenario.

2 Computational Modeling – Strengths and Pitfalls

Computational models simulate the electrical activity and temporal dynamics of neurons and neuronal circuits and can be constructed at

DOI: 10.4324/9781003251392-19

different levels of nervous system organization, from the sub-cellular level of molecular interactions to the level of entire brain regions communicating with each other, and even into the realm of social interactions between brains (Prinz and Hooper 2017).

At all levels, computational modeling complements experimental studies most beneficially if there is a feedback loop between the two: models are constructed based on experimental data, models are used to explore potential mechanisms of brain function and make testable predictions, those predictions are tested in experiments, the experimental results inform refinement of the model – repeat the cycle. The benefits of this iterative process are best captured by the German saying 'Der Weg ist das Ziel' (loosely, 'The journey is the reward'), indicating that much can be learned from models that initially fail to match the ground truth of experimental data, from how they fail, and from how they can be refined.

For the purposes of discussing the dynamic clamp, I will focus now on computational modeling at the scale of individual neurons and small circuits of neurons. At this scale, temporal dynamics of neuronal and synaptic activity can be represented computationally in the form of systems of coupled differential equations that are solved numerically on a computer. Conductance-based models are a particular type of computational model at the cellular and small circuit scale and include differential equations for each neuron's membrane potential, activation of each of the relevant ionic membrane conductances (for example, what fraction of a neuron's sodium channels are open at any given time), and other dynamic variables, such as intracellular calcium concentration and synaptic receptor binding and channel gating.

Conductance-based models can be powerful tools to investigate how the temporal dynamics of a neuronal circuit's activity depend on the circuit connectivity and the intrinsic properties of the neurons and synapses that constitute the circuit. Figure 1 provides an example of such a small circuit model – the neurons and synapses that generate the motor commands that allow the sea slug *Tritonia diomedea* to swim and escape predation through a succession of dorsal and ventral body flexions. Figure 1c shows the output of an early (1980s) computational model of the circuit based on cellular and synaptic information available at the time, which successfully reproduced activation and production of the swim pattern (Getting 1983, 1989) and could be used to investigate how circuit activity depends on cellular and synaptic parameters not accessible to experimental manipulation.

But Figure 1 also illustrates potential pitfalls of computational modeling. The original Getting model of the circuit shown in Figure 1c reproduced the experimentally observed motor pattern so well that researchers were lured into thinking that this seemingly simple circuit was now 'understood'. However, two decades later, newer information on synaptic connectivity and neuromodulation in the circuit was incorporated into

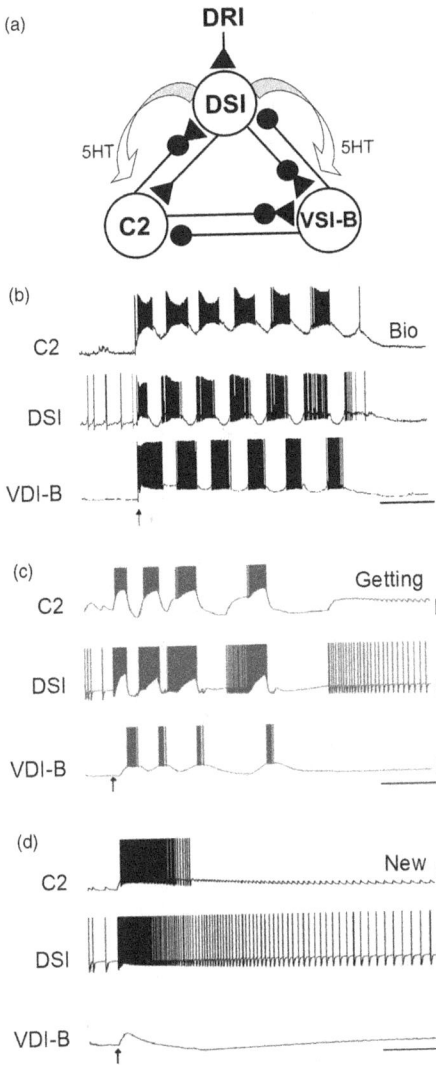

Figure 14.1 Models of the *Tritonia* escape swim circuit. (a) Schematic of the core swim escape circuit, including neurons DRI – dorsal ramp interneuron; DSI – dorsal swim interneuron; C2 – cerebral neuron 2; VDI-B – ventral swim interneuron B. Triangles and circles indicate excitatory and inhibitory synapses, respectively. 5HT indicates circuit-wide serotonin modulation. (b) Escape swim motor pattern recorded from living circuit. Bursts of action potentials in the DSI and VDI-B interneurons correspond to dorsal and ventral body flexions, which alternate to produce swimming. (c) Simulated motor pattern from original Getting model. (d) The updated model based on newer cellular and synaptic information fails to reproduce the motor pattern. Scale bars in (b–d): 10 seconds, 20 mV. Adapted from Calin-Jageman et al. (2007), with permission.

the model and resulted in the failure of the updated model to produce functional motor patterns (Calin-Jageman et al. 2007). This illustrates the importance of constraining a computational model with experimental data as much as possible, and the vagaries of trusting results from models with many cellular and synaptic parameters that are not well constrained by experimental data.

3 Hybrid Living and Model Circuits – Best of Two Worlds

At the cellular and small circuit scale, the dynamic clamp technique provides a complementary approach that can overcome some of the potential pitfalls and uncertainties of computational modeling by combining models with living neural systems in real-time, in a hybrid system configuration (Robinson and Kawai 1993; Sharp et al. 1993a, 1993b; Prinz et al. 2004; Goaillard and Marder 2006; Prinz and Cudmore 2011).

The basic operation of the dynamic clamp is illustrated in Figure 2 for two example applications in which voltage-independent conductances g are inserted into living neurons. A dedicated computer program hosts the equation(s) describing the conductances that the experimenter intends to mimic in a living neuron. The membrane potential (V) of the neuron or neurons to be dynamically clamped is recorded with an electrode, transformed into a digital signal, and fed into the computer in real-time. The computer solves the equation(s) to calculate the ionic current (I) that would be flowing through these modeled (virtual) conductances, and that calculated current I is injected into the living neuron in real-time. The neuron thus receives a dynamically changing current, equivalent to the current it would receive if it actually contained the membrane and/or synaptic conductances that are modeled with the dynamic clamp. As the responses to test pulses in Figure 2b indicate, the dynamic clamp does indeed change the effective input conductance of the living neuron – the dynamic clamp is therefore sometimes referred to as a **conductance clamp**.

While the example applications shown in Figure 2 are simple – dynamic clamp addition of an artificial inhibitory synapse to a living neuron (Figure 2b), and subtraction from a living neuron of a leak conductance introduced by electrode impalement to restore the cell's natural excitability (Figure 2c) – the dynamic clamp can also be used to introduce more complex, but physiologically realistic, conditions and processes into one or several living neurons. For example, the dynamic clamp can be employed to insert or remove one or more types of ion channels with voltage-dependent gating dynamics, as shown in Figure 3. The figure summarizes a study in which dynamic clamp was used to elucidate the cellular mechanisms of spike broadening in the R20 interneuron in the sea hare *Aplysia californica* (Ma and Koester 1996). Because this interneuron can initiate and modulate respiratory activity in the animal depending on spike duration, this example illustrates how the dynamic clamp can complement conventional electrophysiology and

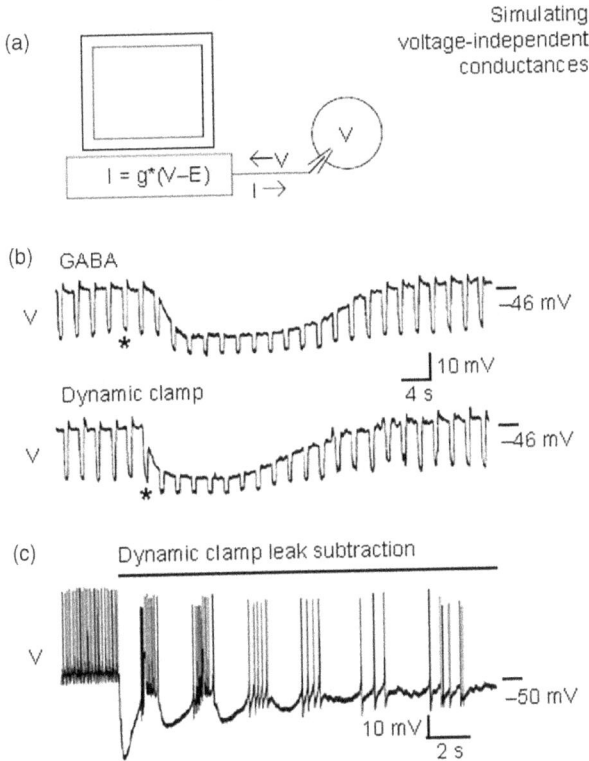

Figure 14.2 Basic dynamic clamp applications: simulation of voltage-independent conductances. (a) Schematic of dynamic clamp configuration. The membrane potential (V) of a living neuron is recorded, digitized, and fed into a computer in real-time. Equations describing the membrane or synaptic currents (I) to be modeled are solved by the computer for every time step to calculate the current I that would flow through these virtual conductances (g), given the momentary value of V and the current's reversal potential (E). The current I is injected into the living neuron, also in real-time. (b) Membrane potential V of a living neuron in response to application of the neurotransmitter GABA (Gamma-aminobutyric acid, top) and in the same neuron in response to application of a virtual synaptic conductance via dynamic clamp (bottom). In addition to the dynamic clamp current I, brief current test pulses are injected throughout both traces; reduced amplitude of the resulting voltage deflections during GABA application and during the virtual synaptic conductance clamp indicates that both manipulations temporarily increase the membrane conductance. Asterisks indicate times of application of GABA and the beginning of dynamic clamp. From (Sharp et al. 1993b), with permission. (c) Dynamic clamp subtraction of the leak conductance introduced by impalement of a living neuron with a sharp electrode. Leak subtraction virtually "repairs" the impalement damage to the membrane, restoring the neuron's intrinsic bursting activity pattern. From Cymbalyuk et al. (2002), with permission.

computational modeling to further our understanding of behaviorally relevant cellular and circuit mechanisms. In the case of dynamic clamp of voltage-dependent conductances as in Figure 3, the equations describing the conductances are systems of coupled differential equations for the gating variables of the corresponding ion channels. In this – more general and versatile – type of dynamic clamp application, the dynamic clamp software and computer therefore must solve differential equations numerically in real-time.

A further example of dynamic clamp versatility is provided in Figure 4, where dynamic clamp is applied to a pyramidal neuron in a slice of rat somatosensory cortex (Chance et al. 2002). Electrical activity in brain slices is often altered compared to activity in the intact brain, and is difficult to control at a millisecond time scale and network-wide level in slice experiments, making studies of the impact of realistic network activity on individual neurons technically difficult. The example application in Figure 4 shows how dynamic clamp can be used to expose neurons in a slice to *in vivo*-like but fully controllable synaptic inputs and conditions. How being embedded in a large network of other neurons affects a neuron's activity and information processing can thus be systematically studied at a physiologically relevant time scale.

While Figure 4 shows how realistic synaptic input from a network can be simulated with the dynamic clamp, the technique can also be used to provide a living neuron with one or multiple synaptic partners in the form of complete model neurons or small circuits simulated by the dynamic clamp software and computer in real-time (Pinto et al. 2001), allowing for the construction of truly hybrid networks.

As these example applications show, in contrast to the less physiological manipulations provided by traditional current clamp or voltage clamp, the dynamic clamp actually mimics in living neurons the presence of ionic membrane channels, synaptic receptors and their associated dynamic conductances, or of an entire surrounding network and the inputs it provides (Figures 2–4). In this sense, the dynamic clamp is akin to pharmacological manipulation or overexpression or mutation of cellular and synaptic conductances, or of embedding of a neuron in a network, but at the flip of a switch, and with full experimental control over the virtual conductance(s) by changing parameters in the dynamic clamp equations.

How, then, does the dynamic clamp approach combine 'the best of both worlds'? The **computational component** of dynamic-clamp constructed hybrid circuits retains the full control that the experimenter has over a purely computational model, because all parameters of the dynamic clamp equations can be changed at will, easily, and over wide ranges, often including parameters that are not – and in many cases will never be – experimentally manipulatable. On the **biological side** of the hybrid circuit, the living neurons in a sense serve as their own model, allowing the experimenter to probe the effect of various manipulations introduced

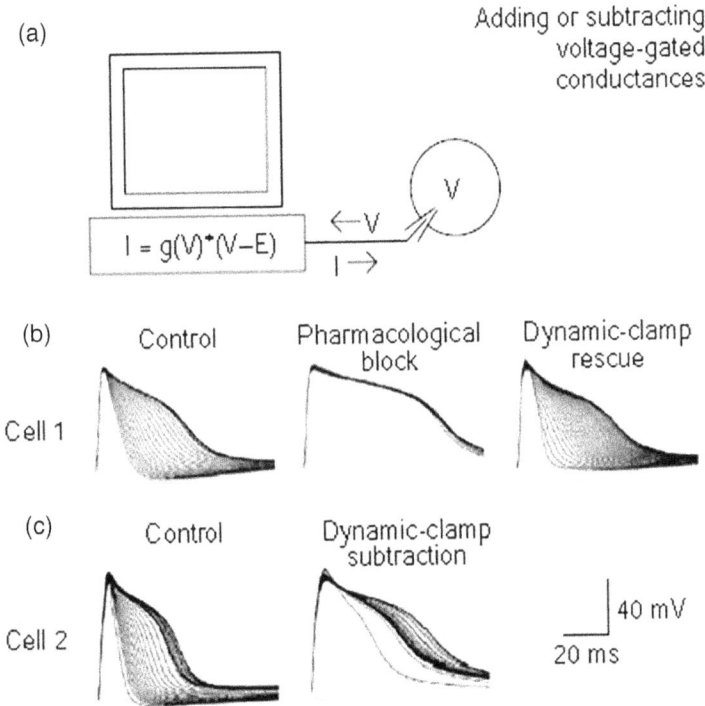

(a)

Adding or subtracting
voltage-gated
conductances

$I = g(V)^*(V-E)$

$\leftarrow V$

$I \rightarrow$

V

(b)   Control   Pharmacological   Dynamic-clamp
                               block   rescue

Cell 1

(c)   Control   Dynamic-clamp
                            subtraction

Cell 2   40 mV
                                              20 ms

Figure 14.3 Dynamic clamp addition and subtraction of voltage-dependent conductances to study spike broadening. (a) Schematic of dynamic clamp configuration. In contrast to Figure 2a, the equations describing the added/subtracted voltage-dependent conductances here are numerically solved differential equations. The impaled neuron is neuron R20 in the sea hare *Aplysia*, which can initiate and modulate respiratory pumping behavior depending on spike duration. (b) Overlaid action potentials recorded from a repetitively stimulated R20 neuron show spike broadening, with narrower spikes for early stimuli and broader spikes for late stimuli (left). Pharmacologically blocking two voltage-dependent potassium currents reveals that they contribute to the initially narrow, then broadening spike shape (middle). Spike broadening is restored by dynamic clamp addition of the same K+ currents (right). (c) Subtraction of the same two currents using dynamic clamp with negative conductance values g mimics their blocking with pharmacology. Adapted from Ma and Koester (1996), with permission.

via dynamic clamp in the context of the living system, without the need for an accurate computational model of the entire neuron or circuit. This eliminates some potential modeling pitfalls, such as the one described in Figure 1. In other words, the dynamic clamp allows the researcher to use computation selectively to control only the modeled aspects of a system,

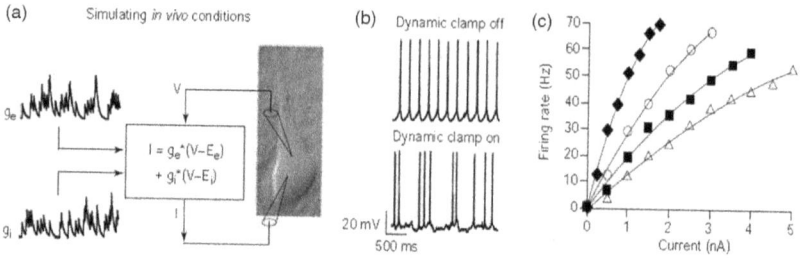

Figure 14.4 Dynamic clamp simulation of *in vivo* conditions in a brain slice. (a) Schematic of dynamic clamp configuration. Simulated excitatory (g_e) and inhibitory (g_i) synaptic conductance traces corresponding to barrages of synaptic inputs from a surrounding network are supplied to the dynamic clamp computer, which calculates the combined excitatory and inhibitory synaptic current and injects it into a pyramidal neuron in a slice of rat cortex in real-time depending on the momentary membrane potential V. (b) Spike pattern of the clamped neuron during simulated *in vivo*-like input barrage (bottom) shows richer and more realistic temporal dynamics compared to the same neuron's spike pattern in response to constant current injection (top). (c) Spike firing rate of the neuron as a function of driving current when dynamic clamp is used to inject zero-fold (diamonds), one-fold (circles), two-fold (squares), or three-fold (triangles) g_e and g_i. Simulated network synaptic input of increasing strength affects the excitability of the neuron, with stronger network input resulting in a smaller gain of action potential firing. Adapted from Chance et al. (2002), with permission.

without having to trust a complex, full computational model that will always only be an approximation of the living system.

4 Circuit Mechanisms of a Learned Behavior – A Dynamic Clamp Study

Figure 5 illustrates how the dynamic clamp can be used to determine cellular and synaptic mechanisms that underlie learning in a behavioral conditioning paradigm. It exemplifies how the dynamic clamp can bridge between different levels of nervous system organization, connecting cellular, synaptic, and small circuit plasticity to whole-animal behavior.

The sea hare *Aplysia californica*, a marine mollusk, is a prime model organism for the study of plasticity mechanisms underlying learning. In particular, *Aplysia* exhibits associative learning in its feeding behavior, which consists of cycles of protraction and retraction of the tongue-like radula rasp to grasp food items (for example, seaweed). In naïve (**control**) animals in the absence of food, spontaneous radula cycles occur with moderate frequency and irregularly. However, after an operant conditioning regimen in which the animal receives a food reward **contingent** on and immediately following each radula cycle, bite frequency is increased and bites (radula cycles) occur at more regular intervals – the

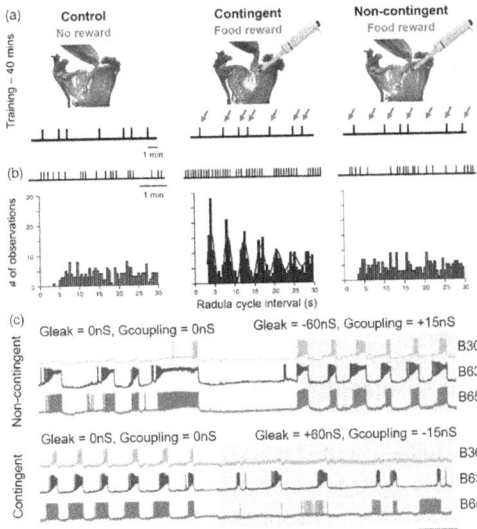

Figure 14.5 Dynamic clamp reveals cellular and synaptic plasticity mechanisms in learning-induced compulsive behavior. (a) Operant conditioning protocol to induce reward learning in *Aplysia* feeding behavior. Images of the sea hare feeding apparatus viewed from the ventral side of the animal, with the radula (tongue-like rasp) protracted (middle) or retracted. Tick marks underneath each image show an example time series of radula protractions during a 40 minute training period in which a seaweed strip (top of frame) was touched to the animal's lip to incite feeding behavior, but not ingested. Control animals received no food reward (left), contingently trained animals received a food reward in the form of a calibrated injection of seaweed juice into the mouth (symbolized by pipette), strictly timed to each radula bite cycle (middle, reward timing indicated by arrows), and non-contingently trained animals received an equal average number of food rewards, but not timed in relation to the bites performed by the animal (right). (b) One hour after the training, contingently trained animals show both increased frequency and increased temporal regularity of radula bite cycles compared to control and non-contingently trained animals, as indicated by the bite cycle interval histogram and fitted line (middle). (a) and (b), adapted from (Nargeot et al. 2007), copyright Society for Neuroscience. (c) In buccal neuronal circuits isolated from contingently trained and non-contingently trained animals, dynamic clamp was used to add/subtract a leak conductance Gleak to/from three bite initiation neurons (B30, B63, B65) that control radula biting. Dynamic clamp was also used to increase/decrease the electrical coupling strength Gcoupling between B30 and B63, and between B63 and B65. The time of dynamic clamp operation is indicated by the shaded area in voltage traces. Subtracting Gleak and increasing coupling strength increased bite command frequency and regularity in buccal circuits from non-contingently trained animals (thus mimicking reward learning, top traces). Conversely, adding Gleak and decreasing coupling strength decreased frequency and regularity in buccal circuits from contingently trained animals, effectively erasing their behavioral learning (bottom traces). Scale bar, 30 seconds.

animal has implicitly learned that radula bites can lead to a food reward, and has adjusted the frequency and regularity (and thereby efficiency) of its feeding motor program (Figure 5a). Animals that receive food rewards not timed to their bite cycles (**non-contingent** training) do not increase the frequency and regularity of their radula cycles (Nargeot and Simmers, 2011).

The small neuronal circuit controlling *Aplysia*'s buccal area, which includes muscles that move the radula, can be isolated from the animal and placed in a dish, where it continues to produce the neuronal bursts of action potentials that in the intact animal would initiate and govern feeding behavior, called a 'fictive biting' motor pattern. Intriguingly, buccal circuits isolated from contingently trained animals continue to produce bite cycle motor patterns with higher frequency and regularity than buccal circuits isolated from non-contingently trained animals or control animals (Nargeot et al. 2007). The neuronal circuit in the dish (*in vitro*) thus retains a circuit-level memory of what the animal learned during training *in vivo*. At the same time, the *in vitro* circuit allows full experimental access to the neurons that form the circuit and can be manipulated with the dynamic clamp.

Important components of the buccal circuit are three bite initiation neurons, B30, B63, and B65, and the electrical synapses between them. In the study summarized in Figure 5c, dynamic clamp was used to tease apart how cellular excitability of B30, B63, and B65 and the strength of the electrical synaptic coupling between them determines the **frequency** and **regularity** of fictive biting (Sieling et al. 2014). The major findings are that

1 increasing neuronal excitability by using dynamic clamp to subtract a leak conductance Gleak from all three neurons increases fictive bite frequency,
2 increasing the strength Gcoupling of the electrical synapses between B30 and B63 and between B63 and B65 with dynamic clamp increases fictive bite pattern regularity,
3 applying both dynamic clamp manipulations simultaneously turns the low frequency, irregular fictive pattern in a buccal circuit isolated from a non-conditionally trained animal into a high frequency, regular pattern (Fig. 5c top), and conversely,
4 applying the reverse dynamic clamp manipulations (i.e., decreasing cellular excitability by adding a leak conductance and decreasing electrical coupling) turns the high frequency, regular fictive pattern in a buccal circuit isolated from a conditionally trained animal into a low frequency, irregular pattern.

Notably, (3) and (4) suggest that learning in the intact animal likely occurs through cellular and synaptic plasticity in the B30, B63, and B65 neurons and can be both mimicked and reversed by appropriately chosen and simple dynamic clamp manipulations in the isolated circuit. This approach and results demonstrate the potential explanatory power of the dynamic clamp technique through bridging between levels of brain organization and function.

5 Dynamic Clamp Constraints and Opportunities – Historically, and Going Forward

Like any other technically cutting-edge tool, the dynamic clamp has limitations and constraints that should not go unmentioned. One of these constraints stems from the fact that in order to be dynamic clamped, neurons must be electrically contacted to record their membrane potential and inject current. This, by definition, limits the number of neurons that can be simultaneously controlled with the dynamic clamp. However, as Figures 4 and 5 illustrate, important questions about the mechanisms of interaction of neurons with their surrounding circuits and networks can nonetheless be studied with carefully crafted dynamic clamp experiments.

Another caveat to dynamic clamp experiments is that current injection usually occurs at the cell body, and that the ions that carry the dynamic clamp current into the cell are not necessarily of the same type as the ions that carry the membrane or synaptic current to be mimicked. For example, while an outward flow of potassium ions might occur in a living neuron far from the cell body in its dendritic tree, the dynamic clamp current injection that is supposed to mimic it occurs at the cell body and might be carried by the injection of chloride ions, dictated by the composition of the electrode solution. It is therefore important for experimenters to keep in mind that the spatio-temporal and chemical nature of the dynamic clamp stimuli they provide to living neurons might not exactly match the nature of the actual *in vivo* events to be simulated.

At the level of day-to-day neuroscience research practice, it should further be noted that the installation, programming, and operation of a dynamic clamp system – precisely because the technique is pushing the envelope of what is technically feasible – requires some computer savvy. However, ongoing efforts continue to make the dynamic clamp more accessible and are lowering the threshold for dynamic clamp experimentation in more and more labs (for example, see http://rtxi.org/).

The update rate of the dynamic clamp – what earns it the label "real-time" – depends on the hardware limitations of the dynamic clamp equipment used, and on the speed with which signals can be digitized and differential equations solved. Modern dynamic clamp systems frequently achieve update rates of 25 kHz or higher, meaning the feedback loop between the living neurons and the equations residing in the computer is completed multiple times per millisecond (Prinz and Cudmore 2011, http://rtxi.org/). Such high update rates are especially important when the conductances to be modeled have very fast dynamics, as is the case for the voltage-gated ionic conductances that underlie action potential generation and operate on sub-millisecond time scales. The dynamic clamp configurations used in the context of such fast dynamics must be able to 'keep up' with the dynamics in the living neurons, lest numerical inaccuracies in the clamped conductances or – even worse – dynamic instabilities of the combined system arise (Preyer and Butera 2009).

Historically, the then novel availability of sufficiently fast digitizing equipment and increasingly powerful computers is likely the reason why the dynamic clamp arose when it did – in 1993 – and that it arose at that time simultaneously and independently in two separate research areas, neuroscience and cardiac physiology (Robinson and Kawai 1993; Sharp et al. 1993a, 1993b). Since its inception, the dynamic clamp has increasingly been adopted as a tool by researchers in both fields (Prinz et al. 2004; Goaillard and Marder 2006; Wilders 2006), as constantly improving hardware, dynamic clamp software, and computer speeds continue to expand its capabilities.

More recently, dynamic clamp systems have been generalized beyond the intracellularly recorded membrane potential as an input to, and the calculated injection current as an output of the dynamic clamp. For example, a recent technological advance uses optogenetics to genetically encode current-generating opsin molecules in targeted cells and light-activate them to produce a dynamic clamp current through the cellular membrane directly, rather than by injecting the current through an electrode into the cell (Quach et al. 2018). While in its current version this novel system still requires an electrode to measure the membrane potential, it is a big step toward contactless, non-invasive dynamic clamp that could in future versions also simultaneously cover larger numbers of neurons (Newman et al. 2015).

In conclusion, the dynamic clamp allows for the construction of hybrid systems that combine and interface living neurons and circuits with computational elements such as numerical models of membrane and synaptic conductances, model neurons, and entire circuits and networks of neurons. It is therefore an important component in the modern neuroscience toolkit.

Acknowledgments

I thank Fred H. Sieling and Romuald Nargeot for providing unpublished data for Figure 5c.

References

Calin-Jageman RJ, Tunstall MJ, Mensh BD, Katz PS, Frost WN (2007). Parameter space analysis suggests multi-site plasticity contributes to motor pattern initiation in *Tritonia*. *Journal of Neurophysiology* 98(4):2382–2398.
Chance FS, Abbott LF, Reyes AD (2002). Gain modulation from background synaptic input. *Neuron* 35:773–782.

Cook SJ, Jarrell TA, Brittin CA, Wang Y, Bloniarz AE, Yakovlev MA, Nguyen KCQ, Tang LTH, Bayer EA, Duerr JS, Buelow HE, Hobert O, Hall DH, Emmons SW (2019). Whole-animal connectomes of both Caenorhabditis elegans sexes. *Nature* 571:63–71.

Cymbalyuk GS, Gaudry Q, Masino MA, Calabrese RL (2002). Bursting in leech heart interneurons: cell-autonomous and network-based mechanisms. *Journal of Neuroscience* 22:10580–10592.

Getting PA (1983). Mechanisms of pattern generation underlying swimming in Tritonia. II. Network reconstruction. *Journal of Neurophysiology* 49(4):1017–1035.

Getting PA (1989). Reconstruction of small neural networks. In: Koch C, Segev I, eds. *Methods in Neural Modeling*. MIT Press, Cambridge, pp. 135–169.

Goaillard JM, Marder E (2006). Dynamic clamp analyses of cardiac, endocrine, and neural function. *Physiology* 21:197–207.

Koppell NJ, Gritton HJ, Whittington MA, Kramer MA (2014). Beyond the connectome: The dynome. *Neuron* 83(6):1319–1328.

Ma M, Koester J (1996). The role of potassium currents in frequency-dependent spike broadening in *Aplysia* R20 neurons: a dynamic clamp analysis. *Journal of Neuroscience* 16:4089–4101.

Nargeot R, Petrissans C, Simmers J (2007). Behavioral and *in vitro* correlates of compulsive-like food seeking induced by operant conditioning in *Aplysia*. *Journal of Neuroscience* 27(30):8059–8070.

Nargeot R, Simmers J (2011). Neural mechanisms of operant conditioning and learning-induced behavioral plasticity in *Aplysia*. *Cellular and Molecular Life Sciences* 68(5):803–816.

Newman JP, Fong MF, Millard DC, Whitmire CJ, Stanley GB, Potter SM (2015). *eLife* 4: e07192.

Pinto RD, Elson RC, Szucs A, Rabinovich MI, Selverston AI, Abarbanel HDI (2001). Extended dynamic clamp: controlling up to four neurons using a single desktop computer and interface. *Journal of Neuroscience Methods* 108:39–48.

Preyer AJ, Butera RJ (2009). Causes of transient instabilities in the dynamic clamp. *IEEE Transactions on Neural Systems and Rehabilitation Engineering* 17(2):190–198.

Prinz AA, Abbott LF, Marder E (2004). The dynamic clamp comes of age. *Trends in Neurosciences* 27:218–224.

Prinz AA, Cudmore RH (2011). Dynamic clamp. *Scholarpedia* 6(5):1470.

Prinz AA, Hooper SL (2017). Computer simulation – power and peril. In: Hooper SL, Buschges A, eds. *The Neurobiology of Motor Control: Fundamental Concepts and New Directions*. Wiley, Hoboken, NJ, 107–133.

Quach B, Krogh-Madsen T, Entcheva E, Christini DJ (2018). Light-activated dynamic clamp using iPSC-derived cardiomyocytes. *Biophysical Journal* 115(11): 2206–2217.

Robinson HP, Kawai N (1993). Injection of digitally synthesized synaptic conductance transients to measure the integrative properties of neurons. *Journal of Neuroscience Methods* 49:157–165.

Sharp AA, O'Neil MB, Abbott LF, Marder E (1993a). The dynamic clamp: artificial conductances in biological neurons. *Trends in Neuroscience* 16:389–394.

Sharp AA, O'Neil MB, Abbott LF, Marder E (1993b). Dynamic clamp: computer-generated conductances in real neurons. *Journal of Neurophysiology* 69:992–995.

Sieling F, Bedecarrats A, Simmers J, Prinz AA, Nargeot R (2014). Differential roles of nonsynaptic and synaptic plasticity in operant reward learning-induced compulsive behavior. *Current Biology* 24(9):941–950.

Sporns O (2010). Connectome. *Scholarpedia* 5(2):5584.

Wilders R (2006). Dynamic clamp: a powerful tool in cardiac electrophysiology. *Journal of Physiology* 576(2):349–359.

Tool Use and Development Beyond Neuroscience

15 Beyond Actual Difference Making
Causal Selections in Genetics[*]

Janella Baxter

1 Introduction

Loss of function studies in genetics are a central experimental approach from which a substantial proportion of gene-centered explanations are derived. Moreover, the gene-centered explanations that are derived from the loss of function studies are crucial data for further research programs such as causal modeling of gene regulatory networks. While previous philosophical discussions have focused on what properties make the gene uniquely significant in biological explanations, this paper has to do with what makes the gene a useful tool for manipulation and control of biological processes in loss of function studies. For, as we'll see, the causal properties that make genes central to loss of function studies are not unique to genes alone but are likely to be shared by other related biomolecules. Nevertheless, the centrality of loss of function studies to contemporary biology and gene-centered explanations requires that our philosophical analyses properly account for the causal and explanatory status of genes in this area. A central aim in the history and philosophy of biology literature has been to reconstruct the underlying justifications for what makes genes explanatorily and experimentally significant. Several, mutually compatible proposals have been made. The history of biology, it turns out, has had more than one operative gene concept. Thus, a common view in the philosophy of biology has been that genes serve a plurality of explanatory and experimental roles in different research programs. Two proposals for the explanatory and experimental significance of genes have recently been articulated – the sequence specificity view and the actual difference making approach (Waters 2007; Weber 2013, 2017).

In this paper, I argue that both the sequence specificity and actual difference making views are inadequate for making sense of the subtle reasoning at play in the loss of function studies. The argument against

* I owe special thanks to Alan Love, John Bickle, Antonella Tramacere, and Carl Craver for their invaluable comments on this paper and to Gabriela Huelga-Morales for welcoming me into her lab at the University of Minnesota, Twin Cities.

DOI: 10.4324/9781003251392-21

the sequence specificity view is easy. It simply involves observing that the gene-centric explanations coming from loss of function studies do not cite the sequence specificity of a gene as the explanatorily significant property. Instead, the explanatorily significant property of genes in such explanations is the pattern of gene expression in a biological system. When it comes to patterns of gene expression, scientists conducting loss of function studies distinguish between switch- and dial-like types of gene expression. Switch- and dial-like gene expression represents two types of causal control that are achievable thanks to recent technological and experimental innovations.

Both switch- and dial-like causal control can be interpreted as more refined concepts of Water's actual difference making view. I embrace this interpretation. However, in embracing this interpretation, I raise reasonable concerns about why philosophers of science should understand the logic of loss of function studies through the lens of switch- and dial-like causation when we already have Waters' actual difference making view. This is when I incorporate a philosophy of technology to help justify preferring the switch- and dial-like account over the actual difference making view.

I argue that the switch- and dial-like causal control represents a "spiral of self-improvement" that is characteristic of scientific progress (Chang 2004, 44). On this view, technological and experimental progress isn't merely an advancement in practical know-how. I argue that this type of progress can also usher forth conceptual change as novel technological and experimental advancements help integrate novel concepts into concrete, empirical practices. In the case of loss of function studies, I argue the novel techniques that make both knockout and knockdown experimental techniques from which biologists may choose help switch- and dial-like causal concepts make contact with the empirical world. Yet, this recent development is not a replacement for the actual difference making concept that characterized earlier stages of inquiry in genetics. Rather, switch- and dial-like causal concepts build upon and refine the older concept.

This account leaves philosophers of science with both the actual difference making and the switch- and dial-like accounts as legitimate ways of understanding the logic of loss of function studies. Nevertheless, I maintain that if our purpose is to understand the subtle reasoning characteristic of loss of function studies, we should prefer the switch- and dial-like account. For one thing, this account helps us track scientific progress in genetics experimentation and theorization. For another, it helps us understand the rationale behind a scientist's choice between switch- or dial-like control in a given experiment. For biologists are often principled in their choice between which type of control they employ in an experiment. They will judge that one type of control is more likely to be illuminating. The switch- and dial-like framework helps us understand their reasoning for doing so.

The structure of my paper proceeds by (Section 2) laying out the sequence specificity and actual difference making accounts that have been proposed in the philosophy of biology literature. Next (Section 3) I introduce the logic of loss of function studies and I argue that dial- and switch-like causal control is what justifies the causal selection of genes in this experimental paradigm. And finally, (Section 4) I argue that for the purpose of understanding loss of function studies we should prefer the switch- and dial-like account over the actual difference making view.

2 Gene-Centered Explanations

It is widely acknowledged that contemporary and classical explanations in the biological sciences often accord a special explanatory status to genes. This is true despite the fact that many causal conditions are relevant to any given effect. A central program in the philosophy of biology literature has been to articulate the underlying rationale of singling out genes in biological explanations that attempt to capture the sort of causal control genes have over biological processes. One proposal, extensively defended by C. Kenneth Waters (1994, 2004, 2006, 2007; Rheinberger and Müller-Wille 2017), is that genes serve as actual difference makers in both contemporary and classical experimental areas of biology. In what follows I distinguish between a narrow and broad sense of actual difference making that is at play in Water's work. Another recent proposal is that genes have sequence specificity with respect to the linear sequences of molecular products (Weber 2006, 2013, 2017; Waters 2007; Woodward 2010; Griffiths and Stotz 2013). I lay out these views in the present section.

The causal selection debate in the philosophy of biology literature has primarily concerned the underlying rationale behind why biologists highlight some causal variables in explanation and background others. In particular, the debate has taken molecular genes and DNA as its central case of causal variables that are frequently privileged in contemporary biological explanations. The debate begins with the observation that any given effect – biological or not – has a large set of relevant causal conditions. For example, green fluorescence in jellyfish requires the presence of the gene for the green fluorescent protein encoded in the jellyfish's genome, the transcription of the gene into messenger RNA (mRNA), and the translation of mRNA into a protein. It also requires the abundance of amino acids and biochemical energy in the form of ATP, as well as viable temperature and pH levels, and so on. Yet, despite this immense causal complexity, biologists often single out the gene for green fluorescent protein when formulating their explanations of why jellyfish fluoresce in the deep sea. Several proposals have been offered as analyses of the underlying rationale for gene selection in many biological explanations – sequence specificity (Weber 2006, 2013, 2017; Waters

2007, 2018; Woodward 2010; Griffiths and Stotz 2013; Griffiths et al. 2015) and actual difference making (Waters 1994, 2006, 2007).

Sequence specificity has to do with the causal control structural genes have over the linear sequences of gene products, like RNA and proteins. Structural genes are sequences of nucleic acid bases – adenine (A), thymine (T)/uracil (U) (for RNA), guanine (G), and cytosine (C) – in DNA that encode other molecular products. Structural genes are conceptually distinct from regulatory genes (Gerstein et al. 2007). Regulatory genes are sequences of nucleic acid bases in DNA that don't have sequence specificity over the linear sequences of other biomolecules. Instead, they enable or inhibit the transcription of structural genes when regulatory factors – proteins and RNA molecules – bind to regulatory modules. Structural genes control the nucleic acid sequences of RNA transcripts by Watson-Crick base pairing rules whereby adenine always specifies uracil, thymine specifies adenine, guanine specifies cytosine, and cytosine specifies guanine. In this way, differences in the nucleic acid sequence of a structural gene produce differences in the nucleic acid sequence of RNA transcripts. In simple cases where there is no alternative splicing, differences in the nucleic acid sequences of structural genes also produce differences in the amino acid sequences of proteins. The nucleic acid sequence of a structural gene determines the amino acid sequence of a protein in units of three nucleic acids at a time or in units of codons. For the most part (with the exception of stop codons – codons that instruct the protein synthesis machinery to "halt" production), each nucleic acid triplet specifies one amino acid type. For example, the codon UGG "codes" only for the amino acid tryptophan. There is some redundancy in the genetic code, meaning that more than one codon specifies the same amino acid, as in the case of ACU, ACC, ACA, and ACG all of which specify threonine. This means that some alternative nucleic acid sequences of a protein coding gene will make no difference to the same amino acid sequence of a protein. However, many differences in the nucleic acid sequence of a protein coding gene will make a difference to the amino acid sequence of a protein.

For some authors, sequence specificity is the primary rationale for the causal selection of genes in contemporary biological explanations. For example, the sequence specificity of structural genes is at the heart of C. Kenneth Waters' account of what makes genetics successful (1994, 2006, 2007, 2018). In Waters' view, the gene concept is flexible and can refer to different entities depending on the purposes of a researcher. For example, when a biologist wishes to explain the linear sequence of a protein, they will appeal to the messenger RNA (mRNA) biomolecule that is read and translated into a sequence of amino acids as the relevant gene. By contrast, when a biologist wishes to explain the linear sequence of an mRNA transcript, they will appeal to the relevant nucleic acid sequence in DNA. In this way, there is no single entity that is a gene for all research purposes. Yet, even on this flexible understanding of the gene concept in contemporary biology, Waters' analysis of contemporary practice focuses entirely on structural genes. At times, Waters writes as if structural genes are the only genes in the game when he writes: "Genes are for linear sequences in products of gene expression" (Waters 1994, 177). This is further illustrated by Waters' account of what has made contemporary genetics successful.

Waters may feel no need to expand his account of the contemporary gene concept because he has another analysis upon which he can fall. This is his actual difference making view (Waters 2007). Like the structural gene concept, the actual difference making concept is also flexible. It can be understood in broad or narrow terms. Broadly, a cause that (1) actually varies relative to an otherwise uniform population and (2) whose varying accounts for an actual difference in an effect variable is an actual difference maker. The broad interpretation of actual difference making makes no reference to any particular scientific paradigm – this is in contrast to the narrow interpretation. All that's required is that conditions (1) and (2) be met. As we'll see below although this can characterize the loss of function studies in contemporary molecular biology, I question the usefulness of this analysis below. The narrow interpretation of actual difference making is specific to classical genetics of the early 20th century.[1] Waters also argues that genes in classical genetics serve as actual difference makers. On this construal, classical genes are actual difference makers with respect to actual differences in a phenotypic trait when they are allowed to actually vary relative to an experimental population (Waters 1994, 2004, 2007) In classical genetics, genes make actual differences to genotype – the genetic composition of an organism – which in turn (can) correlate with actual differences in a phenotypic trait. Classical geneticists exploited both investigative and theoretical principles of inheritance – e.g., independent assortment, segregation, recombination, etc. – to generate lab-raised populations that were (relatively) genetically identical with the exception of a few genes that were permitted to actually vary. So, in a population of fruit flies, some individuals are homozygous – they carry two copies of the same gene – for the wild type eye color (+/+), others are heterozygous for a wild type and a mutant gene, say purple, (+/pr), and still others are homozygous for purple (pr/pr). When phenotypic differences in eye color are obtained – some individuals have red others have purple – classical geneticists inferred that such differences must be due to the genetic differences they were allowed to actually obtain (Bridges and Morgan 1919).[2] Even though classical geneticists knew that other genes – say, the vermillion gene – could make a difference to eye color, Waters insists that it is the wild type or purple genotypes that are explanatorily significant relative to this experimental set-up. The vermillion gene, by contrast, is merely a potential difference maker in this case and, thus, is not privileged in the explanations of classical geneticists.

Actual difference making – in both the broad and narrow senses – as well as sequence specificity are different types of causal control that genes have with respect to biological processes. These accounts have been proposed by various philosophers (notably, Waters 1994, 2004, 2006, 2007; Weber 2006, 2013, 2017) as descriptions of the reasoning behind why biologists systematically privilege genes when formulating their explanations. Waters (1994, 2004, 2006, 2007) and Weber (2004, 2018) both attempt to inform their philosophies by attending to the experimental practices of biologists. However, as I'll argue below, their views on the causal selection of genes have not been attentive to contemporary experimental approaches. For the causal selection of genes at play in the loss of function study fits neither the sequence specificity nor the actual difference making view very well. Experimental practices get better over time as new technologies and experimental techniques are developed. Moreover, explanatory practices often change alongside innovation in experimental approaches. I'll argue below that technological and experimental innovation can justify novel ways of conceptualizing phenomena. As researchers are prompted to justify the inferences they make from experiments, the explanations they formulate often need to invoke novel concepts ushered forth by technological and experimental innovations. Thus, it is likely that sequence specificity and actual difference making may not be up to the task of capturing the causal reasoning at play in novel areas of biology. At least for the purpose of making sense of the subtle logics implicit to loss of function studies – one of the most central experimental paradigms used in contemporary biology – our philosophical analysis should track the conceptual changes at work in these sets of practices.

3 Taking Loss of Function Studies (More) Seriously

Loss of function studies are a central experimental approach to many areas of biology. In what follows, I shall argue that the causal reasoning at play in this sort of experiment isn't adequately captured by the aforementioned literature. Loss of function studies systematically *don't* involve manipulation of a protein coding gene's sequence specificity as a means of manipulating biological processes. Nor do experimentalists carrying out these studies employ the theoretical tenets required of classical geneticists for their explanations. At best, the broad sense of Waters' actual difference making approach best approximates the reasoning at play in this sort of experiment. Yet, as I'll contend in the final section, the broad sense of actual difference making is not a satisfying analysis. In this section, I argue there are two kinds of causal concepts that best characterizes the appeal to genes in many biological explanations – namely, dial- and switch-like control over the concentration of gene products in a living organism (Woodward 2010).

Loss of function studies are perhaps one of the most central experimental techniques to contemporary biology. Not only do these experiments aid crucially in the causal modeling of gene regulatory networks, but – perhaps more modestly – they provide the necessary data for many of the gene-centered explanations contemporary biologists provide. Often the results of these studies inform and are informed by further empirical and theoretical claims, such as causal modeling of gene regulatory networks. However, biologists needn't be constructing causal models when they formulate explanations based on a loss of function study. At a minimum, the sorts of explanations biologists formulate from loss of function experiments can characterize in qualitative terms a causal relationship between a molecular gene (or set of genes) and some phenotypic difference (Barbaric et al. 2007; Housden et al. 2016). The name – "loss of function" – clearly indicates that gene function is at the heart of this sort of experiment. But there can be multiple senses of "function" used in biological vernacular, some of which are the central target of loss of function studies.[3] Perhaps the most appropriate way to interpret functional claims in this sort of experimental program is from the mechanistic tradition (Craver 2007). On this sort of analysis, an entity's activities contribute to the capacity of a more complex system of which the entity is a part. For example, the protein Coronin aids in regulating filament proteins (called actins) that are crucial for cellular movement (Shen et al. 2014).

Loss of function studies exploit sequence specificity as a *means* to manipulating gene expression – but sequence specificity is not the relevant explanans in this sort of experimental approach. Biologists have a host of techniques by which to carry out loss of function studies – ranging from less common methods like small molecule inhibitors and morpholinos to much more pervasive approaches using RNA interference (RNAi) and CRISPR-Cas9 (Housden et al. 2016). Often these techniques do rely on sequence specificity. For example, CRISPR-Cas9 and RNAi have the unique ability to identify and perturb the expression of coding sequences embedded in DNA or RNA. Biologists "program" genes encoding CRISPR-Cas9 or RNAi products so that when they are expressed in an organism, these mechanisms act only on genes with a complementary nucleic acid sequence. In this way, the molecular gene's sequence specificity with respect to the linear sequences of products is both experimentally relevant to loss of function studies and, indeed, explanatory. The precise nucleic acid sequence of CRISPR or RNAi components makes the difference between interference of one gene rather than another. Differences in the CRISPR or RNAi sequences make a difference and thereby explain which gene in an organism's genome is perturbed. But this is not the explanatory target of loss of function studies. The explanatory target of this sort of study is what accounts for some phenotypic differences in the experimental population.[4] The relevant explanans in loss of function studies is gene expression. So, when the interruption of a gene's expression correlates with a phenotypic difference, it is the targeted gene's expression and not the gene sequence that is explanatory. For example, loss of function studies of the Dpy gene in *Caenorhabditis elegans* (or C. elegans) result in dumpy – short and fat – body types (Shen et al. 2014). It is the perturbation of the Dpy gene's expression that biologists single out in explanations of short/fat body types. The intervention made by the loss of function tools, while reliant on the properties characterized in the previous section, does not produce a change in the linear sequence of a gene's products. Instead, when successfully utilized, these tools introduce changes that produce changes in the expression of a gene.

Loss of function studies proceed by manipulating the concentration of a gene's product in an organism; however, this type of study encompasses two related types of causal control – dial- and switch-like. Dial-like control is a type of INF (short for influence)-specificity (Woodward 2010). Causes with INF-specificity can take a range of alternative values, each of which (ideally) determines one and only one value from a range of alternatives that an effect variable can take. INF-specificity is often analogized to the tuning dial on a radio. Tuning dials often have many alternative values they can take. Tuning the dial to one setting correlates with one radio station playing over the speakers, while tuning to another setting correlates with a different radio station playing, and so one for each possible setting of the dial. This is very much like the dial-like control some kinds of loss of function interventions have over phenotypic traits. An important exception is that the alternative settings of a radio station dial correlate with discrete, alternative output values for the effect variable; whereas, dial-like control in loss of function studies needn't. Instead, the alternative values a dial-like cause can take can correlate with continuous values in the effect variable. In this way, a causal variable is analogous to the modulation of brightness in a room by means of a light dimmer. A light dimmer can be turned up or down to increase or decrease the brightness of a room in a continuous way. This sort of control is often achieved by means of gene knockdown approaches in loss of function studies (O'Malley et al. 2010). For example, the amount of a fluorescent protein in a biological population can be increased/decreased by administering more or less of the gene knockdown technology, RNAi (Baggs et al. 2009). RNAi interferes with a gene's expression by targeting and degrading its mRNA transcripts.[5] The more RNAi reagent added, ideally, the greater amount of a gene's product is eliminated. Sometimes this corresponds to a phenotypic difference. Experimental investigation of how dial-like control of various genes make differences to mammalian circadian rhythm cycles found that depleting the Bmal1 gene by about 40% corresponded to a slight increase in luminescence, while a 60% decrease corresponded to an even greater increase. This kind of causal control manipulates the concentration level of a gene product in a matter of amounts – say, micromolars. Distinguishing between one causal value from another is, in this sort of case, determined arbitrarily. The researchers could have just as easily tested a 38.76% (rather than 40%) depletion in the Bmal1 gene product and discovered that some change in the degree of luminescence obtains. What matters is that some change in the causal variable corresponds to some change in the effect variable. Any changes in the causal variable that fail to do this don't count as distinct values that the causal variable can take. Distinct values correspond to changes that do make a difference to the value of the effect variable.

A puzzling feature of knockdown experiments is that biologists use the language of genes in their explanations of the phenotypic differences that occur and not the language of mRNA. Baggs et al., for example, write:

> The depletion of only three genes...*Clock*, *Bmal1*, and *Per1*...disrupted robust circadian oscillations in bioluminescence.
> (Ibid, 0565)

The study from which this claim comes involves RNAi knockdowns of several mRNA products involved in mammalian circadian rhythm cycles. And yet, these authors speak of "the depletion of...genes..." This is an illustration of how flexible the molecular gene concept is in contemporary biology. Waters (1994) has argued that a common gene concept underlies the immensely diverse range of biochemicals to which biologists apply the term. Since nucleic acid sequences in DNA and RNA often determine the linear sequences of other downstream products, the word "gene" may properly apply to either type of biomolecule. Thus, the molecular gene concept can be ambiguous when it is not specified what product the gene is for and at what stage of gene expression. In this case, the relevant gene refers to the mRNA transcripts that are the target of RNAi. The nucleic acid sequences of the mRNA transcripts are genes *for* the amino acid sequence of a protein during the stage of gene expression called translation. Of course, there are genes for the mRNA transcripts that are the target of the knockdown intervention. These are the Clock, Bmal1, and Per1 nucleic acid sequences encoded in the organism's DNA, which determine the nucleic acid sequences of mRNA products during the stage of gene expression called transcription. What this shows is that sequence specificity plays a crucial role in the identification and individuation of genes in biology; however, this should not be mistaken for the causal significance of a gene. Loss of function studies intervene at various stages of gene expression – knockdown experiments intervene on mRNA, and (as we'll soon see) knockout experiments intervene directly on DNA – and it is the various ways gene expression can be manipulated that is conceptually relevant to the explanations biologists formulate.

Dial-like causal control differs from other types of loss of function interventions in that it leaves some amount of gene product in the organism's cellular environment. Gene knockout studies are an increasingly pervasive experimental approach to the loss of function studies. This sort of intervention involves switch-like causal control. Instead of there being a range of many values a causal variable can take, each of which associates with a different value in the effect variable, switch-like causal control is all or nothing. On this sort of experimental approach, the contrast focus is between the presence or absence of a gene product in a biological population. This sort of control is best achieved by gene-editing techniques like CRISPR-Cas9, which break and rejoin DNA strands at a precise site where a protein coding gene is encoded. When the broken strands are rejoined, cellular repair mechanisms can replace a codon that specifies an amino acid with a stop codon. Ideally, the insertion of premature stop codons in all redundant copies of a gene throughout an organism's genome will ensure that no protein is synthesized. When a stark phenotypic difference between a knockout and control population is achieved by means of a knockout intervention, the target gene often becomes a standard test case by which to determine whether other knockout interventions are successful. For example, knockout studies of the Dpy gene in *Caenorhabditis elegans* (or C. elegans) result in dumpy – short and fat – body types and are often used to test whether CRISPR-Cas9 reagents target a gene of interest (Shen et al. 2014). In knockout studies, biologists privilege the absence of a gene whose DNA sequence *would* determine the amino acid sequence of a protein in their explanations of any phenotypic differences that might obtain. In the case of Dpy knockouts, biologists highlight the absence of the Dpy nucleic acid sequence in DNA to explain the phenotypic difference between the knockout and control population – in this case, short and fat versus normal body types respectively.

One might object that either the narrow or broad construal of Waters' actual difference making approach adequately captures the causal reasoning of loss of function experiments. On the narrow construal, loss of function studies reason about the actual differences molecular genes produce in ways that are similar to the reasoning strategies employed by classical geneticists. For example, both strategies appeal to genes to explain phenotypic differences when the genes are allowed to actually vary relative to an otherwise genetically and environmentally uniform population. Although it's true that important conceptual and experimental parallels can be found between contemporary and classical genetics (Vance 1996; Waters 2004, 2009), the causal reasoning strategies are not the same. An important difference is the role dominant and recessive traits played in the reasoning of classical geneticists (Bridges and Morgan 1919). In diploid organisms – or organisms carrying two copies of each gene – dominant traits are produced by either homo- or heterozygosity for a dominant allele. That is, either a dominant trait, such as the red eye color, is caused by either a genotype with two copies of the red eye gene (+/+) or a genotype with one copy of the red eye gene and one copy of a mutant gene, like purple (+/pr). By contrast, recessive genotypes require homozygosity of a mutant gene (pr/pr). For classical geneticists to explain the difference between some phenotypic traits that emerged in their experimental populations, say red and purple eyes, they had to appeal to the actual differences in genotypes with different dominant and recessive alleles. Dominant and recessive traits are not a feature of the causal reasoning in loss of function studies. What matters is that phenotypic differences correlate with an experimenter's intervention on a gene product. Contemporary biologists do without the theory of dominant and recessive traits to explain differences in their populations. An adequate account of the experimental and explanatory strategies of classical and contemporary geneticists ought to be sensitive to this subtle difference.

Perhaps a further objection is that Waters' broad construal of actual difference making adequately captures the causal reasoning of loss of function studies. On this proposal, scientists attribute any actual differences that might obtain in a (relatively) uniform population to causal variables that they allow to actually vary. This reasoning appears to capture the causal reasoning of contemporary biologists conducting loss of function studies. Indeed, biologists attribute actual phenotypic differences that obtain in their experimental populations to the actual differences they induce in molecular genes. Yet I caution against embracing this characterization. For it is too crude of an analysis to differentiate between actual difference making practices that biologists recognize as being illuminating (or, at least, have the promise of being illuminating) and ones they don't. As I'll argue below, contemporary biologists can make actual *many* types of differences when studying the functions of a gene. Yet, biologists are systematic about the sorts of experiments they conduct and the sorts they don't. The broad construal of actual difference making cannot account for this. I'll argue instead that we characterize the causal reasoning at play in the loss of function studies in terms of dial- and switch-like causal control.

Technical and experimental innovation can stimulate explanatory innovation. Loss of function techniques like RNAi and CRISPR-Cas9 with their respective types of causal control exerted over genes give scientists a way to make specific causal concepts operational (Chang 2014). That is, these tools make the integration of dial- and switch-like causal concepts with concrete empirical practices possible. While for some authors, technological innovation is itself "conceptually impoverished" as it is merely the application of already developed conceptual frameworks from pure science (Bunge 1966), technological innovation for loss of function studies (and perhaps many other experimental paradigms) suggests otherwise. Rather, knockdown and knockout approaches provide scientists with justification for conceptualizing phenomena in one way rather than another. As novel concepts are introduced by means of novel technological and experimental innovations the logic of the explanations scientist formulate changes as well. Scientists are often confronted with the need to explain the reasoning behind the inferences they draw from the experiments they conduct. In the cases I am discussing, the inferences drawn are often rather modest – concerning things like what is causally responsible for some observable effect in a particular population in a particular environment. Nonetheless, the techniques employed in a particular experiment shape significantly the conceptual framework implicit to the explanations biologists formulate. Depending on whether a scientist uses a knockdown or knockout approach, this will determine whether they will conceptualize the cause and effect variables in terms of a dial- or switch-like way.

4 Selecting the Right Intervention for the Job

So far I've argued that the kind of causal control exploited in loss of function studies is not captured by either the sequence specificity account or Waters' narrow sense of actual difference making approach. But what about the broad sense of actual difference making? By showing that experimentalists are principled about when they use dial-like and switch-like causal control over genes, I'll argue that the broad sense of actual difference making cannot distinguish between actual difference making strategies that they regard as illuminating and ones they don't. I advocate that we instead embrace dial- and switch-like causal control as a more nuanced analysis of the causal reasoning biologists employ when singling out genes in explanations that draw from loss of function experiments. Richer and more nuanced concepts are what we should expect from technological and experimental innovation.

Experimentalists working in areas of genetics and molecular biology have a host of interventions by which to make actual differences in living systems as a means to studying how they work; however, a host of constraints steer them towards particular tools for particular tasks. As I've shown, a primary epistemic aim of many biologists is to produce observable phenotypic differences in experimental populations by perturbing gene expression. For many biologists it is also crucial that they can attribute phenotypic differences to functions that a gene (and its products) have as a result of its evolutionary history – not as a result of the biologist's intervention. Furthermore, it is often important that any phenotypic differences that may obtain as a result of an intervention help illuminate how a gene's functions contribute to the maintenance of an organism's life. These aims can constrain which experiments a biologist selects. And finally, an intervention must hold the promise of illuminating a phenomenon within a time scale that is practical for the researcher.

As the techniques and methods of contemporary biologists continue to improve, biologists now have many ways to exploit the actual difference-making capabilities of genes – not all of which they employ. One way has to do with a gene's sequence specificity with respect to the linear sequences of the products they encode. Modern gene-editing tools have recently provided researchers with the power to intervene directly on the nucleic acid sequence of a gene in such a way as to make actual (almost) any possible gene sequence. This would count as an actual difference making approach to the study of gene function. In this sort of experiment, researchers make an actual difference in the nucleic acid sequence of a gene and associate any phenotypic differences that might actually obtain in the population to their intervention. Yet, this is not a common approach that illuminates the kind of phenomena many researchers working in areas of molecular biology are studying. And for good reason. Whether an alternative nucleic acid sequence of a molecular gene will produce an observable phenotypic difference is an empirical matter that biologists are often not able to know prior to the experiment. At the level of individual proteins, scientists have only a piecemeal understanding of how changes in the nucleic acid sequence of a protein coding gene will influence the protein's structure and function. At a more global systems level, the phenotypic characteristics of a living system can remain undisturbed despite point mutations in genes (Kitano 2004). Furthermore, the number of possible gene sequences an experimentalist might have to test to determine which actually make a phenotypic difference can be quite large – for an average size gene of 900 base pairs, the number of possibilities can be 4^{900} (since there are four alternative bases for each position in the sequence). Experimentally testing each of these can be quite inefficient for a researcher. Perhaps more problematic is the possibility of creating a gene with novel functions – functions it would not otherwise have were it not for human intervention. So, even if such an intervention were to produce a phenotypic difference, a researcher cannot know whether the phenotypic difference is due to an artificial function they themselves created or to a function that the gene has acquired over evolutionary history. The broad sense of actual difference making would count among the illuminating actual difference making practices, manipulation of a gene's sequence specificity. Yet, this is only an illuminating experimental approach for some types of investigative questions. When it comes to uncovering a gene's functions, the biological community generally pursues a very different investigative path.

Achieving observable phenotypic differences that a biologist may attribute to a gene's evolved functionalities is no trivial matter. The phenotypic characteristics of living systems can display little to no differences despite changes in the underlying processes that cause them (Kitano 2004; Barbaric et al. 2007). This can be due to a host of reasons. Protein functions are often undisturbed by point mutations in the structure (Castagnoli et al. 2004). The presence of complex gene regulatory networks can (sometimes) mean that changes in the rate and duration of a gene's expression make no difference to the biological processes in which the gene participates. It is also common for living systems to encode gene products capable of similar functions, which can compensate for other gene products in their absence (Mitchell 2009). While some changes in the underlying processes of a living system can produce no phenotypic differences, others can outright be unilluminating for other reasons. For example, intervention on genes that are necessary for maintaining the life of a biological organism can be lethal. Despite these challenges, biologists nevertheless conduct loss of function studies instead of other types of experiments to uncover gene function.

While it is common for researchers to use both dial- and switch-like interventions to study a gene's expression, biologists are often principled about which sort of intervention they conduct. If a researcher has reason to believe a gene's function will be compensated for by the functions of other genes, they may avoid manipulating gene expression in a switch-like way. This is the reasoning behind the dial-like control used in the circadian rhythm study by Braggs et al. Instead of eliminating a gene's product(s) from a living system entirely, dial-like control allows for some product to be present. Ideally, this sort of intervention will produce a significant reduction in the amount of gene product to generate an observable phenotypic difference in the experimental population, but it is an empirical matter as to whether the reduction in product will trigger other compensatory mechanisms that prevent any phenotypic difference from occurring. Complete elimination of a gene product from a biological system that encodes compensatory mechanisms may not produce observable phenotypic differences. However, dial-like control over a gene's expression may. By contrast, switch-like causal control over a gene's expression is often preferable to dial-like control when the gene of interest has subtle phenotypic effects. For example, small amounts of the neurofibromatosis type 2 gene are sufficient to maintain toxin sensitivity in cancer cell growths (Shalem et al. 2014). Dial-like control on this gene's expression rarely shows any phenotypic difference. Switch-like control, by contrast, shows a significant difference in toxin sensitivity. By turning this gene's expression from "on" to "off," researchers are able to achieve a clear phenotypic difference that is otherwise masked. Thus, in an effort to exaggerate a gene's phenotypic differences, thereby making its contribution more easily observable, biologists are more likely to prefer interventions that eliminate a gene product from a living system entirely.

Switch- and dial-like causal concepts are recent refinements of Waters' broad actual difference making concept. Technological and experimental progress often involves the innovation of novel concrete, empirical practices that enable scientists to probe new and sometimes increasingly subtle questions. This kind of progress doesn't just represent innovation in practical know-how (though I by no means with to diminish this kind of knowledge). Often, with technological and experimental innovation comes conceptual innovation as new practical innovations help put more abstract concepts into contact with the empirical world. In the case of loss of function studies, switch- and dial-like causal control achieved by means of different experimental techniques have given biologists novel and more subtle ways of probing the genotype's relationship to the phenotype. With the ability to ask new and increasingly subtle questions about the genotype's relationship to the phenotype, techniques such as RNAi and CRISPR-Cas9 have also given scientists new and increasingly subtle ways to conceptualize the genotype's relationship to the phenotype. So, while the broad interpretation of the actual difference making view can absorb switch- and dial-like causal concepts, this doesn't mean doing so is illuminating for the purposes of philosophy of science. For one thing, the broad interpretation of the actual difference making view cannot account for the judgments scientists make about which sorts of experimental interventions they deem likely to be illuminating in a particular context and which they deem likely to be unilluminating. For another, progress in scientific inquiry often proceeds by means of what Hasok Chang calls a "spiral of self-improvement" whereby later stages of scientific inquiry build upon and refine previous ways of investigating and thinking about phenomena (Chang 2004, 44). What this shows is that philosophers of science have more than one way to make sense of the underlying rationale biologists have for singling out genes for explanatory purposes in loss of function experiments. We can think of the rationale in terms of Waters' broad sense of actual difference making or in terms of the dial- and switch-like concepts I've articulated here. In one sense, both ways of understanding loss of function studies are appropriate. However, we should prefer one way over the other for specific kinds of purposes. I've argued that if our purpose is to understand the subtle causal reasoning at work in one of the most widely conducted experiments in contemporary biology, we should prefer the switch- and dial-like account. Switch- and dial-like accounts help us track practical and conceptual progress in biology. Moreover, this more refined set of concepts helps us capture the logic behind the choices biologists make when conducting knockdown or knockout experiments.

5 Conclusion

The gene is a central explanatory variable in much of classical and contemporary biology. I have argued that the rationale behind the widespread causal selection of molecular genes varies depending on the type of tools scientists use to manipulate and control genetic processes. This is significant not just because it represents progress in practical know-how. It's significant because novel technologies and techniques can also play a role in conceptual change as they make novel concepts operational. The story I am telling about the loss of function studies is a story about how gene concepts have become increasingly sophisticated as biologist's experimental tools have increased in number and power. This means that the switch- and dial-like account defended in this paper is a recent refinement of the broad interpretation of Waters' actual difference making view. Yet this doesn't mean that the actual difference making view is adequate for our purposes. If our purpose is to understand the subtle reasoning at play in the loss of function studies – and I believe philosophers of genetics should have this purpose – we should prefer the switch- and dial-like account. This account better accommodates the nature of technological and conceptual progress in the history of genetics and it helps us appreciate the judgments biologists make about which type of causal control is likely to be more illuminating.

Notes

1 By classical genetics, Waters really has in mind the system of practices and theories of the American geneticist, Thomas Hunt Morgan and his lab. If by "classical genetics," one simply means the system of practices and theories aimed at understanding genetics in the early 20th century, then Waters' account only captures a subset of the science going on at the time. Different laboratories around the world studying genetics operated by distinct styles of thought at the time (see Harwood 1993).

2 Difference making alone cannot explain which genotype aligns with which phenotypic difference. This required theoretical knowledge about dominant and recessive traits as well as extensive empirical knowledge about which act as dominant/recessive. Waters acknowledges this, however, it is noteworthy his actual difference making approach cannot fully account for this aspect of the reasoning at play in the experiments of classical genetics.

3 See Millikan (1989), Neander (1991a, 1991b), Wouters (2003), Walsh and Ariew (2013) for a brief survey of the numerous function concepts in the life sciences.

4 Some molecular tools do indeed produce phenotypic differences, however. For example, genetic markers such as fluorescent proteins are an illustrative example. Yet this sort of tool differs importantly from the loss of function tools presently discussed. Genetic markers are often used as an assay technique to help researchers detect the presence of a gene product; whereas, loss of function techniques are methods for interrupting causal relationships.

5 Dial-like control over the concentration of a gene product can be achieved with a variety of methods including small molecules. Even gene-editing techniques such as CRISPR-Cas9 can achieve this sort of control by targeting only some copies of the same gene in a genome or by targeting all copies of a gene at a particular stage of development. RNAi is by far the most popular method.

References

Baggs J., T. S. Price, L. DiTacchio, S. Panda, G. FitzGerald, J. Hogenesch. 2009. "Network Features of the Mammalian Circadian Clock." *PLoS Biology*, 7(3), pp. 0563–75.

Barbaric I., G. Miller, T. N. Dear. 2007. "Appearances Can be Deceiving: Phenotypes of Knockout Mice." *Briefings in Functional Genomics and Proteomics*, 6(2), pp. 91–103.

Bridges C. B., Morgan T. H. 1919. *The Second-Chromosome Group of Mutant Characters*. Carnegie Institution of Washington Publication 278. Washington, DC: Carnegie Institution, pp. 123–304.

Bunge M. 1966. "Technology as Applied Science." *Technology and Culture*, 7(3), pp. 329–47.

Castagnoli L., A. Costantini, C. Dall'Armi, S. Gonfloni, L. Montecchi-Palazzi, S. Panni, S. Paoluzi, E. Santonico, G. Cesareni. 2004. "Selective Promiscuity in the Interaction Network Mediated by Protein Recognition Modules." *FEBS Letters*, 567, pp. 74–9.

Chang H. 2004. *Inventing Temperature: Measurement and Scientific Progress*. New York: Oxford University Press.

Chang H. 2014. *Is Water H$_2$O? Evidence, Realism and Pluralism*. Boston Studies in the Philosophy of Science, Volume 293. New York: Springer Science & Business Media.

Craver C.F. 2007. *Explaining the Brain: Mechanisms and the Mosaic Unity of Neuroscience*. New York: Oxford University Press.

Gerstein M. B., C. Bruce, J. S. Rozowsky, D. Zheng, J. Du, J. O. Korbel, O. Emanuelsson, Z. D. Zhang, S. Weissman, M. Snyder. 2007. *What Is a Gene, Post-ENCODE? History and Updated Definition*. Cold Spring Harbor, NY: Cold Spring Harbor Laboratory Press.

Griffiths P., K. Stotz. 2013. *Genetics and Philosophy: An Introduction*. New York: Cambridge University Press.

Griffiths P., A. Pocheville, B. Calcott, K. Stotz, H. Kim, R. Knight. 2015. "Measuring Causal Specificity." *Philosophy of Science*, 82(4), 529–55.

Harwood J. 1993. *Styles of Scientific Thought: The German Genetics Community, 1900–1933*. Chicago, IL: The University of Chicago Press.

Housden, B., M. Muhar, M. Gemberling, C. Gersbach, D. Stainier, G. Seydoux, S. Mohr, J. Zuber, N. Perrimon. 2016. "Loss-of-Function Genetic Tools for Animal Models: Cross-Species and Cross-Platform Differences." *Nature*, 18, 24–40.

Kitano H. 2004. "Biological Robustness." *Nature Reviews*, 5, pp. 826–37.

Mitchell S. 2009. *Unsimple Truths: Science, Complexity, and Policy*. Chicago, IL: University of Chicago Press.

Millikan R. G. 1989. "In Defense of Proper Functions." *Philosophy of Science*, 56(2), pp. 288–302.

Neander K. 1991a. "Functions as Selected Effects: The Conceptual Analyst's Defense." *Philosophy of Science*, 58(2), pp. 168–84.

Neander K. 1991b. "The Teleological Notion of Function." *Australasian Journal of Philosophy*, 69(4), pp. 454–68.

O'Malley M. A., K. C. Elliot, R. M. Burian. 2010. "From Genetic to Genomic Regulation: Iterativity in microRNA Research." *Studies in History and Philosophy of Biological and Biomedical Sciences*, 41, pp. 407–17.

Rheinberger H.-J., S. Müller-Wille. 2017. *The Gene: From Genetics to Postgenomics*. Chicago, IL: University of Chicago Press.

Shalem O., N. E. Sanjana, E. Hartenian, X. Shi, D. Scott, T. Mikkelsen, D. Heckl, B. L. Ebert, D. E. Root, J. G. Doench, F. Zhang. 2014. "Genome-Scale CRISPR-Cas9 Knockout Screening in Human Cells." *Science*, 343, pp. 84–87.

Shen Z., X. Zhang, Y. Chai, Z. Zhu, P. Yi, G. Feng, W. Li, G. Ou. 2014. "Conditional Knockouts Generated by Engineered CRISPR-Cas9 Endonuclease Reveal the Roles of Coronin in *C. elegans* Neural Development." *Developmental Cell*, 30, pp. 615–36.

Vance R. 1996. "Heroic Antireductionism and Genetics: A Tale of One Science." *Philosophy of Science*, 63, pp. 36–45.

Walsh D. M., A. Ariew. 2013. "A Taxonomy of Functions." *Canadian Journal of Philosophy*, 26(4), pp. 493–514.

Waters C. K. 1994. "Genes Made Molecular." *Philosophy of Science*, 61, pp. 163–185.

Waters C. K. 2004. "What was Classical Genetics?" *Studies in History and Philosophy of Science*, 35, pp. 783–809.

Waters C. K. 2006. "A Pluralist Interpretation of Gene-Centered Biology." In *Scientific Pluralism, Minnesota Studies in the Philosophy of Science*, Volume XIX, edited by S. H. Kellert, H. E. Longino, C. K. Waters. Minneapolis: University of Minnesota Press, pp. 190–214.

Waters C. K. 2007. "Causes That Make a Difference." *Journal of Philosophy*, 104(11), pp. 551–579.

Waters C. K. 2009. "Beyond Theoretical Reduction and Layer-Cake Antireduction: How DNA Retooled Genetics and Transformed Biological Practice." In *The Oxford Handbook of Biology*, edited by M. Ruse. New York: Oxford University Press, pp. 238–62.

Weber M. 2004. *Philosophy of Experimental Biology*. Cambridge: Cambridge University Press.

Weber M. 2006. "The Central Dogma as a Thesis of Causal Specificity." *History and Philosophy of the Life Sciences*, 28, pp. 595–610.

Weber M. 2013. "Causal Selection vs Causal Parity in Biology: Relevant Counterfactuals and Biologically Normal Interventions." In *Causation in Biology and Philosophy*, edited by C. K. Waters, M. Travisano, J. Woodward. Minneapolis: University of Minnesota Press.

Weber M. 2017. "Discussion Note: Which Kind of Causal Specificity Matters Biologically?" *Philosophy of Science*, 84(3), pp. 574–85.

Weber M. 2018. "Experiment in Biology." *The Stanford Encyclopedia of Philosophy*. https://plato.stanford.edu/entries/biology-experiment/.

Whittaker S., J.-P. Theurillat, E. Van Allen, N. Wagle, J. Hsaio, G. S. Cowley, D. Schadendorf, D. Root, L. Garraway. 2013. "A Genome-Scale RNA Interference Screen Implicates NF1 Loss in Resistance to RAF Inhibition." *Cancer Discovery*, 3, pp. 351–62.

Woodward J. 2010. "Causation in Biology: Stability, Specificity, and the Choice of Levels of Explanation." *Biology and Philosophy* 25, pp. 287–318.

Wouters A. 2003. "Four Notions of Biological Function." *Studies in History and Philosophy of Biological and Biomedical Sciences*, 34, pp. 633–68.

Contributors

Nina A. Atanasova, Ph.D. is Lecturer of Philosophy at the Department of Philosophy and Religious Studies at The University of Toledo. She began her career in 2014 after receiving her Ph.D. in Philosophy (Philosophy and the Life Sciences Track) from the University of Cincinnati the same year. While a graduate student, she rotated in the Vorhees/Williams Neurology Lab at Cincinnati Children's Research Foundation. She joined the International Association for Science and Cultural Diversity as an Assistant Secretary General in 2015 and has been its Secretary General since 2017. Her research centers on epistemology and methodology of neuroscience.

Ann-Sophie Barwich is Assistant Professor at Indiana University, Bloomington, Department of History and Philosophy of Science and Medicine and Cognitive Science Program. Her research specializes in olfaction as a model for theories of cognition and the brain. She is the author of *Smellosophy: What the Nose Tells the Mind* (Harvard University Press, 2020).

Janella Baxter is Lecturer in the Department of Philosophy at Washington University, St. Louis. Her area of research is philosophy of biology and technology. She is one of the co-founders of the Biological Engineering Collaboratory, an interdisciplinary network for historians, social scientists, and philosophers working at the intersection of biology and engineering.

John Bickle is Professor of Philosophy and Shackouls Honors College Faculty at Mississippi State University and Affiliate Faculty in the Department of Neurobiology and Anatomical Sciences at the University of Mississippi Medical Center. His area of research is philosophy of neuroscience, especially neuroscience-in-practice. He is the author of four academic books, 100 articles and chapters in philosophy and neuroscience journals and volumes, and he edited *The Oxford Handbook of Philosophy and Neuroscience*.

Daniel Burnston is Associate Professor of Philosophy at Tulane University, director of the Tulane Cognitive Studies Program, affiliate faculty member in the Tulane Brain Institute, and co-editor of the Brains Blog. He works on topics in philosophy of cognitive science and philosophy of science, focusing primarily on the organization of the brain and mind. He has published in top philosophy of science journals, including *Philosophy of Science, BJPS*, and *Biology and Philosophy*, as well as in interdisciplinary venues in cognitive science and neuroscience.

David Colaço is Humboldt Postdoctoral Fellow at the Munich Center for Mathematical Philosophy of LMU Munich. He is a historian and philosopher of science who addresses reasoning and experimental practices in scientific research, with a focus on cognitive science and neuroscience. He has published a number of papers, including *Philosophy of Science, Biology and Philosophy* and *Analysis*.

Carl F. Craver is Professor in the Philosophy Department and the Philosophy-Neuroscience-Psychology Program at Washington University. He specializes in the philosophy of science, with particular expertise in neuroscience and cognitive science. He is the author of *Explaining the Brain: Mechanisms and the Mosaic Unity of Neuroscience* (Clarendon; 2007) and the co-author with Lindley Darden of *In Search of Mechanisms: Discoveries across the Life Sciences (Chicago; 2013)*.

Luis H. Favela is Associate Professor of Philosophy and Cognitive Sciences at the University of Central Florida. He has been a Fellow at the University of Pittsburgh's Center for Philosophy of Science and Duke University's Summer Seminars in Neuroscience and Philosophy, as well as Visiting Researcher at Indiana University Bloomington's Computational Cognitive Neuroscience Laboratory in the Department of Psychological and Brain Sciences. His interdisciplinary research at the intersection of philosophy and the mind sciences applies complexity science, dynamical systems theory, and ecological psychology to investigations of behavior, cognition, and consciousness in diverse systems at various spatial and temporal scales.

Stuart Firestein is Professor of Neuroscience in the Department of Biological Sciences at Columbia University. His research focuses on the vertebrate olfactory system, perhaps the best chemical detector on the planet. Dedicated to promoting the accessibility of science to a public audience Firestein serves as an advisor for the Alfred P. Sloan Foundation's program for the Public Understanding of Science. He is an AAAS Fellow, a Guggenheim Fellow and has written two books on science for a public audience *Ignorance, How It Drives Science* and *Failure, Why Science Is so Successful*.

Valerie Gray Hardcastle is the St. Elizabeth Healthcare Executive Director of the Institute for Health Innovation and the Vice President for Health Innovation at Northern Kentucky University. An internationally recognized scholar, Hardcastle is the author of five books and over 210 essays. She studies the nature and structure of interdisciplinary theories in cognitive science and has focused primarily on developing a philosophical framework for understanding conscious phenomena responsive to neuroscientific and psychological data. Most recently, she is investigating how the nature of addiction can shed light on what it means to be human.

Gregory Johnson is Instructor of Philosophy at Mississippi State University. His area of research is philosophy of psychology and neuroscience. He has published in *Philosophical Psychology, Minds and Machines*, and other journals. He is the author of *Argument and Inference: An Introduction to Inductive Logic* (MIT Press, 2016).

Marco J. Nathan is Associate Professor and Chair in the Department of Philosophy at the University of Denver. His research focuses on the philosophy of science, with particular emphasis on biology, neuroscience, cognitive neuropsychology, and economics. He is the author of *Black Boxes: How Science Turns Ignorance Into Knowledge* (OUP, 2021) as well as numerous articles in both philosophical and scientific venues.

David Parker is University Senior Lecturer in the Department of Physiology, Development and Neuroscience, University of Cambridge (UK). His research focuses on neural circuits and neuromodulation, specifically on electrophysiological analyses of neuronal interactions and how they contribute to the generation of spinal cord locomotor rhythms. He has also examined how changes in spinal cord circuits could contribute to functional recovery after spinal cord injury, research that has included collaborative computational analyses. His work has been published in the *Journal of Neuroscience*, the *Journal of Neurophysiology, Neuroscience*, and *Frontiers in Neural Circuits*.

Astrid Prinz is Associate Professor in the Department of Biology at Emory University. Coming from a background in Physics, she uses computational modeling to study rhythmic pattern generation and homeostatic regulation in small neural circuits, currently in the mouse and fruit fly. She is the Past President of the International Organization for Computational Neurosciences.

Alcino J. Silva is Director of The UCLA Integrative Center for Learning and Memory and is Distinguished Professor in the Departments of Neurobiology, Psychiatry & Biobehavioral Sciences and Psychology at UCLA. He pioneered the field of Molecular and Cellular Cognition, and in 2002 founded and became the first President of the Molecular and Cellular Cognition Society, an organization with more than 8,000 members and chapters in North America, Asia, and Europe. His laboratory is searching for the mechanisms that underlie the allocation, encoding, and storage of information in the brain. Additionally, insights into mechanisms of memory are being used by his lab to unravel the causes and develop treatments for cognitive deficits associated with aging, intellectual disabilities, and autism, as well as to enhance recovery after brain injury. A key effort in his lab involves the development of computational tools to integrate and summarize large amounts of causal information with a searchable, graphical format (researchmaps.org).

C. Matthew Stewart is Associate Professor of Otolaryngology, Head and Neck Surgery at Johns Hopkins University, School of Medicine. His research focuses on sensorimotor integration of the vestibular and visual systems and his clinical practice expertise is in surgical restoration of hearing as well as surgical management of tumors of the ear and skull base. Most recently, he has been examining the human host cell mechanisms of infection by the SARS-CoV-2 virus to explain the long-term recovery syndromes affecting the peripheral and central nervous systems. He received an MD/PhD from the University of Texas Medical Branch Galveston and is a Fellow of the American College of Surgeons.

Antonella Tramacere carries out research in the fields of philosophy of comparative and evolutionary psychology, neuroscience, and cognition. She has published in important neuroscientific journals, such as *Trends in Cognitive Science, Biological Reviews* and *Neuroscience*, as well as in philosophy journals, such as *Topoi, Synthese* and *Biology and Philosophy*. She is engaged in international collaborations and projects with the Max Planck for the Sciences of Human History in Leipzig (Germany), with the Center for Mind and Cognition of the University of Bochum (Germany), with the Laboratory of Symbolic Communication of Riken in Tokyo (Japan), and with the Department of Philosophy and Religion at Mississippi State University (USA). Currently at the Department of Philosophy and Communication Study of the University of Bologna, she is leading a theoretical and experimental project concerning emotions and mentalizing in the visual perception of oneself.

Charles V. Vorhees, Ph.D. is Professor of Pediatrics at the University of Cincinnati College of Medicine and Division of Neurology, Cincinnati Children's Hospital Medical Center. He is co-director of the Animal Behavior Core and program director of the Teratology Training Program. He is graduate faculty in the Neuroscience and Molecular and Developmental Biology (MDB) graduate programs. He served as MDB Program Director for six years and as an officer for another nine. He has been a member of the Neuroscience Program Admission Committee for ten years. He was Editor-in-Chief of *Neurotoxicology and Teratology* for nine years. He is a founding member of the Developmental Neurotoxicology Society and was president in 1984–1985 and 2012–2013. He was an Eli Lilly Distinguished Lecturer in 1990, and a Society for Neuroscience Grass Foundation Lecturer in 2002. He has served on scientific advisory committees for the Food and Drug Administration, the Environmental Protection Agency, the National Institutes of Health, CalEPA, and the National Academy of Sciences.

Michael T. Williams is Associate Professor at the University of Cincinnati Department of Pediatrics and Cincinnati Children's Research Foundation Division of Neurology. Currently, he is co-director of the Animal Behavioral Core at Cincinnati Children's along with Charles Vorhees. His research interests are broad within the realm of developmental neurotoxicology and include the effects of manganese, proton particle therapy, PCBs, pyrethroids, drugs of abuse, hydrocephalus, stress, as well as the genetic models of developmental disorders. He has over 155 published manuscripts. He is a member of Society for Neuroscience, International Behavioral Neuroscience Society (IBNS), Developmental Neurotoxicology Society, and Society of Toxicology. He was made a fellow of IBNS in 2009 and won the Patricia Rodier Mid-career Award for Research and Mentoring in 2020 (delayed until 2021). He is a current member of the Neurotoxicology and Teratology editorial board.

Lu Xu is Postdoctoral Research Scientist in the Firestein lab at the Department of Biological Sciences, Columbia University. She is currently studying olfactory coding using a combination of physiological, molecular, and imaging techniques.

Index

For Product Safety Concerns and Information please contact our EU
representative GPSR@taylorandfrancis.com
Taylor & Francis Verlag GmbH, Kaufingerstraße 24, 80331 München, Germany

www.ingramcontent.com/pod-product-compliance
Lightning Source LLC
Chambersburg PA
CBHW061620220326
41598CB00026BA/3825